BREAST RECONSTRUCTION - CURRENT PERSPECTIVES AND STATE OF THE ART TECHNIQUES

Edited by **Aldona J. Spiegel**

Breast Reconstruction - Current Perspectives and State of the Art Techniques
http://dx.doi.org/10.5772/56873
Edited by Aldona J. Spiegel

Contributors

Jesse Selber, Sean Boutros, Jason J Hall, Jules Walters, Scott Reis, Stefania Tuinder, Rene Van Der Hulst, Marc Lobbes, B Versluis, Arno Lataster, Rachel Wellner, Corinne Becker, Joseph Disa, Katie Weichman, Constance Chen, Bob Allen, Maria LoTempio, Egidio Riggio, Maurizio Nava, Jose Ma Serra-Mestre, Jose Ma Serra-Renom, Francesco D'Andrea, Zachary Menn, Aldona Spiegel, Joshua Levine, Julie V. Vasile, Heather A. Erhard, John J. Ho, Hakan Usal, Lan Mu, Senkai Li, Rebecca Studinger

Published by InTech

Janeza Trdine 9, 51000 Rijeka, Croatia

Publishing Process Manager Viktorija Zgela
Technical Editor InTech DTP team
Cover InTech Design team

Additional hard copies can be obtained from orders@intechopen.com

Breast Reconstruction - Current Perspectives and State of the Art Techniques, Edited by Aldona J. Spiegel
p. cm.
ISBN 978-953-51-1181-8

For EU product safety concerns:
IN TECH d.o.o., Prolaz Marije Krucifikse Kozulić 3, 51000 Rijeka, Croatia,
info@intechopen.com or visit our website at intechopen.com.

Meet the editor

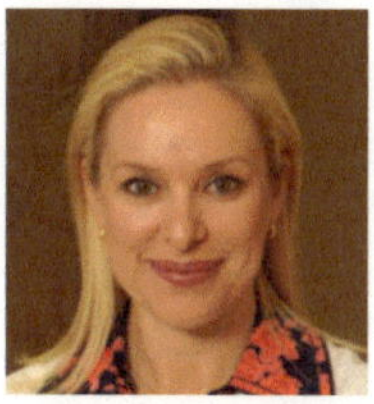

Dr. Aldona Spiegel is Director of the Center for Breast Restoration with the Institute for Reconstructive Surgery at The Methodist Hospital in Houston, Texas (2005) and is Associate Professor in the Division of Plastic Surgery of Weill Medical College at Cornell University (2012). She earned her undergraduate and medical degrees from the University of Ottawa (1990, 1994) and completed her general surgery training at Johns Hopkins Hospital in Baltimore, Maryland (1997). She completed a microsurgery fellowship (1998) and plastic surgery (2001) training at Baylor College of Medicine, Houston, Texas where she was a faculty member (2001–2005). Dr. Spiegel is a member of several committees and Editorial Review Boards and has contributed numerous journal articles and book chapters to scholarly publications. Her primary fields of interest include microsurgery, breast reconstruction, and reinnervation.

Contents

Preface

The Group for Advancement of Breast Reconstruction (GABRs) was organized as a way to advance the specialized field of Perforator Flap Reconstruction. It began as an outgrowth of a stimulating discussion between Dr. Robert Allen and colleagues at the 6th International Course on Perforator Flaps (2002) in Taipei, Taiwan. Since then, biannual meetings have been held around the world. The first meeting was hosted by Dr. Allen in Charleston, S.C. (2006), followed by a meeting at Chateau Villette in France (2007). The third meeting was hosted by Dr. Lan Mu in Beijing, China (2008), and most recent meeting was in Kenwood, California (2012).

Many of the chapters of this book are written by GABRs members, and some of the book's content was presented at the last meeting. Some of the most interesting parts of this book can be found in the important ideas, tips, tricks and personal advice shared during these discussions. Authors have been given flexibility to include this interesting information in their individual chapters. Since there is very limited exposure to these ideas within scientific journals that require rigorous statistical data, this book will be an excellent source for additional information in this highly specialized field.

In breast reconstruction, flap based procedures and implant based procedures are the two major modalities that have emerged as surgical options for patients. These are both continuing to evolve as new, innovative techniques help to improve outcomes and patient satisfaction. This book is divided into four sections. The first section includes overviews of mastectomy options and considerations in breast reconstruction procedure selection. The next section comprises non microsurgical reconstruction options which include implant based reconstruction refinements, the emerging role of fat grafting, as well as a novel technique of robotic latissimus flap harvesting. The third section is devoted to microsurgical reconstruction including flap refinements, tips and tricks, as well as advice on handling difficult situations. The final section includes the growing field of lymphedema surgery which is an important addition to breast reconstruction.

Surgeons specializing in breast reconstruction are challenged by the need for both artistic and technical skills. This very specialized field requires that the surgeon understands the patient's emotional needs and guides her in choosing from among the many techniques available. True success is measured in the eyes of the patient.

The field is evolving as new technically challenging microsurgical procedures are being developed including smaller caliber vessels being transferred from new areas of the body and a more "free" style dictated by patient body habitus, while preserving the donor site aesthetics as much as possible. Implant-based reconstruction is also advancing, with development of new devices, the addition of acellular dermal matrix, and new fat grafting techniques.

New mastectomy techniques have recently allowed more patients to be candidates for nipple-sparing mastectomy, which has permitted some patients to choose prophylactic mastectomy more freely. While maintaining the life of the tissue, reconstructive breast surgery is also challenged with the need to maintain the individual aesthetics of each patient's individual breasts. To maintain balance and symmetry, and to return the breast to a natural state of, hopefully, "better than the original" takes the hand of a well-trained, compassionate, thoughtful artist. In the reconstruction process, which involves much problem solving, there is room for constant innovation which keeps this emerging field challenging. Surgeons are forever making strides to enable patients burdened with breast cancer to regain their femininity and, as much as possible, leave their burden behind.

Aldona J. Spiegel
Director, Center for Breast Restoration, Institute for Reconstructive Surgery,
The Methodist Hospital, Houston, Texas
Associate Professor, Division of Plastic Surgery,
Weill Medical College, Cornell University
USA

Section 1

Oncology and Breast Reconstruction

Chapter 1

Oncoplastic Surgery

Rachel Wellner

Additional information is available at the end of the chapter

http://dx.doi.org/10.5772/56639

1. Introduction

The evolution of breast cancer management, following an arc of scientific discovery, is steeped in rich tradition and sacrament. A basic historical understanding of key discoveries in oncology sets the framework for our modern standards in cancer management, including our various applications in the field of breast oncology, breast reconstruction, and the "marriage" of the two, aptly named "oncoplastic surgery".

Cancer was first described by Hippocrates, the ancient Greek physician considered the father of medicine, who observed that malignant tumors resembled crabs (Gr. karkinos), with its mass-like center and appendages arching outward. [1] Cancer is an age-old disease that has continued to elude mankind for centuries. The process of uncontrolled cell division, cancer refers to a process by which the hosts own cells divide rapidly in a seemingly chaotic, haphazard way, but, in actuality, is the result of complex genetic and environmental factors that "program" a person's own normal cells to acquire a malignant quality, ultimately leading to the infiltration of normal organs by these masses of abnormal cells. [1]

Breast cancer is the world's leading cancer in women second to all skin malignancies. [2] Behind lung cancer, breast cancer is the second leading cause of cancer mortality in women. [2] It affects approximately one in eight women over a lifetime, translating into roughly over 230, 000 new cases of invasive breast cancer and over 50, 000 cases of non-invasive breast cancer per year in the country alone. About 40, 000 people die of breast cancer annually in the U. S. It continues to be a major cause of mortality world-wide, particularly in developing countries, where access to prevention, screening, and even appropriate management might be scarce. [2]

Breast cancer incidence increased in the 1980s and 1990s, a trend that was multifactorial, largely attributable to the increase in screening mammography, but also associated with reproductive risk factors and environmental risks such as the widespread use of hormone replacement therapy. The incidence has remained relatively stable in recent years, reflecting a decline in the use of exogenous hormones in post-menopausal women and a stabilization in numbers of women undergoing screening. [2]

Breast cancer incidence is strongly related to age, peaking in the later decades. Other risk factors implicated in the development of breast cancer include genetics (strong family history of breast or other related malignancies), hormonal and reproductive risk factors such as early menarche, late menopause, late onset of first pregnancy, hormone replacement therapy, and environmental risk factors including obesity, excess alcohol, high-dose radiation, and possibly nutritional factors. People at high risk for breast cancer include those previously diagnosed with breast cancer, those with atypical cells on a breast biopsy, and patients with mammographically dense breasts. [2]

Paralleling our improved understanding of breast carcinogenesis, risk factors, and improved surveillance are a multitude of advances in treatments.

The first loosely documented case of treated breast cancer was in 550 B. C. in the Persian Queen Atossa, who commissioned her slave Democedes to perform a primitive lumpectomy, essentially coring out her tumor, and allowing closure via secondary intention. [1] Treatments in centuries to follow ranged from drainage of "black bile, " salves, prayer, various home remedies, breast amputation, and treatment of depression. In the early 19th Century, William Halsted first described his radical mastectomy. The Halsted radical mastectomy involved removal of the entire breast gland, axillary lymph nodes, and chest wall muscles. Along with myriad other advances, with the advent of Joseph Lister's antiseptic techniques and general anesthetic developments discovered at the turn of the century, a surgical endeavor that would have been considered almost universally fatal was now conceivable. [1]

1.1. Images

At the time, the Halsted mastectomy was believed to offer a true cure for the breast cancer patient, given that she survived surgery. The theory of breast cancer representing a systemic disease had been washed away with Galen's black bile. A local disease required radical local treatment, regardless of physical deformity and lack of functionality. As such, the results were uniformly disfiguring but accepted as the singular option for survival. During this period, cancer was believed to be a local disease that spread in a predictable, time dependent fashion, therefore enlisting a massive operation to remove all cancer cells in order to render a patient cured. This procedure represented the standard of care for the next century, despite many patients presenting with small cancers not requiring such a radical approach.

Despite the improved short-term survival in patients undergoing maximal debulkment, long term results of this approach did not fare as well. By the mid 20th Century, the National Surgical Adjuvant Breast and Bowel Project (NSABP) had been conceived. [5] In 1971, Drs. Bernard and Edwin Fisher conducted animal studies that demonstrated metastases of tumor cells to both the lymphatics and the circulation, thereby laying question to Halsted's model of breast cancer as a "local" disease. In a trial of 1600 women undergoing Halsted radical mastectomy versus the less invasive total mastectomy, which spared lymph nodes and chest wall muscles, outcomes were comparable for the two groups, leading to the abandonment of the Halstead

http://dx.doi.org/10.5772/56639

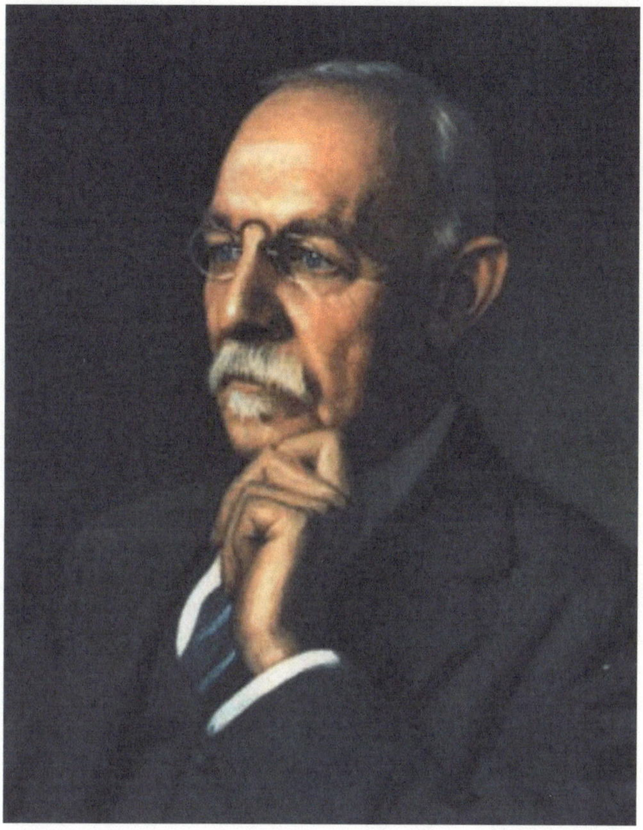

Figure 1. Dr. William Halsted [3]

radical mastectomy. This development heralded a new era of "minimally invasive" breast surgery. [5] Shortly, the same group was comparing lumpectomy to a modified radical mastectomy, learning that lumpectomy with the addition of breast irradiation demonstrated equivalent survival rates despite a slight increase in local recurrence rates. [6] Next, a series of trials adding systemic therapy to surgical treatment, ranging from chemotherapy to specialized hormonal treatments, were conducted, showing a further improvement in survival and local recurrence rates in select patients. [7] Advances in modern chemotherapy have significantly influenced the landscape of breast cancer treatment. The survival rate for early-stage breast cancer is greater than 90 percent, and even many patients with Stage IV breast cancer, the most advanced stage indicating wide-spread disease, can expect a longer survival on systemic therapies. [2] These treatments range from traditional chemotherapy to targeted agents such as anti-hormonal drugs (tamoxifen, aromatase inhibitors) and Herceptin (traztusimab). Newer techniques in radiation therapy have also made lumpectomy exceptionally safe while lowering recurrence rates significantly.

Currently, breast conservation (lumpectomy), skin- and nipple-sparing mastectomies, and less radical lymph node resections all constitute oncologically sound procedures with minimal

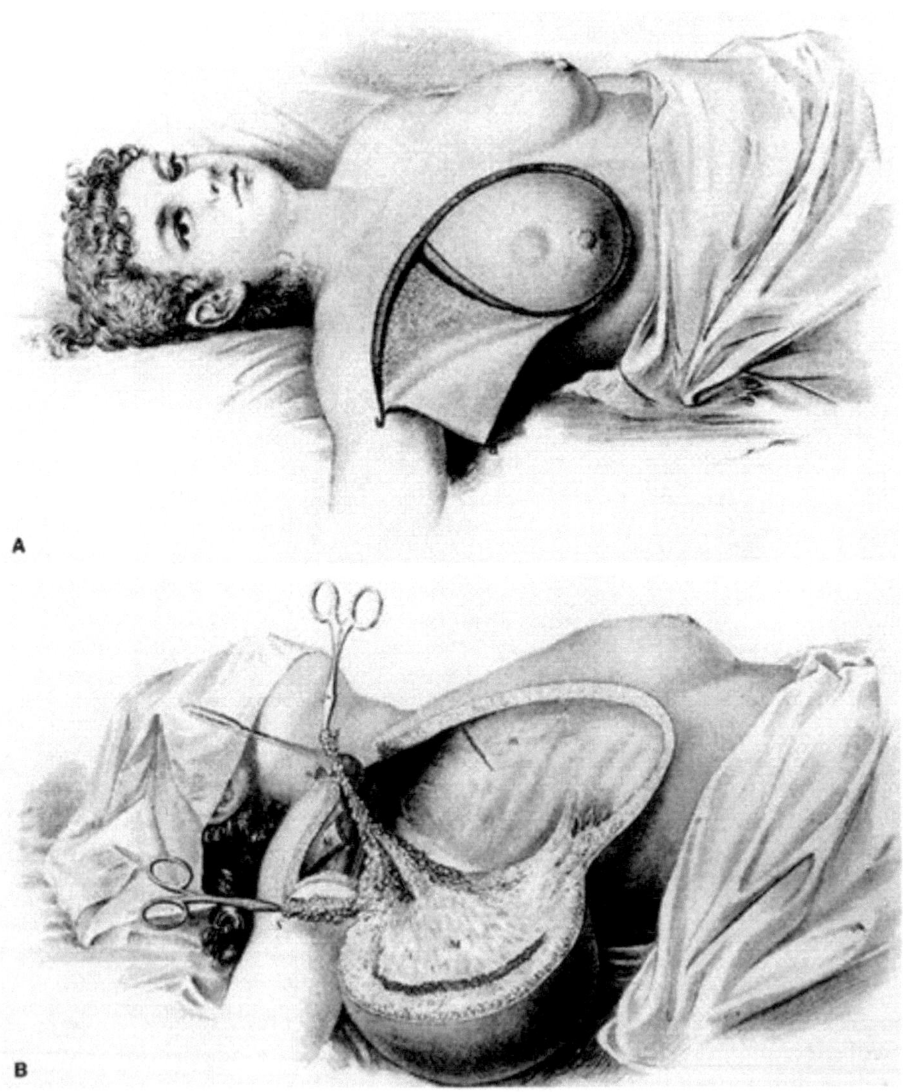

Figure 2. The Halsted Radical Mastectomy [4]

alteration of a patient's natural breast. Furthermore, advances in breast reconstruction, including "oncoplastic" surgery (the restoration of tissue contours while removing all cancer), afford women the opportunity to restore their bodies.

2. Defining oncoplastic surgery

In its simplest terms, oncoplastic surgery refers to combining a surgery used to treat or prevent breast cancer with a reconstructive procedure that will ultimately enhance cosmetic results. [8]

http://dx.doi.org/10.5772/56639

This undertaking must be accomplished while adhering to strict oncologic principles. The components of oncoplastic surgery include:

1. Excision of cancer with adequately wide free margins to achieve locoregional control, immediate remodeling of defect

2. Contralateral symmetrization/reconstruction

3. Immediate and late reconstruction after mastectomy

4. Breast Conserving Surgery (BCS) with volume replacement or volume displacement

In this chapter each of these components will be described in detail. Some surgical techniques will be presented, but this chapter is intended as a framework to present the principles of oncoplastic surgery. The creativity and controversy that surrounds this burgeoning field will make for exciting future trends in breast surgery.

3. Oncoplastic Breast Conservation Surgery (BCS)

Techniques for oncoplastic BCS are both innovative and varied. As discussed previously, whole breast radiation added to BCS offers equivalent overall survival to mastectomy. [7] In general, BCS is sssociated with superior cosmetic outcomes, and patients report greater satisfaction with body image and less psychological distress. The two major types of breast conservation include lumpectomy and quadrantectomy. Quadrantectomy was popularized in Europe and is still used there frequently. Quadrantectomy adheres to segmental anatomy of the breast. Components of quadrantectomy include resection of anterior skin and inclusion of pectoralis fascia. The goal in a quadrantectomy is to obtain a 1-2 cm margin. The wide margin is cited as one of the main benefits of quadrantectomy, with a local recurrence rate around 3-4% at 20 years. [9] However, inferior cosmetic results stemming from resecting an entire quartile of the breast lead to lower overall satisfaction. [10]

Lumpectomy was popularized in the United States, largely in response to the cosmetic limitations of the quadrantectomy, but this more limited resection carried with it problems of having a lower negative margin rate and a slightly higher local recurrence rate. The lumpectomy is a conservative resection. Skin is generally not included. Pectoralis fascia is not always included. The goal in a lumpectomy is a small margin (>1mm), although there is no consensus of what number represents a negative margin. The lumpectomy operation is supported by NSABP-B06, which a 14% local recurrence at 20 years for invasive disease [6]. Enhanced cosmetic results were reported with this technique.

Milan II, a large randomized trial comparing lumpectomy with quadrantectomy, compared lumpectomy to quadrantectomy. Tumors up to 2. 5cm in size were included, and both patient groups received adjuvant radiation therapy. The overall survival for the two groups was equivalent, but the local recurrence risk at 5 years was slightly superior in the quadrantectomy group. [10]

Oncoplastic BCS emerged as a way to reconcile the higher local recurrence rate seen with lumpectomy versus quadrantectomy and the inferior cosmetic results seen with quadrantectectomy versus lumpectomy. Oncoplastic BCS was first described by Audretsch in 1998 and emerged as a specialty in Europe. [8] It evolved specifically to address the dissatisfying cosmetic results of partial breast resections. Up to 30% of patients that undergo either type of BCS have a residual deformity, nipple distortion, or asymmetry, a problem that oncoplastic surgery aimed to mitigate. By definition, oncoplastic BCS combines a breast conserving resection of cancer with well-established plastic surgery techniques that remove breast tissue encompassing the known cancer.

The indications for oncoplastic BCS include patients considering a reduction mammaplasy/pexy at time of diagnosis, patients with an expected poor cosmetic outcome after standard BCS, patients with free or involved margins seeking correction of defect, or requiring an oncologic re-excision, patients with unfavorable tumor to breast size (>10-20% volume), and patients with unfavorable tumor location (inferior, medial, central quadrants). Contraindications include inflammatory breast cancer, no tumor-free margins obtained, multicentric carcinoma (relative), no adjuvant XRT (relative), no response to or progression of disease on neoadjuvant chemotherapy. [11]

There are two major classifications of oncoplastic BCS, volume replacement and volume displacement. [12] Volume replacement involves transposition of autologous tissue into the segmental mastectomy defect. This technique maintains the original size and shape of the breast, therefore not obviating the need for contralateral surgery for symmetry. The second type, volume displacement, involves permanently removal of breast tissue. The breast is "reshaped" with residual breast tissue. With this technique, the original size & shape is altered, and a contralateral procedure to restore symmetry is generally required. [12]

The various different types of volume displacement oncoplastic BCS are depicted pictorially (Figs 3-14). [13]

Several series over past decade demonstrate over a 90% survival rate for early breast cancers undergoing oncoplastic BCS and an acceptable low local recurrence rate (highest 9. 4%, Clough et. al.). [Table 1] [11, 14, 15]

Author	Year	Number of subjects	Weight (g)/Volume of specimen	Close/Involv. margins (re-excision/mastectomy)	Local recurrence rate	Survival rate	FU period (mths)
Clough et al.	2003	101	222		9.4%	95.7%	44
Kaur et al.	2005	30	200	16%			
Rietjans et al.	2007	148	198	2.02%	3%	92.47%	74
Giacalone et al.	2007	31	190	21%			
Ballester et al.	2008	86	150	12.7%	2%		20
Meretoja et al.	2010	90		12.2%	0%		26
Fitoussi et al.	2010	540	187.7	18.9%	6.8%	92.9%	49

Table 1. Outcomes of oncoplastic BCS

http://dx.doi.org/10.5772/56639

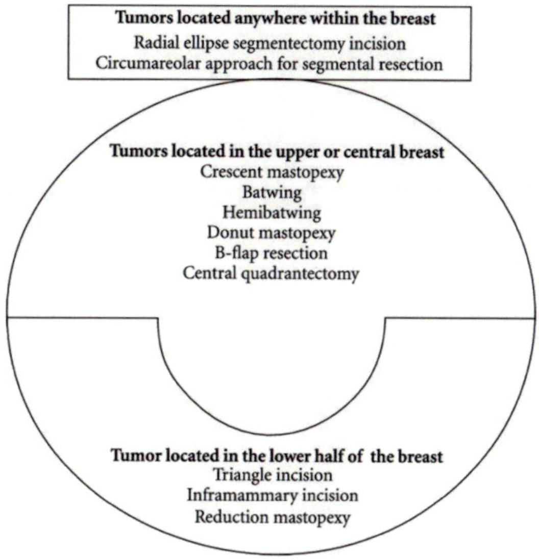

Figure 3. Types of volume displacement based on tumor location

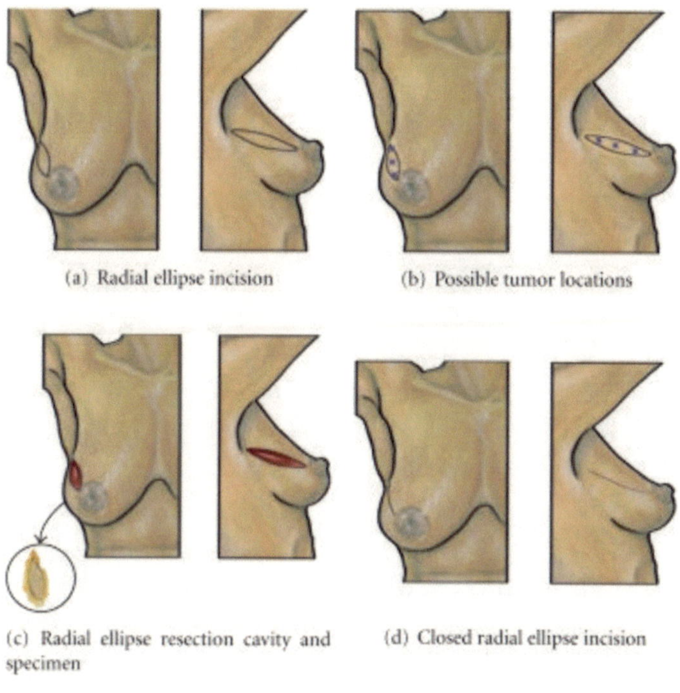

Figure 4. Radial ellipse incision for all tumor locations

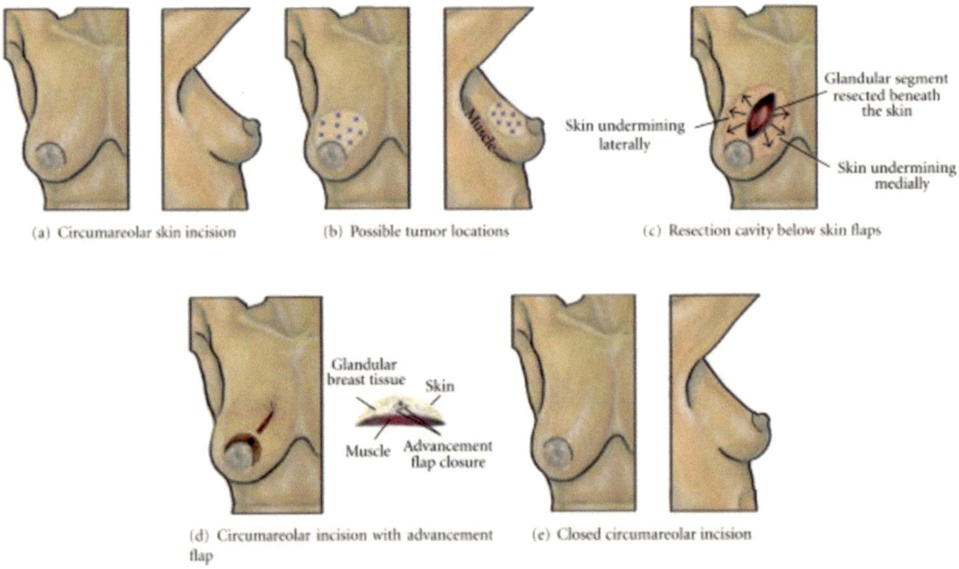

Figure 5. Circumareolar incision for all tumor locations

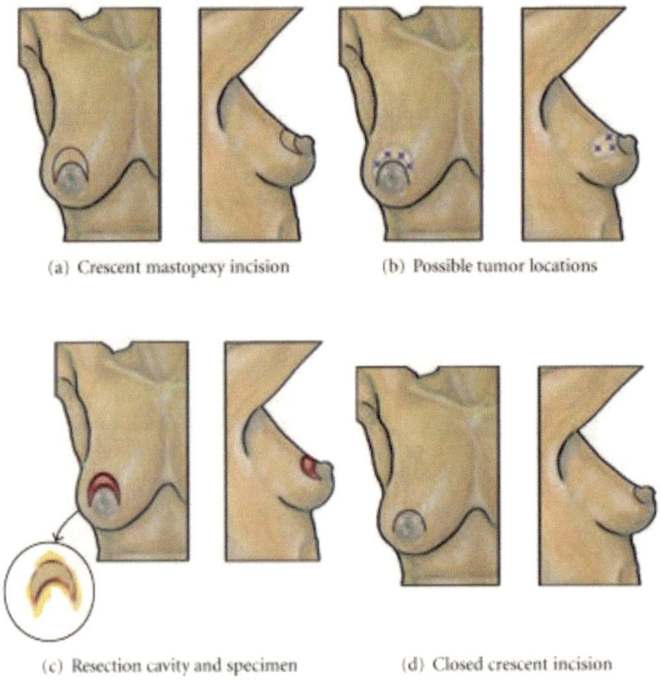

Figure 6. Crescent mastopexy for upper-pole or central tumors

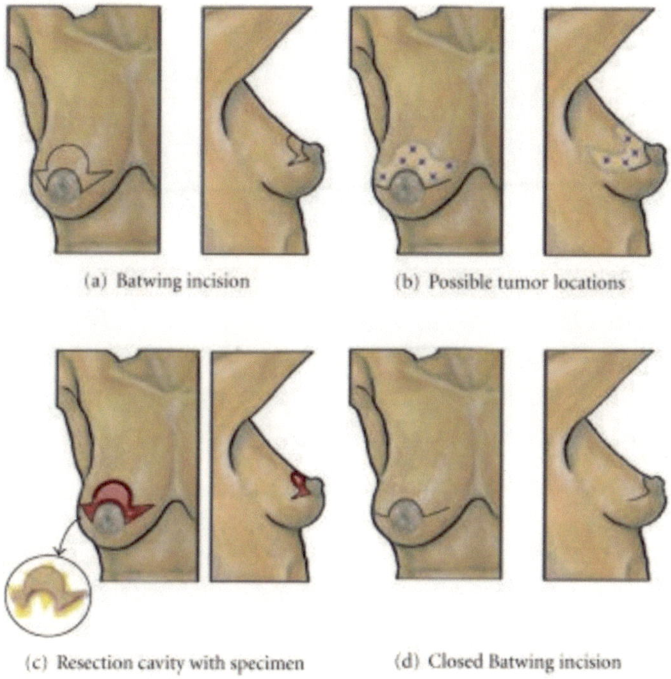

Figure 7. Batwing incision for upper-pole or central tumors

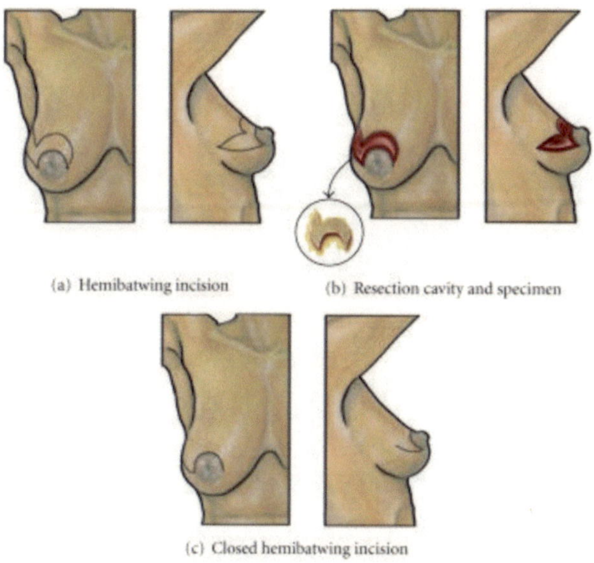

Figure 8. Hemibatwing incision for upper-pole or central tumors

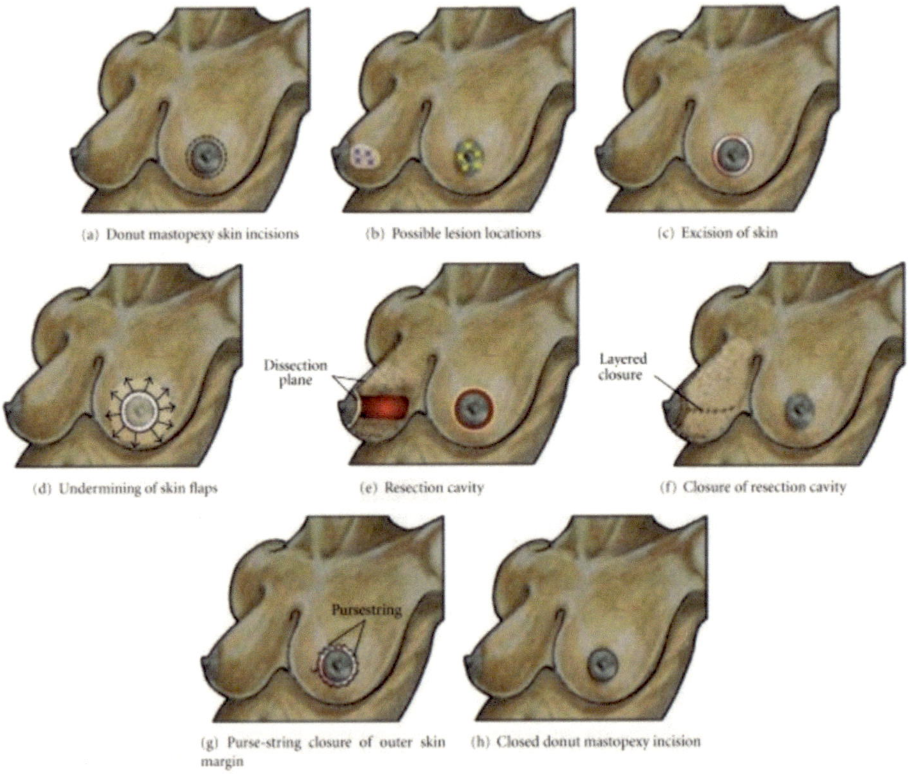

Figure 9. Donut mastopexy for upper-pole or central tumors

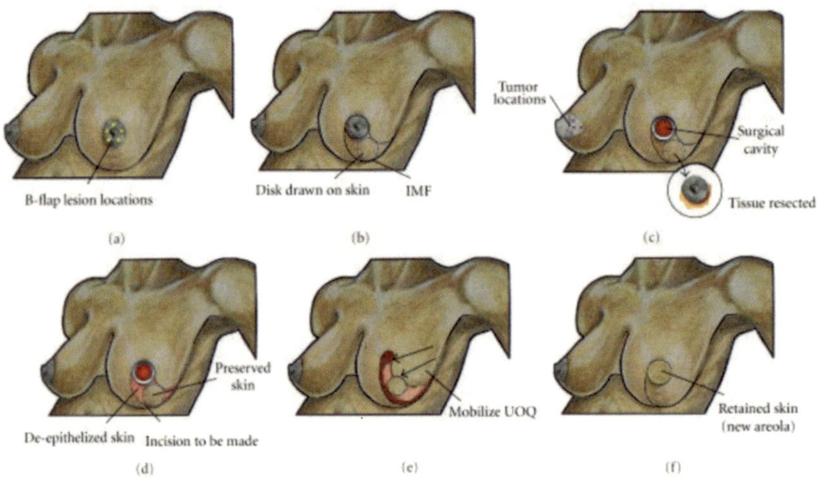

Figure 10. B-flap for central tumors

http://dx.doi.org/10.5772/56639

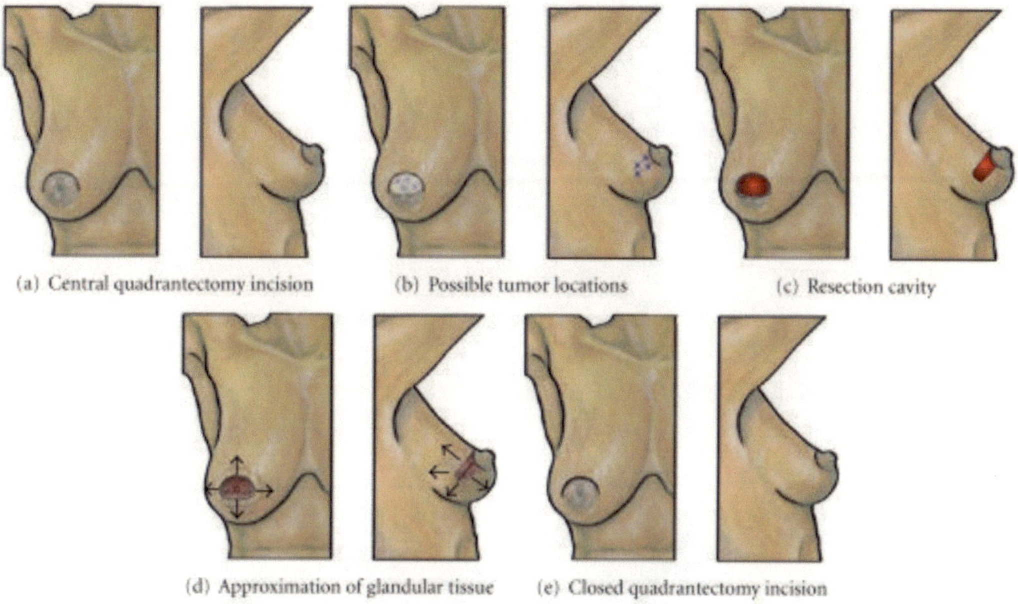

Figure 11. Central quadrantectomy for central tumors

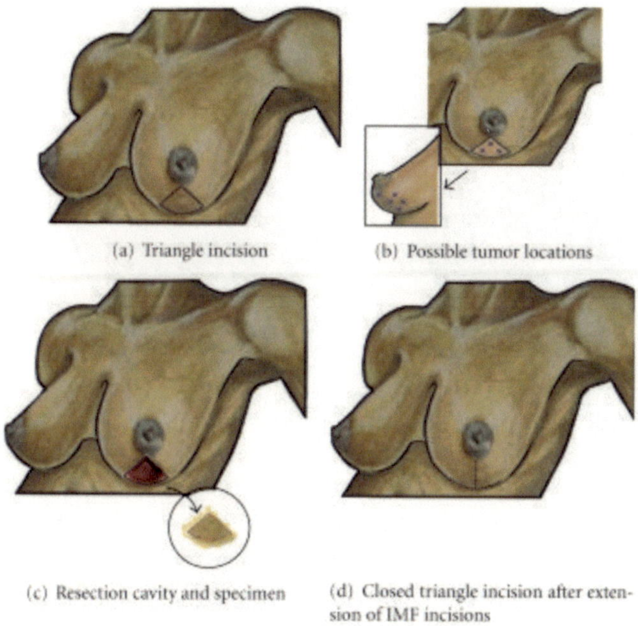

Figure 12. Triangle incision for lower pole tumors

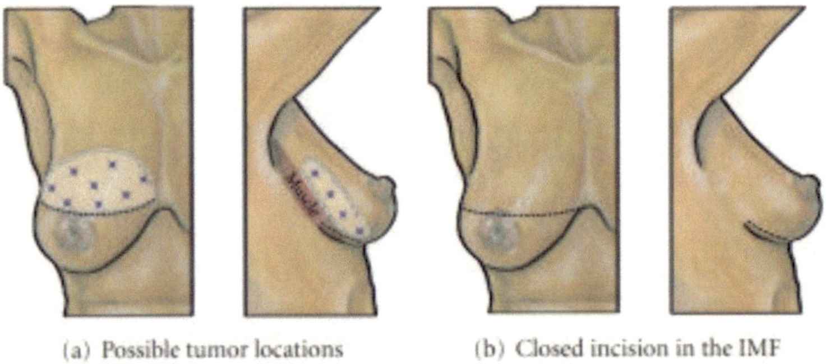

Figure 13. Inframammary incision for lower pole tumors

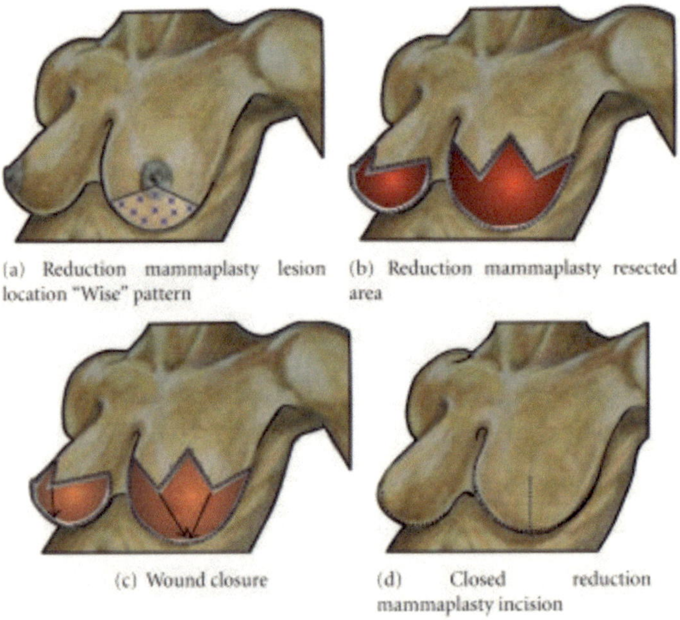

Figure 14. Reduction mastopexy for lower pole tumors

The proponents of oncoplastic BCS site the larger volume resections performed given the large degree of freedom for the deliberate creation of defects, theoretically improving the oncologic safety of the procedure. Inherently, wider margins are generally achieved and whole breast radiation can be applied more liberally and uniformly without significant risk to the breast contour. Furthermore, oncoplastic BCS can be applied to larger tumors, making breast conservation available to more women. Finally, many patients and practitioners report superior cosmetic results with oncoplastic BCS. [11, 14, 15, 16]

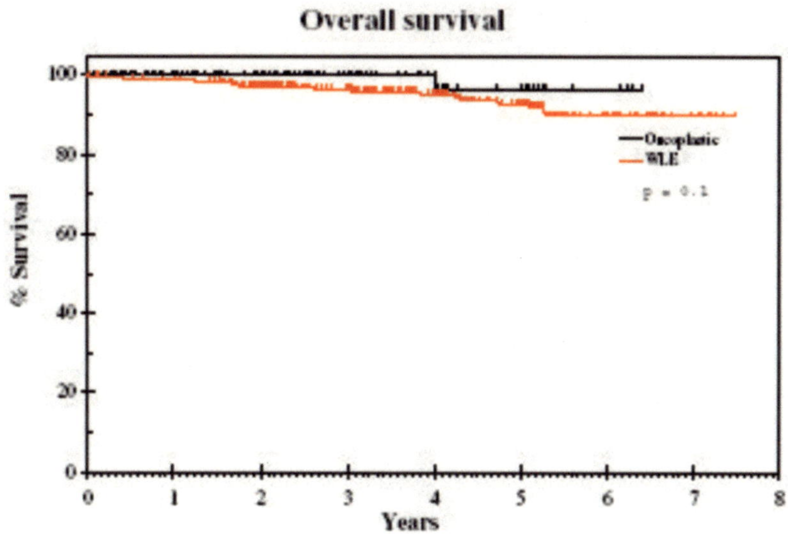

Figure 15. Overall survival oncoplastic BCS versus standard lumpectomy [11]

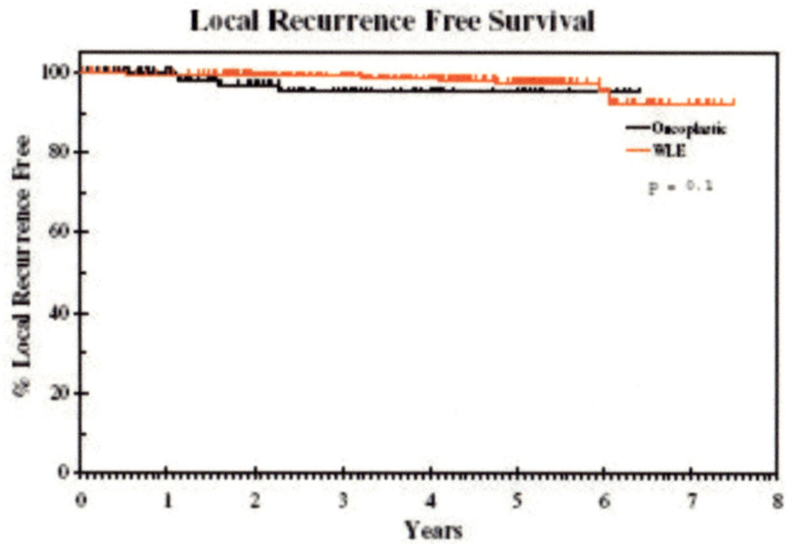

Figure 16. Local-recurrence free survival oncoplastic BCS versus standard lumpectomy [11]

Criticism for oncoplastic BCS includes the fact that most data are from single institution series with short follow up. Furthermore, there have been no formal studies showing that oncoplastic surgery changed management from mastectomy to less invasive breast conservation, despite the theoretical benefits listed above for patients with larger tumors. Studies have not yet demonstrated higher patient satisfaction with oncoplastic BCS versus standard BCS. Finally, oncoplastic techniques are generally creative and challenging. While some embrace the innovative concept, others are resistant to changing tried and tested standard techniques.

4. Oncoplastic mastectomy

Oncoplastic mastectomy follows the same principle as oncoplastic breast conservation, that is, the restoration of natural breast contour following resection for cancer. An oncoplastic mastectomy is indicated for any patient who is a candidate for immediate reconstruction following total mastectomy. Contraindications include inability to obtain free margins, inflammatory breast cancer, post-operative XRT (relative and becoming largely outdated as a contraindication), and concomitant physical/psychological illness prohibiting reconstruction.

Traditional extended transverse mastectomy incisions yielded modest results in clothing at best. Earlier breast cancer detection has allowed for increased flexibility in skin preservation during mastectomy and reconstruction. Modern mastectomy incisions follow current principles of aesthetic breast surgery. As such, scars on the medial and upper poles are often avoided. Furthermore, in the 1980s, the non-elliptical incision was introduced, resulting in a considerable improvement in the nature of the original deformity created. It is accepted that the original deformity made during initial incision significantly influences the eventual cosmetic outcome, the preservation of native skin envelope being paramount to achieving favorable results.

The skin-sparing mastectomy (SSM) incorporates an anatomic incision with preservation of skin envelope. Other considerations in the SSM include removal of the nipple areolar complex (NAC) except in the specialized nipple-sparing version of the SSM, removal of initial biopsy site, and adequate exposure to allow for possible axillary dissection. Reconstructive considerations that come into clinical decision-making include breast size, degree of ptosis, general health of the patient, patient preference, and history of active tobacco use. Contraindications to SSM include extensive skin involvement and inflammatory breast cancer.

Results of SSM are favorable, demonstrating a risk of local failure of approximately 6. 2% with the exclusion of extensive inflammatory component. [17] Simmons et al (*ASO* 1999) conducted a retrospective review of 231 patients, showing local and distant recurrence rates following SSM to be 3. 90% and 3. 90% respectively (no significant difference vs. traditional mastectomy). [18] A lack of prospective data is limiting.

Nipple areolar complex sparing mastectomy (NSM) is the most recent incarnation of the SSM. In its early evolution, the NSM faced considerable opposition. Early studies of mastectomy specimens showed occult tumor in proximity to the NAC. Furthermore, in the 1960s, a series of high risk patients undergoing prophylactic subcutaneous mastectomy, during which a rim of tissue was deliberately left beneath the nipple areolar complex for perfusion, developed breast cancer, putting the oncologic safety of the modern NSM in question. Other considerations include avoidance of necrosis of the NAC, satisfactory NAC position, and implant preservation in the case of an implant-based reconstruction. Avoidance of necrosis hinges upon careful planning of incision and preservation of skin and intercostal perforators (see Figure 17 for examples of skin incisions). [19]

http://dx.doi.org/10.5772/56639

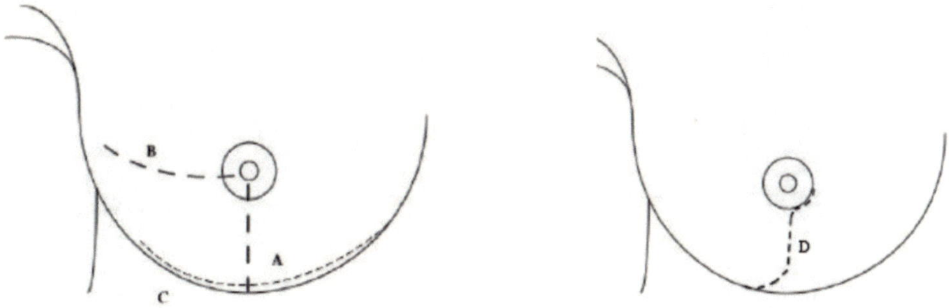

Figure 17. Examples of skin incisions for optimal NAC perfusion in NSM

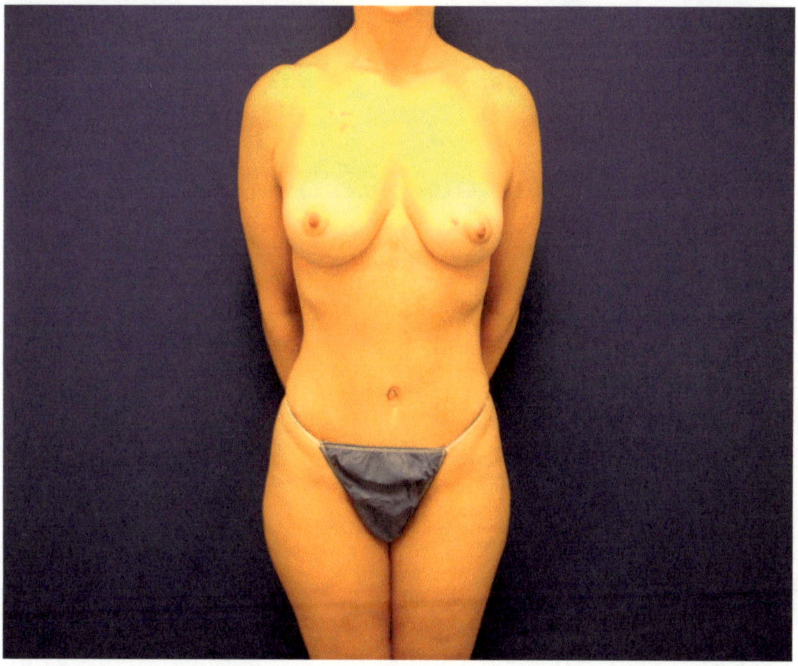

Figure 18. Preoperative BRCA positive patient

The principle upon which NSM is based is that NAC involvement occurs in relatively few patients with favorable tumor characteristics. Unfavorable tumor characteristics that suggest the potential presence of cancer cells in the NAC include subareolar or multicentric tumors, positive nodal status and extensive intraductal component. Inclusion for NSM (varies between authors) is generally: tumor ≤ 3- 4. 5 cm in size, tumor ≥ 1-2. 5 cm from areola, ≥ 4 cm from center of nipple, no gross involvement of the NAC (bloody discharge, Paget's), and retroareolar tissue sampling negative. Additional relative inclusion criteria include no to minimal lymph node involvement, uni-focality, and ptosis less than Grade 4. [20]

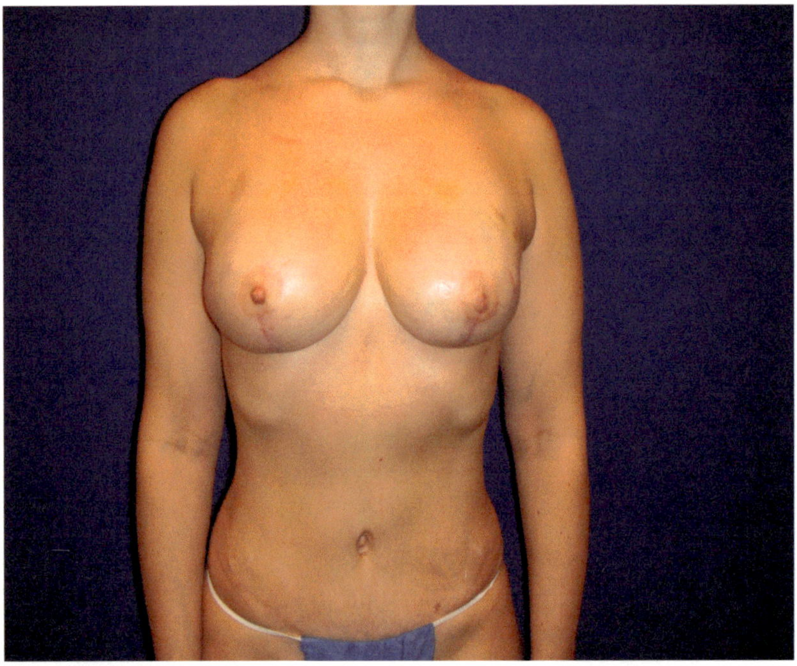

Figure 19. Post-operative BRCA patient status post NSM, PAP reconstruction

Large studies report occult nipple involvement with cancer between 5. 6 and 31% of the time with a local recurrence rate of < 5%. Cancer has been found in the retained nipple after risk-reducing mastectomy in the prophylactic setting <1% of the time. Nipple necrosis rates have been reported to be between 8 and 16%. Reconstructive factors including large breast size and excessive ptosis are associated with nipple necrosis and frank nipple loss. [21, 22]

5. Conclusions

Oncoplastic Breast Surgery represents an attractive and creative alternative to traditional methods. Despite barriers to its adoption, all evidence points to the oncologic safety and efficacy of oncoplastic surgery with improved patient satisfaction. Further prospective study is needed as we enter into the unique era of combining surgical disciplines.

Author details

Rachel Wellner*

Hackensack University Medical Center, Hackensack, NJ, USA

References

[1] Libuti, Steven. "Cancer. " In *Greenfield's Surgery: Scientific Principles and Practice*, 4th Ed. Eds. Mulholland, Lillemoe, 2006: 292-293.

[2] The American Cancer Society: www. cancer. org

[3] Figure 1: http://www. surgical-tutor. org. uk/default-home. htm?surgeons/halstead. htm~right

[4] Figure 2 http://edgeofthewest. files. wordpress. com/2008/07/halsted_drawing. jpg

[5] Fisher B, Jeong JH, Anderson S, Bryant J, Fisher ER, Wolmark N. Twenty-five-year follow-up of a randomized trial comparing radical mastectomy, total mastectomy, and total mastectomy followed by irradiation. *N Engl J Med.* 2002 Aug 22;347(8): 567-75.

[6] Fisher B, Anderson S, Bryant J, Margolese RG, Deutsch M, Fisher ER, Jeong JH, Wolmark N. Twenty-year follow-up of a randomized trial comparing total mastectomy, lumpectomy, and lumpectomy plus irradiation for the treatment of invasive breast cancer. *N Engl J Med.* 2002 Oct 17;347(16):1233-41.

[7] Early Breast Cancer Trialists' Collaborative Group. Polychemotherapy for early breast cancer: an overview of the randomised trials. *Lancet.* 1998 Sep 19;352(9132): 930-42.

[8] Clough KB, Kroll SS, Audretsch W. An approach to the repair of partial mastectomy defects. *Plast Reconstr Surg.* 1999 Aug;104(2):409-20.

[9] Veronesi U, Cascinelli N, Mariani L, Greco M, Saccozzi R, Luini A, Aguilar M, Marubini E. Twenty-year follow-up of a randomized study comparing breast-conserving surgery with radical mastectomy for early breast cancer. *N Engl J Med.* 2002 Oct 17;347(16):1227-32.

[10] Veronesi U, Luini A, Galimberti V, Zurrida S. Conservation approaches for the management of stage I/II carcinoma of the breast: Milan Cancer Institute trials. *World J Surg.* 1994 Jan-Feb;18(1):70-5.

[11] Clough KB, Lewis JS, Couturaud B, et. al. Oncoplastic techniques allow extensive resections for breast-conserving therapy of breast carcinomas. *Ann Surg* 2003; 237:26-34.

[12] Anderson BO, Masetti R, Silverstein MJ. Oncoplastic approaches to partial mastectomy: an overview of volume displacement techniques. *Lancet Oncol* 2005; 6: 145-57.

[13] Holmes, Schooler, Smith. Oncoplastic Approaches to Breast Conservation. *Int J Breast Cancer.* 2011; 2011: 303879.

[14] Chakravorty, Shrestha, Sanmugalingam, et. al. How safe is oncoplastic breast conservation?: Comparative analysis with standard breast conserving surgery. *EJSO* Volume 38, Issue 5, May 2012, Pages 395–398.

[15] Kaur N, Petit JY, Rietjens M, et. al. Comparative study of surgical margins in oncoplastic surgery and quadrantectomy in breast cancer. *Ann Surg Oncol* 2005; 12: 539-45.

[16] Lebovic. Anderson. Oncoplastic Breast Surgery: Current Status and Best Candidates for Treatment. *Current Breast Cancer Reports,* 2009.

[17] Singletary SE, Robb GL: Oncologic safety of skin-sparing mastectomy. *Ann Surg Oncol* 2003; 20: 95-7.

[18] Simmons RM, Adamovich TL. Skin-sparing mastectomy. *Surg Clin North Am.* 2003 Aug;83(4):885-99. Review.

[19] Stolier, Levine. Reducing the Risk of Nipple Necrosis: Technical Considerations in 340 Patients. *The Breast Journal.* Jan 2012.

[20] Voltura AM, Tsangaris TN, Rosson GD, Jacobs LK, Flores JI, Singh NK, Argani P, Balch CM. Nipple-sparing mastectomy: critical assessment of 51 procedures and implications for selection criteria. *Ann Surg Oncol.* 2008 Dec;15(12):3396-401. Epub 2008 Oct 16.

[21] Jensen, Orringer, Giuliano. Nipple-Sparing Mastectomy in 99 Patients with a Mean Follow-up of 5 Years. Ann Surg Onc 2011 (18): 1665-1670.

[22] Sacchini, Pinotti, Barros, et. al. Nipple-Sparing Mastectomy for Breast Cancer and Risk Reduction: Oncologic or Technical Problem? *Journal of the American College of Surgeons,* Volume 203, Issue 5, Pages 704-714.

Chapter 2

Selection of an Appropriate Method of Breast Reconstruction: Factors Involved in Customizing Breast Restoration

Zachary Menn and Aldona Spiegel

Additional information is available at the end of the chapter

http://dx.doi.org/10.5772/56333

1. Introduction

When considering breast reconstruction, the patient's perception essentially determines the success, or failure, of the reconstruction. It is important for the surgeon to ask questions and listen to the patient to determine what expectations the patient has for the final results. In the past, the goal of breast reconstruction was to help a patient look "normal" in clothing. With the advancements in technique and technology, we have raised the bar so that patients look good not only in clothing, but also when they see themselves undressed in the mirror. In this chapter we will discuss how to match a breast reconstruction candidate with the procedure that will provide the best result.

2. The defect

As with any reconstructive procedure, the first step is the evaluation of the defect to be reconstructed. The size, shape, and quality of the defect are all important factors and are resultant from the type of mastectomy performed. Radical, modified radical, skin sparing, areolar sparing, and nipple sparing mastectomies all create a different defect with different requirements for reconstruction. It is important to determine if the defect simply requires volume replacement or if there is a component of skin that needs to be replaced. It is vital to examine the skin flaps remaining after the mastectomy for any damage from radiation or the surgery. If the skin is not viable or has radiation damage it may be unusable in the reconstruction and require resection. The amount and type of volume replacement needs to be estimated by determining the final preference for breast size of the patient.

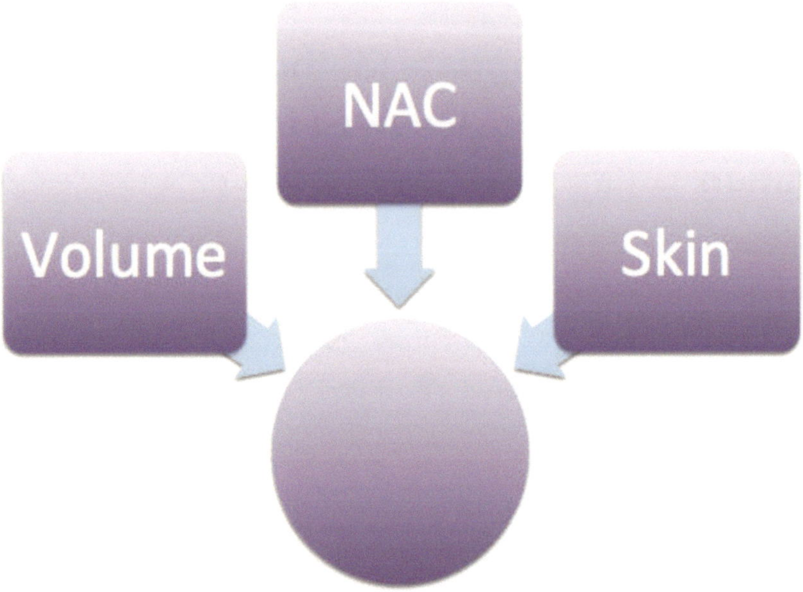

Figure 1. The type of reconstruction should be chosen based upon what is missing following mastectomy including breast volume, nipple-areolar complex and/or skin.

3. The patient

3.1. Patient assessment

During the patient assessment at the initial visit, there are many important pieces of information that should be gathered during the history and physical.

Physical Exam: The size of the breast(s) to be reconstructed needs to be considered in your planning, as well as whether the reconstruction will be unilateral or bilateral. Bilateral reconstruction and larger breasts will require a larger volume of donor site tissue which may limit some reconstructive options. Examine the breasts for scars, asymmetry, ptosis, nipple position and skin quality making sure to point out any irregularities to the patient. The distribution and amount of excess soft tissue should also be noted. First, examine the abdomen for adipose tissue volume. Next examine the back, buttocks and inner thighs for laxity and soft tissue volume.

Oncologic status: The patient's oncologic status should be requested to determine what prior treatments they already completed and if there is a future need for radiation. It is also important to determine if the prior treatment was adequate, particularly if the patient was referred from an outside facility. Additional radiologic studies may be necessary to make this determination. If the patient has not received adequate treatment, there may be future need for radiation, which might change the approach to reconstruction.

Medical history: A thorough medical history is important before considering a type of reconstruction because some medical and social issues may be contraindications to certain reconstructive procedures. Some contraindications to free flaps include: smoking, diabetes, obesity, peripheral vascular disease, clotting disorders, and advanced age. Breast implant manufacturers caution that the safety and effectiveness of these devices have not been established in patients with autoimmune diseases (such as lupus and scleroderma), a compromised immune system (receiving immunosuppressive therapy) or patients with conditions or medications which interfere with wound healing ability (such as corticosteroid therapy or poorly controlled diabetes) or blood clotting (such as coumadin therapy).[1] Each of these factors should be inquired about, as they have an impact on procedure selection.

Surgical history: Surgical and obstetric history should be taken. All C-sections, abdominoplasties, liposuction procedures, traumas, abdominal surgeries, and any scar severing the blood supply to specific areas of excess soft tissue (abdomen, buttock, back and thigh) should be noted as this will determine which body areas are available as a donor site for reconstruction.

Family and Social history: Age, marital status, family history and social support may greatly impact the decision of which type of reconstruction best fits a specific patient. A young, thin patient with a strong family history of breast cancer, BRCA positive, having prophylactic nipple sparing mastectomies, may be more suited for an implant only reconstruction due to possible lack of excess soft tissue that may be seen more prominently in an older individual. Social support is also important to consider as well as activity level requirements in employment, allotted time off work, and home responsibilities. This is why it is important to discuss the patient's social situation and support network before deciding on a type of breast reconstruction.

3.2. Patient expectations and goals

A conversation with the patient should be had to determine the size of the breast(s) to be reconstructed and decide whether it will be a unilateral or a bilateral reconstruction. At this time, it is also important to assess the patient's perception of the contralateral breast. Some patients may need bilateral reconstruction due to the spread of the disease and require a mastectomy, while others may opt for a prophylactic mastectomy due to a genetic predisposition for breast cancer. Others may not need a mastectomy on the contralateral breast, but some symmetry surgery may still be necessary. Autologous reconstruction can typically match the contralateral breast, while implant only reconstruction makes matching the native breast more difficult. The patient should be counseled at the initial visit about the possibility of surgery on the contralateral breast even though it is unaffected by the cancer. Another patient factor, possibly the most important to consider, is the patient's preference of reconstruction. It is the surgeon's job, as the expert, to explain the reconstructive options, educate the patient as to the best option for their specific situation, and ultimately let the patient decide upon the option with which they are most comfortable.

3.3. Patient commitment

It is vital that patients who expect to undergo autologous reconstruction commit to a healthy lifestyle and prepare their body for the major surgery that is breast reconstruction. Smoking secession and weight loss are important, if necessary. There is also a commitment after the surgery to follow up at least once and restrict activities for four to six weeks after autologous reconstruction.

4. The surgeon

The surgeon plays the major role in the success of the surgery. As the choices for breast reconstruction have evolved, it has been noted that specialized microsurgical procedures have a "learning curve" and are more successful when performed by a surgeon or team with a higher volume of cases. [2]

4.1. Types of reconstruction

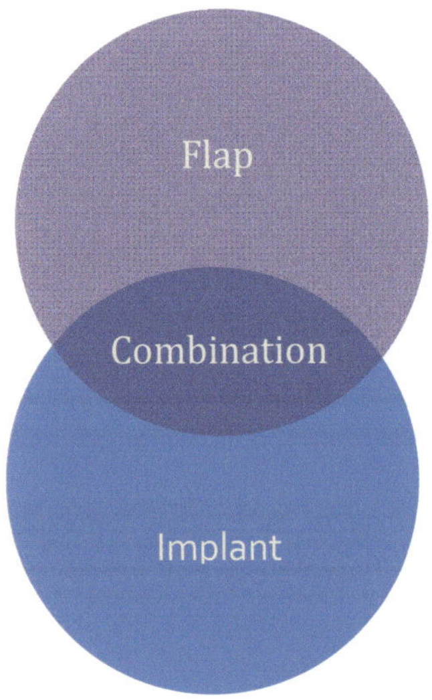

Figure 2. Breast reconstruction can be broken down into two categories: autologous flap reconstruction and implant-based reconstruction. However, in some cases, a combination of the two may provide the best result.

4.2. Tissue expanders/implants

This is a popular choice for breast reconstruction; it involves no donor site incision and minimal recovery time. There is no need for a donor site, so this type of reconstruction is suitable for patients who may have been ruled out for other reconstructions due to an insufficient donor site. This type of reconstruction is also preferable for older and less healthy patients who may not be able to tolerate a lengthier, flap-based reconstructive procedure. The surgeon needs to consider the timing of implant placement if future radiation therapy is required. The sequence and timing of implant placement after radiotherapy influences the complication rate. Reconstructive failure is significantly higher if the time between completion of radiotherapy and implant exchange is less than 6 months.[3] In many cases where the mastectomy has been radiated, implant only reconstruction is not an option due to higher complication rates and the need for skin replacement. The use of acellular dermal matrices can be helpful with implant only reconstruction, but in the end it is the surgeon's preference. With this option, the patient needs to be counseled about the risk and benefit of implants versus autologous flap reconstruction. The short term risks are reduced since the recovery does not involve a donor site. However, long term risks are higher as inherent to the implant device.

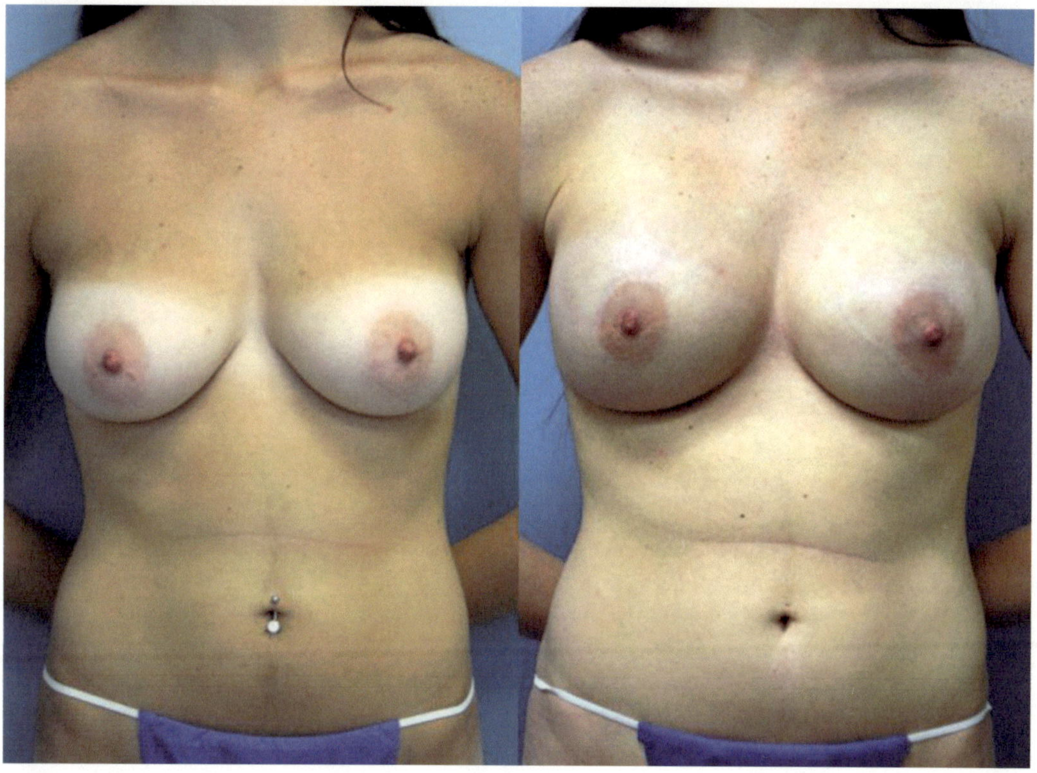

Figure 3. Preoperative and postoperative views of a bilateral tissue expander and implant based breast reconstruction.

4.3. Autologous flaps

4.3.1. Abdominal flaps

When examining a patient for breast reconstruction, a pinch test will help to estimate the amount of excess tissue available. In general, an average patient with a BMI greater than 20 and a history of at least one pregnancy should have enough abdominal tissue for a unilateral B to C cup breast reconstruction. The most important requirement for this flap is patent vessels in the lower abdomen. Previous abdominoplasty and extensive liposuction are contraindications to these flaps due to the disruption of the underlying blood supply. On examination, look for any abdominal scars. Scars may indicate a previous severance of the subcutaneous vasculature. Vessel patency can be determined by CTA or use of Doppler ultrasound.

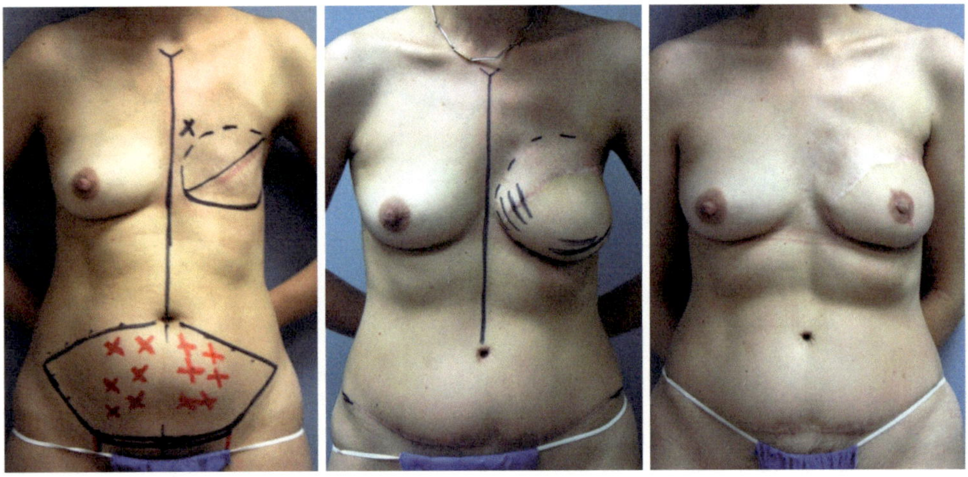

Figure 4. Preoperative markings and postoperative views of an abdominal perforator-based free flap breast reconstruction.

4.3.1.1. DIEP

This is the first choice for autologous reconstruction in our Center. The indications for the DIEP are similar to the indications for SIEA and TRAM as far as the need for excess lower abdominal tissue. Optimal perforator selection is key, as it impacts flap perfusion and muscle preservation. Imaging is helpful to determine if blood supply is patent and to map out the best perforator vessels. The DIEP flap may be combined with an implant to increase volume for a better size match with the contralateral breast or to improve the aesthetic outcome.

4.3.1.2. SIEA

Much like the DIEP flap, the SIEA flap requires excess lower abdominal tissue but is not a perforator flap. The difference between the two flaps is the blood supply with the SIEA using the superficial inferior epigastric artery to perfuse the flap. The availability of the SIEA has been shown to be variable. Drs Taylor and Daniel demonstrate that the SIEA was not present in 35% of their 100 cadaveric dissection specimens.[4] More recent literature by Stern and Nahai showed that 87% of subjects had an identifiable SIEA, while Reardon et al found the SIEA in 90% of subjects. [5-7] Specific to the survival of the SIEA flap is the need for a donor artery of 1.5 mm diameter or greater described by Spiegel et al.[8] This study found that in 278 clinical dissections over a 3 year period, approximately 31% of cases had identifiable superficial inferior epigastric arteries that were larger than 1.5 mm in diameter. The infrequent availability of a sufficiently sized artery limits the use of this type of reconstruction.

4.3.1.3. TRAM

The TRAM flap can be used as a pedicled or free flap. The use of this flap depends on the surgeon and the situation. Preserving the muscle has become more ubiquitous. The DIEP flap has become more of the standard of care as more residents are being taught this procedure. The use of a pedicled TRAM flap may be appropriate if a free flap is not possible in the selected patient.

4.3.2. Latissimus flap

The latissimus dorsi flap is a good second choice flap if the lower abdomen is inadequate, unavailable, or if the patient is opposed to an abdominally-based reconstruction. The volume of this flap is dependent upon the amount of soft tissue available on the back and skin laxity. Skin laxity is important for creating a skin island with the flap to replace skin deficit left from the mastectomy.

The latissimus dorsi flap may be muscle and soft tissue alone, or if skin is needed, it can be taken as a musculocutaneous flap. If a large amount of soft tissue is needed, an extended latissimus myocutaneous flap can be used in order to include more fat with the flap. Due to the limited volume that is provided, even with the extended latissimus dorsi myocutaneous

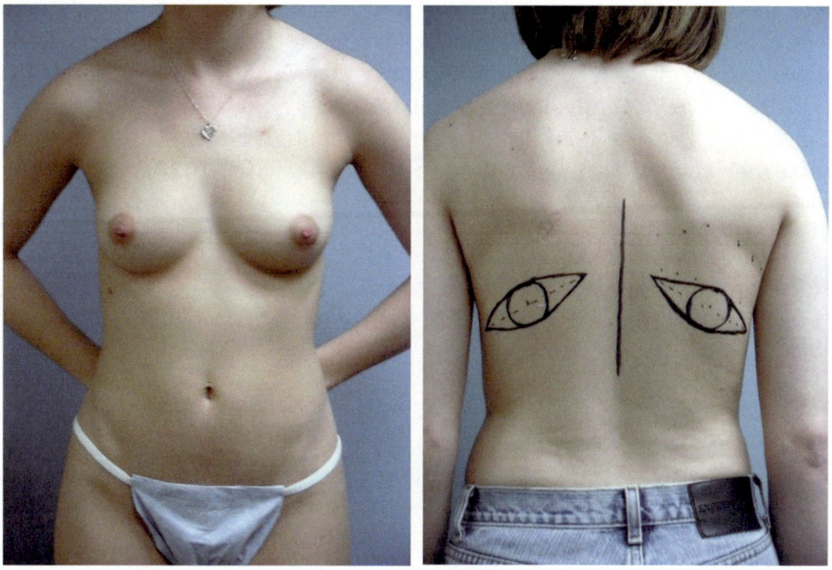

Figure 5. Anterior and posterior views of a preoperative bilateral latissimus dorsi breast reconstruction patient with markings.

flap, these flaps are usually combined with an implant to produce an adequate breast size. This flap generally provides donor site scars that are easily hidden in clothing.

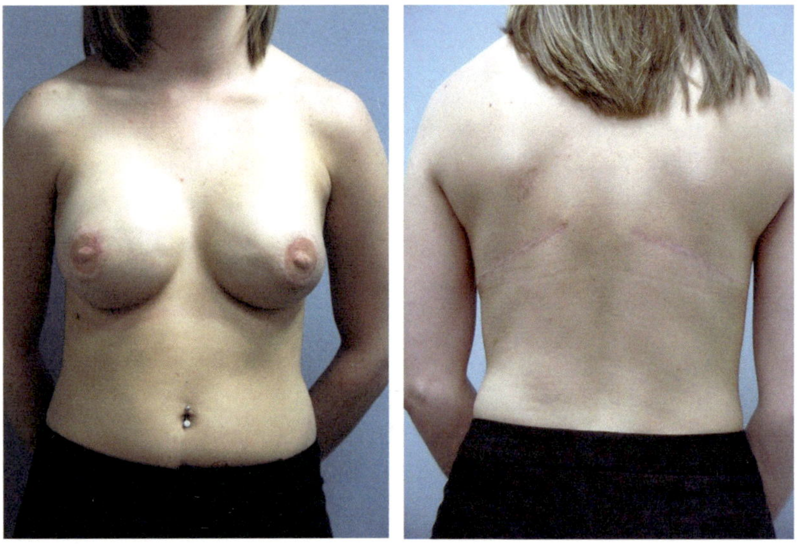

Figure 6. Anterior and posterior views of a postoperative bilateral latissimus dorsi breast reconstruction patient.

4.3.3. Gluteal flaps

Gluteal flaps are an alternative choice for autologous reconstruction when an abdominal donor site has been ruled out due to insufficient tissue or compromised blood supply from previous surgery or scarring. Another reason for choosing this flap is simply an excess amount of available soft tissue in the gluteal region. Patient preference plays a significant role in the selection of this flap because even if the patient has enough gluteal tissue to create a breast, they may like their current gluteal shape and may not be willing to change it.

The gluteal myocutaneous flap was described for breast reconstruction by Fujino in 1981.[9] Since that time, the gluteal flap has evolved into the SGAP, IGAP, and scGAP flaps. These perforator flaps are far more popular now due to the decreased donor site morbidity. Gluteal artery perforator flaps have become a well-liked alternative when the first line abdominal flaps are not available.

The choice of the SGAP and IGAP flaps depend on the patient and surgeon. Patients who wish to get rid of "saddlebags" while maintaining superior fullness of the buttocks may benefit from the IGAP which hides its scar in the inferior gluteal fold; however some reports state that the lateral edge of the scar may be visible in a bathing suit. The SGAP on the other hand, conceals its scar within most bathing suit bottoms at the expense of removing some of the superior fullness of the buttocks. The surgeon must decide which area has sufficient tissue to reconstruct the breast. The patient must also decide which scar/volume deformity they prefer. Working together the surgeon and patient must come to an agreement as to what would be best for the patient.

http://dx.doi.org/10.5772/56333

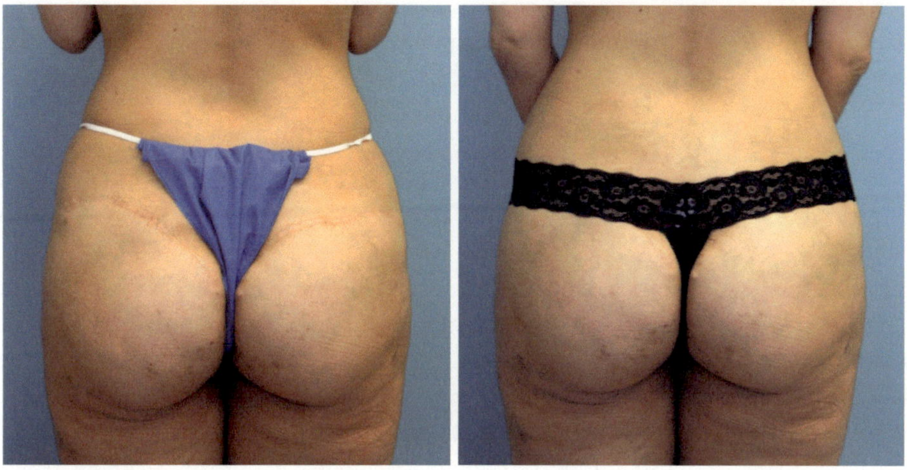

Figure 7. Postoperative view of the donor site scar from a superior gluteal artery perforator (SGAP) flap and a view showing the scar easily concealed by the patient's underwear.

4.3.4. Other flaps

4.3.4.1. TUG Flap

The TUG flap is best for patients with excess soft tissue in the medial thigh. This flap is indicated when other, more popular, flap donor sites have been ruled out due to insufficient tissue, compromised blood supply from previous surgery or scarring, or patient preference. This flap provides a well hidden donor site scar in the groin crease. This flap requires a surgeon familiar with this procedure.

4.3.4.2. PAP Flap

The PAP flap uses excess soft tissue of the medial thigh. This flap provides a well hidden donor site scar in the infragluteal fold. This flap is indicated when other donor sites have been ruled out due to insufficient tissue, compromised blood supply from previous surgery or scarring, or patient preference. Patient preference for this site is not the overall deciding factor as this flap also requires a surgeon who is familiar with this relatively new technique.

5. Other breast reconstruction techniques

5.1. Lipomodeling

Lipomodeling can be a sole mode of reconstruction for some surgeons who perform total breast reconstruction with ATF (autologous fat transfer) with or without the addition of an external tissue expander device; however, most surgeons use lipomodeling as an adjunct. It is useful for correcting of size mismatch and contour deformities, as well as the improvement of aesthetics. It can also be used to improve the quality of skin if the breast has been previously irradiated.

6. Summary

A focus on aesthetic refinements beyond flap survival is important for optimal breast reconstruction results. Good communication with general surgeons during mastectomy planning helps to provide a better cosmetic result and can make a reconstructive surgeon's life a lot easier. Additionally, the development of the Breast Q has allowed us to better analyze these results by quantifying the patient's opinion of the outcome. By selecting a method of breast reconstruction that best fits an individual patient, a surgeon can improve his/her odds of great results, from both the surgeon's and the patient's point of view, before the first cut is made.

Author details

Zachary Menn and Aldona Spiegel

Weill Cornell Medical College, The Methodist Hospital, Houston, Texas, USA

References

[1] Mentor CorpMemoryGel Breast Implants Product Insert Data Sheet. August 2010. (Web site) Available at: www.mentorwwllc.com/Documents/gel-PIDS.pdf.Accessed November 6, (2012).

[2] Massey, M. F, et al. Perforator flaps: recent experience, current trends, and future directions based on 3974 microsurgical breast reconstructions. Plast Reconstr Surg. (2009). Sep; , 124(3), 737-51.

[3] Peled, A. W, et al. Increasing the time to expander-implant exchange after postmastectomy radiation therapy reduces expander-implant failure. Plast Reconstr Surg. (2012). Sep; , 130(3), 503-9.

[4] Taylor, G. I, & Daniel, R. K. The anatomy of several free flap donor sites. Plast Reconstr Surg. (1975). Sep; , 56(3), 243-53.

[5] Stern, H. S, & Nahai, F. The versatile superficial inferior epigastric artery free flap. Br J Plast Surg (1992). May-Jun; , 45(4), 270-4.

[6] Reardon, C. M, Ceallaigh, O, & Sullivan, S, O. ST. An anatomical study of the superficial inferior epigastric vessels in humans. Br J Plast Surg. (2004). Sep;, 57(6), 515-9.

[7] Wolfram, D, Schoeller, T, Hussi, H, & Wechselberger, G. The superficial inferior epigastric artery (SIEA) flap: indications for breast reconstruction. Ann Plast Surg. (2006). Dec;, 57(6), 593-6.

[8] Spiegel, A. J, & Khan, F. N. An intraoperative algorithm for use of the SIEA flap for breast reconstruction. Plast Reconstr Surg. (2007). Nov;, 120(6), 1450-9.

[9] Fujino, T, Abe, O, & Enomoto, K. Primary reconstruction of the breast by free myocutaneous gluteal flap. Int Adv Surg Oncol. (1981). , 4, 127-43.

Section 2

Non Microsurgical Reconstruction

Chapter 3

Implant-Based Dual-Plane Reconstruction of the Breast Following Sparing Mastectomy

Egidio Riggio and Maurizio B. Nava

Additional information is available at the end of the chapter

http://dx.doi.org/10.5772/56466

1. Introduction

The immediate restoration of the breast is considered as the most favourable treatment for women undergoing a primary mastectomy since many years, but it is is not always true as it can occur in case of radiation therapy. Nowadays many patients care the aesthetics of the breast more than only ten years ago. An immediate definite reconstruction is unfrequently achievable using flaps or implants due to both clinical and surgical reasons. In our institution, a one-stage reconstruction embraces a minor part of patients. The first improvement of the cosmetic outcome starts with the preservation of native skin envelope in the immediate breast reconstruction (IBR) when this event is followed by less visible scars and reduced risk for skin necrosis. Toth and Lappert [1] described a skin-sparing mastectomy in 1991. The reconstructions without nipple are less pleasant as already suggested by Wellisch et al. [2] Furthermore the nipple is often difficult to be restored with the same charactheristics present before a skin-sparing mastectomy (SSM). Moreover preserving nipple and areola is much more grateful for the patients.The problem can arise if the breast is ptotic or large breast where the maintainance of redundant skin and nipple is risky. A moderate periareolar deepithelization or a skin-reducing mastectomy would be helpful trying to maintain more blood supply to the nipple-areola complex and skin around. [3] By the way, apart of the plastic surgery's implications, nipple-sparing mastectomy (NSM) is already the gold standard in the women at high genetic risk (BRCA1-2) as risk-reducing mastectomy. [4-6] Based on the expectations of more conservative approaches, NSM is progressively extending the indications in the treatment of the breast cancer, such as multifocal IDCS, T1-T2 IDC, T3 after tumor regression by neoadjuvant therapy. [7] The local recurrence risk is acceptable after peripheral tumors smaller than 3 cm. [8-11]

The challenging goal of any IBR is given by the chance for a one-stage procedure with the same complication rate and aesthetic outcome as the two-stage reconstruction. In the past the single-stage reconstruction with implants was consistently considered more complicated and risky than the reconstruction with autologous flap. [12] However complications were reported in all the immediate reconstructions, not only using permanent implants. [13] In addition poor IBR results were strictly related to both the inadequate surgical skill and the unsatisfactory selection for the right patient or breast implant as well. [14] Also the permanent expander alone or combined to the latissimus dorsi flap was extensively considered in some institutions as demonstrated by Gui et al. [15] The current standard for the implant reconstruction after mastectomy is the two-stage reconstruction with temporary expander followed by permanent implant, and secondarly the reconstruction using autologous free and pedicled flaps.

In the last decade the Acellular Dermal Matrix (ADM) has been used and successfully reported into the expander-based reconstruction especially in US, even if associated to higher incidence of seroma (3.9%), infection (2.7%) and total failure (3.0%) as underlined in a meta-analysis of complications recently published. [16] Moreover ADM significantly adds a cost to the two-stage IBR and hence but only few publications suggest single-stage implant-based IBR with ADM in a positive way. [17, 18] Theoretically it would be expected that ADM can facilitate the IBR in one stage, i.e. without using temporary expander. The oncoplastic surgeons that are still using successfully the two-stage reconstruction with expander but with no kind of mesh, frequently occurring in Europe, cannot understand the real advantage of ADM in two steps. The need for ADM or synthetic mesh in case of expander-based reconstruction may be due to the behaviour of the breast surgeon that does not spare both muscular fascia and a strip of soft tissues along the submammary fold during mastectomy. The one-stage procedure offers significant advantages: reducing recovery costs, avoiding the fixed second operation, decreasing the days of convalescence (including the series of tissue expansion) and achieving a more prompt restoration of body image and perception. [19]

The key point of any single-step IBR is the correct selection of patients where a satisfactory grade of symmetry can be reached. The patient expectations for the best and most prompt cosmetic result have greatly increased compared to only ten years ago. Nevertheless the ideal procedure is still far from being found.

In the meantime, based on the refusal for dermal matrix derived by cadaver human-tissue like Alloderm (Lifecell Corp., Branchburg NJ USA) mainly in Europe, the marketing system is proposing new biomeshes [20-22], like the Strattice (Lifecell Corp., Branchburg NJ USA) and the Meso Biomatrix (Kensey Nash Corp. Exton PA USA) derived by porcine dermis and mesothelium respectively as well as alloplastic meshes, i.e. the TiLOOP made of titanized polypropylene (Pfm medical titanium, GfE Medizintechnik GmbH, Nurnberg Germany) or the Seriscaffold of biodegradable silk (Allergan Inc. Irvine CA USA).

In our opinion far from commercial inputs, on the contrary, the breast meshes should have a limited use in case of IBR while a well-tailored surgical technique can still achieve more physiological outcomes. The dual-plane technique here illustrated is an example how a feasible autologous pocket for silicone implant allows to reach the goal of a breast reconstruction in a single procedure.

2. Immediate reconstruction after primary breast cancer

Breast reconstruction should ideally be both immediate and definitive so as to avoid patients undergoing further surgery later. It is generally considered, from an oncological and psychological point of view, that there are no contraindications to immediate reconstruction excepting particular cases but it is not so clear about the definite single stage, whereas it is already established for the breast cancer conservative treatment. [23]

One-stage reconstruction after skin-sparing-mastectomy and specially nipple-sparing mastectomy (NSM) is performed thanks to several procedures: a) autologous flaps (DIEP, TRAM, Latissimus dorsi + implant); b) autologous preparation of the pocket used for permanent implant (saline or silicone)/expandable permanent implant (Becker or other types), c) preparation of an implant pocket with support of eterologous (tissue biomatrix) or alloplastic meshes tailored for breast surgery. The one-stage IBR might not always be indicated, e.g. in presence of local radiated tissues where a delayed reconstruction is often formerly discussed with the patient. The example of the autologous flaps may be paradigmatic. Flaps have the great benefit of restoring the breast with soft and well-vascularized tissues, and this advantage becomes essential when breast tissues were before irradiated. Nevertheless when reconstruction is immediate, there are side effects that withdraw from the elective choice of a distant flap for several reasons: a) longer operation and recovery time with all the related medical complications; b) misunderstanding of the real implications of that kind of surgery in patients much more worried of cancer implications at the moment of the pre-op consultation; c) higher hazard for postponement of the oncological care (chemotherapy or irradiation) in case of flap failure and wound complications, that are more severe if compared with reconstruction by silicone implant, although their occurrence is infrequent. Flap failure after IBR strongly compromises patient body image and self-esteem, and moreover complicates any further reconstruction. Some review studies recommend delayed flap reconstruction in patients at high risk for adjuvant radiation therapy. [24, 25] On the contrary, in case of expander or protsthesis, also the worst complication could be treated by an easier removal of the device, with a limited delay of the cancer therapy. Moreover this failure can be solved afterward by using a flap or a tissue expander another time.

IBR does not interfere with the progress of the disease but it should be chosen the less risky procedure to reconstruct the breast. The ideal treatment must reduce at a minimum the occurrence of major surgical complications that can significantly delay the following chemotherapy and/or radiotherapy in breast cancer patients. In such a way, also the ADM, the other kinds of biomatrix, and in particular the alloplastic meshes can conceal higher incidence of complications, seroma and implant extrusion as first, then extreme thinning of the lower pole soft tissue above the implant compared with an autologous IBR performed only through a special preparation of the muscular and fascial pocket for implant.

We believe that the permanent implant pocket must retain these special features to have a final success: a) to be well vascularized, b) to be resilient, pliable, and adequately large; c) to be separated from the subcutaneous mastectomy pocket and the axillary cavity, as to decrease the risk for seroma or infection; to be partially free of the active contractions and reactive stiffness of the pectoralis maior muscle but contemporarily avoiding any malposition and malrotation of the implant.

Since mastectomy interferes with the psychologic, social, and sexual well-being of the women, it should be proper that the final statement about the kind of breast reconstruction is going to be realized by a well-informed patient. She must have the right of opting for both the immediate and easiest type of reconstruction, also the patient with a radiation to be post-operatively planned or that with a poor cancer prognosis. In that case she may promptly have something looking like a breast. It does not matter if the implantable device will be a permanent implant or a "temporary" saline expander as well.

3. Planning for the one-stage implant-based breast reconstruction

Contrary to prior surgical approaches to implant-based IBR and without use of dermal matrix and alloplastic mesh, the technique here described permits to extend the one-stage reconstruction to patients with larger breast or minimal ptosis, even satisfying the demand of bilateral enlargement of the breast. The technique is easier to be used in bilateral mastectomies either for those sparing the nipple or those sparing only skin, in unilateral mastectomy, preferably if nipple-sparing.

3.1. Clinical fundamentals

Some of the patients undergoing skin- or nipple-sparing mastectomy can be eligible for this kind of IBR, nearly the 30%. The ideal breast is the breast without ptosis, with weight less than 500 g, with good skin elasticity or at least moderate redundancy as occurring in the skin after pregnancy. The last is the most favourable condition in order to plan augmentation of the prior breast size. Women with large breast (D/DD breast cup size) or severe ptosis and the obese patients must be excluded. Cautious contraindications are given by the heavy smoker patient (>30 cigarettes a day) or by the breast with multiple prior scars. However the primary evaluation is addressed towards the expectations of the single women about the breast shape and size. It is not psychologically easy to explain all the plastic and cosmetic aspects to a women often worried by the cancer just discovered and distressed thinking about the incoming oncological treatments. The mood of many patients may not allow good understanding of some among the following queries: 1-stage vs. 2-stage reconstruction; implant vs. autologous flap; expander vs. permanent implant; best shape vs best symmetry of the breast; timing of the complimentary contra-lateral surgery and hence choice for augmentation, mastopexy or reduction respectively.

Immediate aesthetic correction of the healthy breast is suggested in the majority of the patients requiring total augmentation. On the contrary, if required, pexy is much better to be carried out at a second stage. Adequate symmetry is very difficult to be attained in case of contralateral reduction as well as pexy alone or with augmentation. The nipple-areola position and breast size cannot be well planned during mastectomy because the definitive shape of the new breast and the same nipple/areola position are to be evaluated after healing. The risk for asymmetric displacement is real in case of every nipple-sparing mastectomy. Moreover, it is well known that the nipple/areola complex can be barely placed in another position after mastopexy or breast reduction. For this type of patients the contralateral surgery should be delayed regardless of the possibility of IBR in a single step. The decision to plan a larger implant size and also decide the ultimate augmentation of the healthy breast can be taken at the time of the pexy or reduction as well.

On the other hand, permanent implant can also be changed with another of better shape and volume corresponding to the contra-lateral breast at a second stage that becomes possible, but not necessary, if symmetry is already satisfactory following the previous immediate reconstruction. It should be clear to the patient that the one-stage reconstruction with a permanent implant gives a prompt and definitive result but is not unchangeable. In fact a surgical revision may always take place improving all the breast, if the result is not satisfactory.

Another preoperative valuation regards the preservation of soft tissues in the lower section of the breast, which means not only in the inner plane but also in the outer, i.e. the skin. The dual-plane technique cannot match up with those surgical approaches planning inframammary or vertical incision for the mastectomy. [26] These incisions can compromise any natural refilling of the lower breast, and hence lead to the insertion of expander instead of permanent implant, or to the aid of ADM with higher costs for the hospital. The overall preference for a lateral radial, even in presence of previous areola scars, is supported by data reported in literature, Riggio et al. [27] reported 1% of areola necrosis in a preliminary clinical study. Garwood et al. [28] decreased the same risk to a 5% rate, and pointed out that the incision of at least 30% of areola circumference is already to be considered as independent risk factor for necrosis. Of course, the lateral radial incision is preferred because of lower risk of skin ischemia and of more accurate dissection behind nipple and areola, but it is not enough if the mastectomy does not spare the whole subcutaneous layer and its vascular network. Sometimes incision can include earlier lumpectomy scars and partial areolar incision are performed in presence of prior scars. The periareolar deepithelialization is rarely carried out if there is vertical skin excess.

3.2. Anatomical fundamentals

Any preparation for a full-coverage autologous pocket, i.e. made of local tissues of the breast, first bases on the thorough preservation of the inframammary fold frame during mastectomy. The real anatomy of the superficial fascial system inside the submammary fold unit was finely described by Riggio et al. (2000), Fig.1. [29]

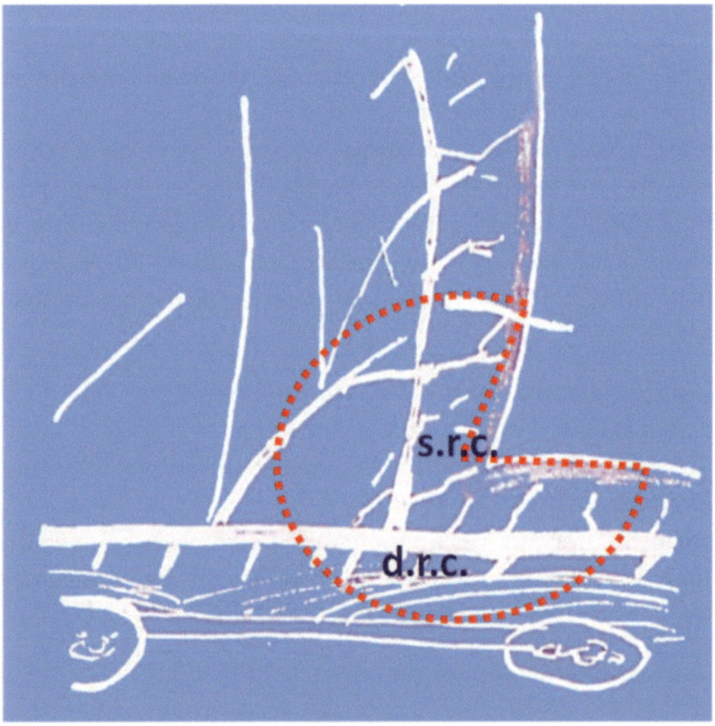

Figure 1. The inframammary fascial system: *s.r.c.,superficial retinacula cutis* into the superficial subcutaneous (adipose) layer between skin and superficial fascia and its annex (the breast gland envelope); *d.r.c., deep retinacula cutis* into the deep subcutaneous (areolar/adipose) layer between superficial fascia and deep fascia (the musculo-fascial plane). The density and thickness of the connective frame is here particular, *the dotted red encircle*. There is also thin areolar tissue between muscle and rib cage.

The fine anatomy is made of multiple subcutaneous attachments, i.e. thickened retinacula between the superficial and deep fascia (zone of adherence), where contiguous connective micro-frames of the superficial and deep subcutaneous layers persist as different anatomical microunits of the same fascial frame, as according to the functional concept of skin-superficial fat-superficial fascial system described by Lockwood in the trunk and extremities (1991) and to the study of Nava et al. (1998) that already explained the fascial system in the surgical reconstruction of the inframammary fold. [30, 31]

Maintaining the attachments of the inframammary fascial system at the deep plane (fascio-muscular layer) is mandatory along all the inframammary contour (Fig.2). The breast surgeon has to avoid any cut or undermining at the submammary level, in both the superficial and deep subcutaneous layers. Maintaining a few millimeters of soft tissues above the inframammary line can totally spare the connections, also called (deep retinacula) between the superficial system and muscular plane. This care allows the mastectomy field to be maintained far from the submuscular pocket for implant.

The preservation of the pectoralis fascia is viable and its resection is not justified by any evidence-based oncological reason in routine modified radical mastectomy for invasive breast

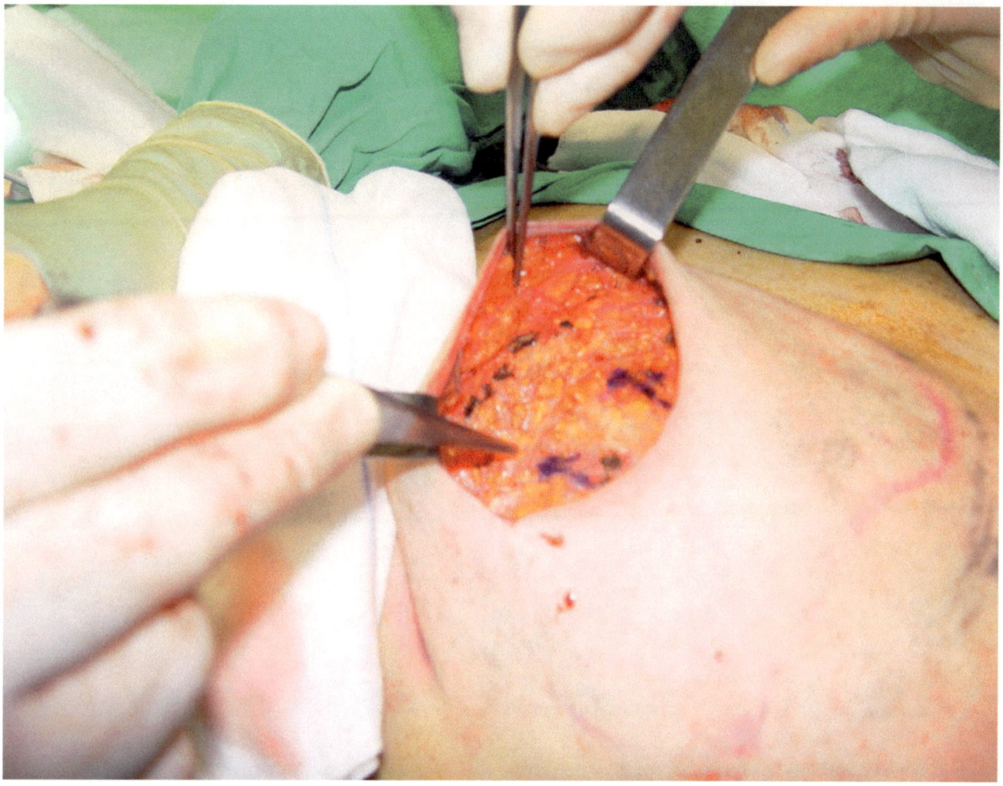

Figure 2. The inframammary superficial fascia, direct prolongation of the abdominal fascia (Scarpa's fascia), extends to the retromammary space and properly links the superficial connective frame to the deep fascia (the pectoralis maior and serrate anterior muscular plane) along all the inframammary fold. The mastectomy must preserve this strip of soft tissue after dissecting off the breast gland. *Intra-operative view.*

cancer. [32] On the other hand, sparing this fascia is also important that occurs at two levels: 1) at the inferomedial portion because it allows to release the muscle insertions preserving the stability of the implant coverage; 2) close to the free border of the pectoralis maior and above the serratus anterior because it allows correctly to suture the pocket above the implant without dehiscence.

Before starting with reconstruction (Fig.3), the plastic surgeon must check the following topics: a) the anatomical quality of the surgical field (some conditions interfere with the pocket preparation, e.g. cranial insertions of the pectoralis maior muscle far from the inframammary level); b) a prior mastectomy dissection carefully preserving both the inframmamary fascial system and the deep fascia along the lower border of the pectoralis maior muscle. Any leakage should be sutured using vicryl 2/0 stitches but, if the musculofascial layer is going to tear again, the plan for permanent implant must be discontinued pro expander, avoiding the saline inflation intra-operatively. All patients have before to be warned that the insertion of a permanent implant is not sure until the end of the surgical procedure.

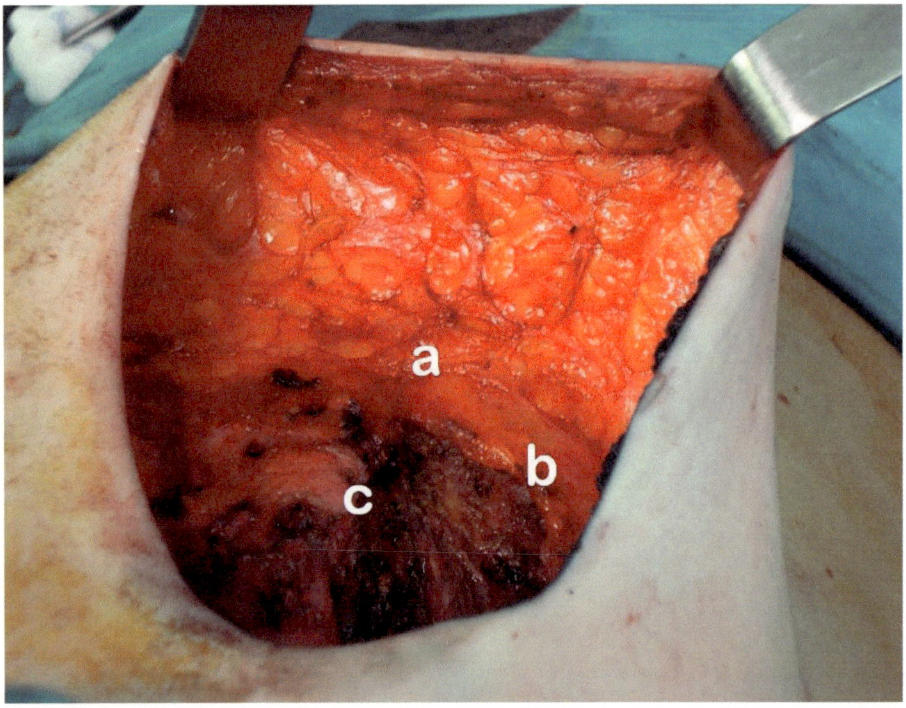

Figure 3. The surgical field of the submammary zone after radical modified mastectomy with preservation of: *a)* the inframammary unit, made of subcutaneous fatty tissue, superficial fascia and related retinacula; *b)* both aponeurosis of the pectoralis maior and serratus anterior muscle and likely the fascia between the two muscles (this layer, if discontinued by the prior dissection must be rebuilt using some stitches or occasionally a small patch of absorbable material; *c)* the muscles and proper fascia (deep fascia). The surgeon that destroys the submammary fascial frame precludes the immediate chance for any satisfying 1-stage reconstruction with silicone implant.

4. The dual-plane pocket for 1-stage immediate reconstruction with highly-cohesive implants

The best presentation in IBR is given by the aesthetic preservation of the nipple-areola complex when oncologically safe. The removal of skin around the nipple limits the use of the same technique in the skin-sparing group of mastectomy. Maintaining all the breast skin envelope results in skin redundancy which becomes too wide in case of larger or pendant breast. The skin, after the Cooper's ligaments resection, is free to extend, especially when skin is less elastic (after weight loss, pregnancy, aging). Side effect of the skin excess is the growing risk for the necrosis of the inner skin. This complication is uncommon if patient selection and subcutaneous dissection are correct whilst, on the other hand, other complications are common as skin folding, scar retraction, and NAC displacement. They are difficult to be solved secondarly and really compromise breast aesthetics and body perception. IBR gives an answer to this problem related to skin excess and tries immediately to replace as much as possible the volume loss after parenchyma excision with larger implants. A prompt expansion volume is able of filling, or better overfilling, the skin envelope and stabilizing the nipple position. The cutaneous envelope of the breast is consistently major than the respective volume breast only except the teenager's breast. On the contrary, a T-inverted skin reduction together with the nipple preservation, jeopardize the vascular supply to the same nipple and areola apart from the implant dimensions. Breast shape can be outlined by a tear-drop device with high-cohesive silicone and then better maintained through the gel memory. Highly cohesive implants generate a certain strain strength on the envelope at the same way as a rapid expansion does. This is more stable than the strenght produced by saline expander or low-cohesive gel devices. Highly cohesive gel withstands external pressures, e.g. muscular strenght or scar-tissue retraction, with poor inner displacement of the filling gel. Bio-mechanics of the forces acting on the female breast and the physical properties of breast tissues are strictly related to every plastic surgery procedure but, unfortunately, their knowledge is still less than average. [33, 34] We can take advantage from the bio-mechanical properties of the high-cohesive gel, soft tissue and muscle too, preparing a full-vascularized, partially sub-muscular, complete coverage for the implant. The pocket must not be the same as the pocket prepared for an expander to be inflated progressively after surgery and then substituted. Surgical refinements must be maximized in a single-stage reconstruction. In addition, the planning for implant size and shape is more and more challenging in IBR in order to achieve the best symmetrical outcome.(Fig 4)

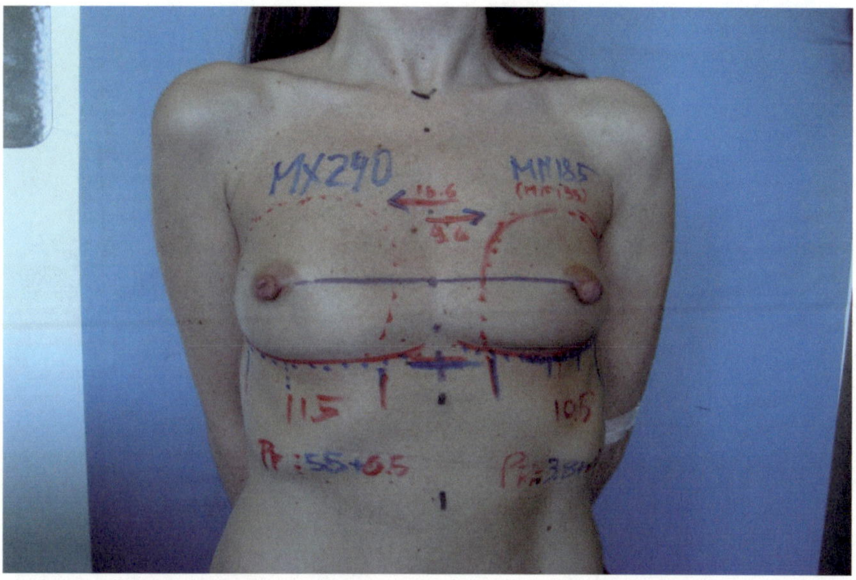

Figure 4. Preoperative planning for nipple-sparing mastectomy (DCIS) + IBR with anatomical implant (natrelle high-cohesive 410MX 290g) in the right breast and submuscular augmentation (natrelel high-coesive 410MM 185g)

The selection for tear-drop implants will depend on the anatomic landmarks of breast and chest wall in the same way as planned in aesthetic surgery. Width, height, and projection are to be measured choosing shape and size of the implant. Here width and height of implant are difficult to be planned accurately compared to the selection for a temporary expander or to the 2-stage reconstruction (expander substitution). Only bilateral reconstruction makes easier the choice, here the preliminary indications are consistently maintained during surgery. Intra-operatively plastic surgeon must evaluate the limits of breast removal and the remaining soft-tissue thicknesses in order to change the implant in width or height usually by about 0.5-1 cm more or less. It is also recommended to weigh the specimen after mastectomy and compare the breast weight with the implant weight taking into account that is better to choose an implant a little bigger than the breast weight. Soft-tissue retraction and atrophy can occur after normal healing or radiotherapy. When contemporary enlargement of the contralateral breast is planned, augmentation is preferably sub-muscular with the aim of improving implant symmetry and better screening of the healthy breast.

4.1. Submuscular preparation of the pocket: Part I

After harvesting the free edge of the pectoralis maior muscle, with identification of the deeper pectoralis minor muscle (Fig. 5), dissection begins from the lateral part of the proper fascia of pectoralis minor and carries below the of the serratus anterior muscle and proper fascia laterally and downward (Fig. 6).

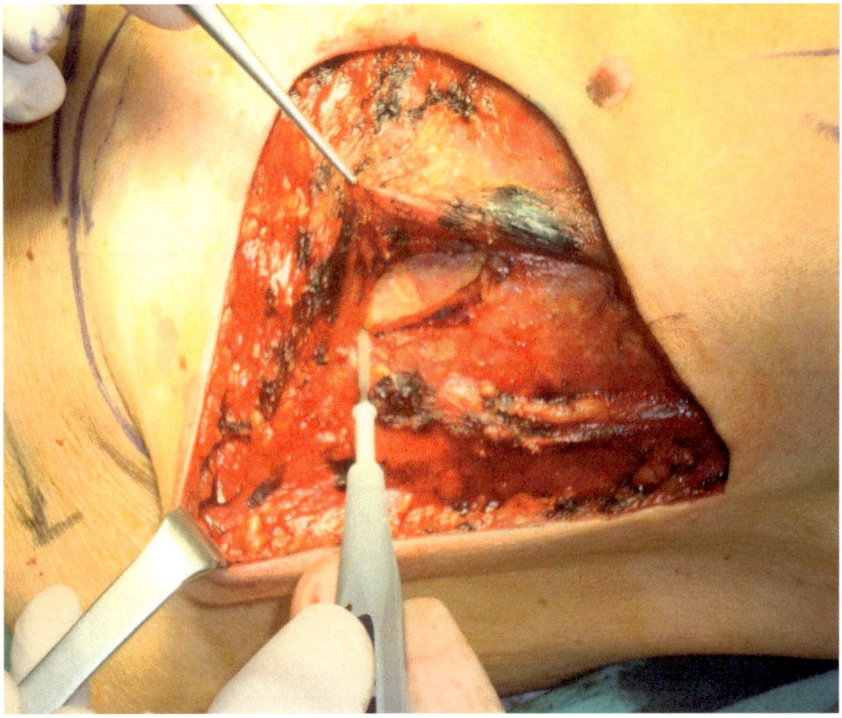

Figure 5. Along the upper lateral border of the pectoralis maior muscle, scoring the deep muscular fascia towards the pectoralis minor muscle.

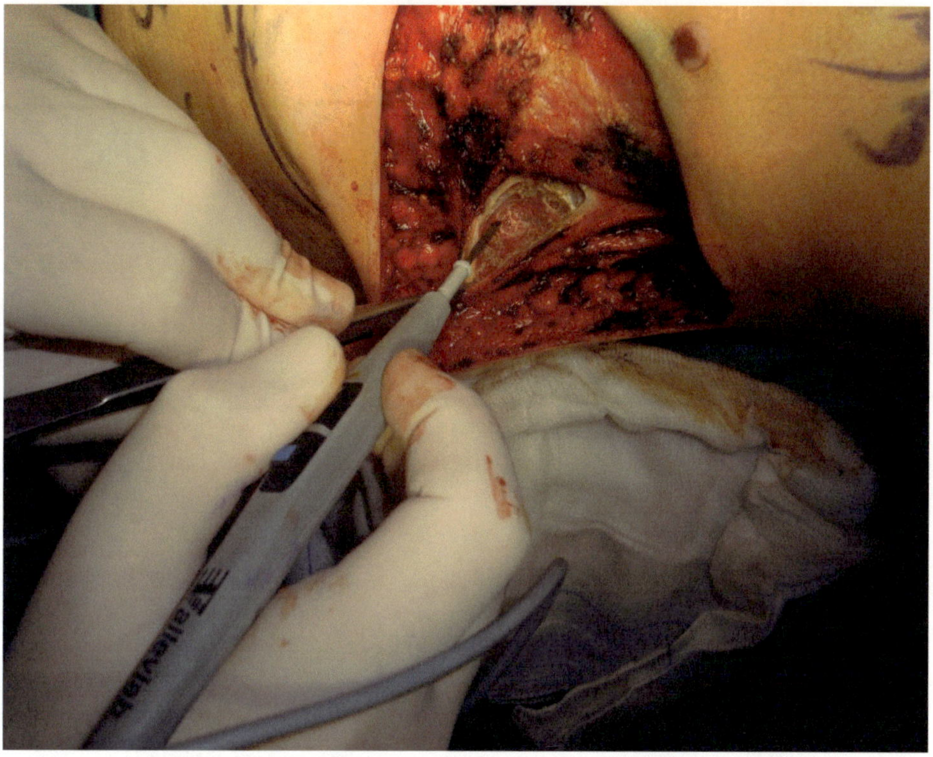

Figure 6. Harvest of the serratus anterior fascia and muscle, never only fascia, but trying to split the muscular fibers

Serratus anterior muscle can be split using an intramuscular dissection when the thickness is adequate and the proper fascia has been spared during mastectomy. The aim is leaving a layer of muscle fibers above the rib cage with the following effects: a) a more pliable coverage in the lateral side of the device pocket; b) maintenance of some active work of the deeper part of the muscle; pain reduction after surgery. The lateral limit of the pocket must exactly correspond to the implant width at the aim of avoiding implant malposition.

Then the upper and medial undermining is carried out under the pectoralis maior muscle and the extension will depend on the implant size. The pocket width must precisely correspond to the device width in order to avoid any lateral malposition (Fig. 7)

Dissection carries on towards the lower fibers of the serratus anterior and the lower insertions of the pectoralis maior and (Fig.8). As usual in breast surgery, the lower medial insertions of the pectoralis muscle are scored. The submuscular undermining reaches the visible submammary line (Fig.9).

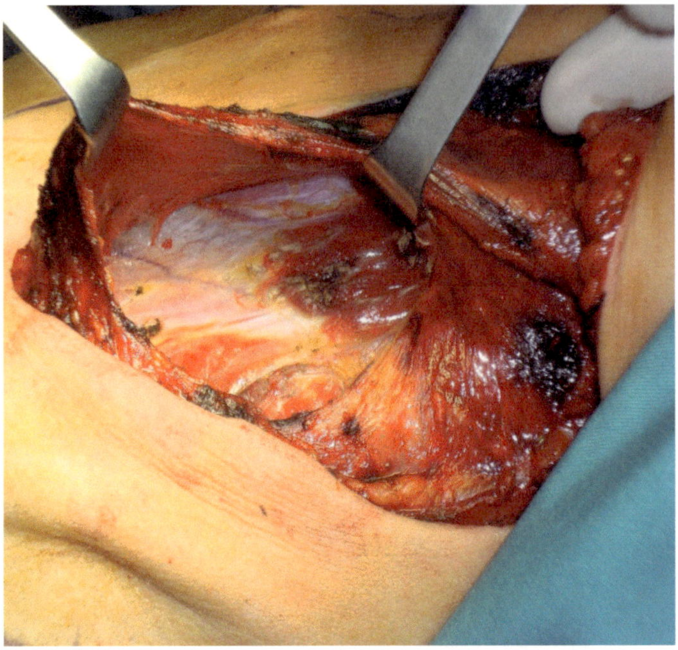

Figure 7. The submuscular dissection in the midpart of the implant coverage

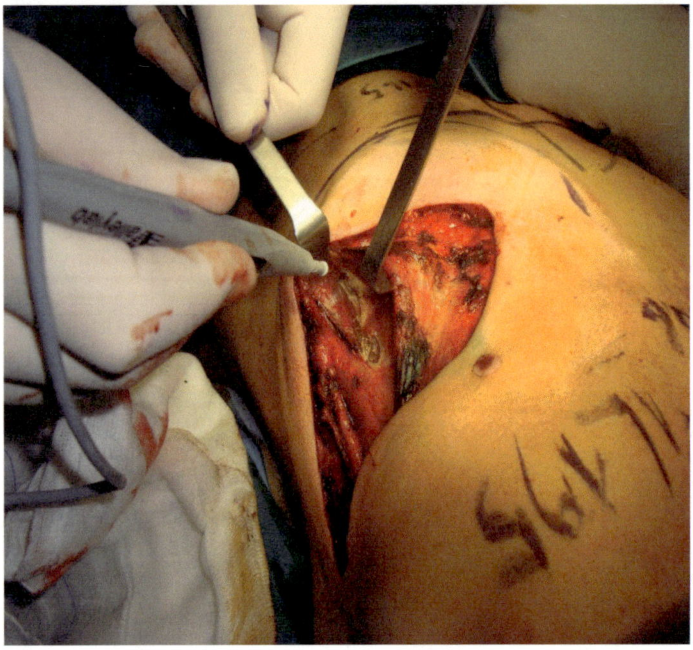

Figure 8. Scoring fibers and insertions of the muscles towards the inframammary zone

http://dx.doi.org/10.5772/56466

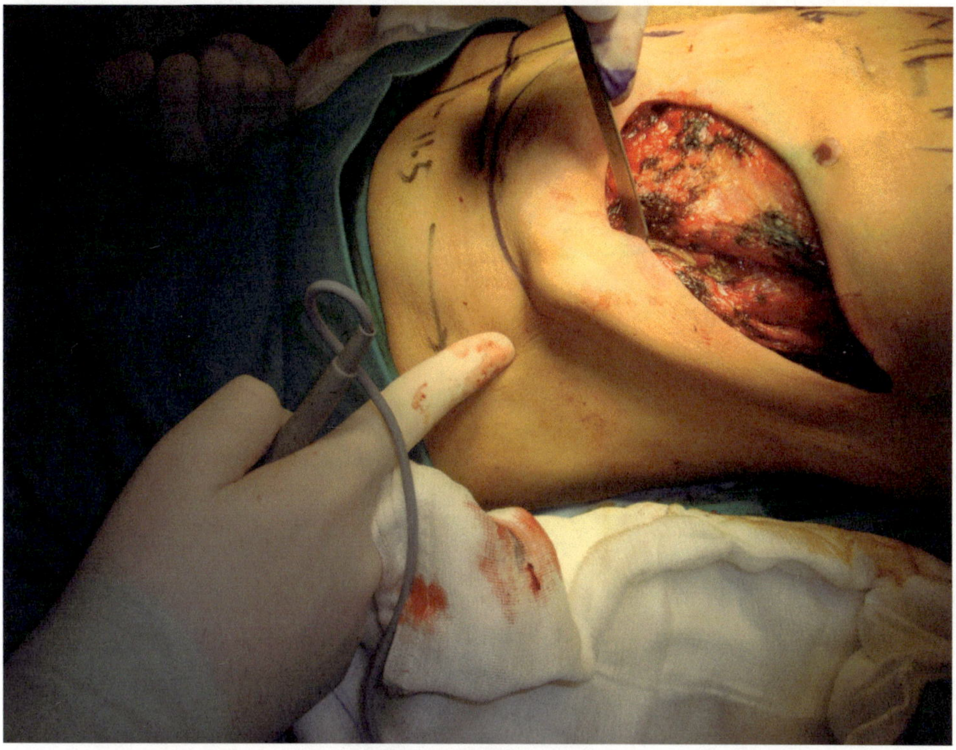

Figure 9. The submuscular pocket ends into the inframammary fold, any downward over-dissection should be avoided.

In a two-stage reconstruction with tissue expander, the submuscular pocket is complete when partial or total release of the deep fascia is performed at the same inframammary line, also called pectoralis fascia or muscular fascia, overlaying the muscles (Fig.10, 11). The superficial fascia must be preserved because it will expand progressively and physiologically. Also the deep fascia, if thin, can expand as well. On the other hand, in case of ADM-based IBR, the deep fascia is totally dissected just above the inframammary level and then the lower edge of the biomatrix is sutured along the inframammary fold.

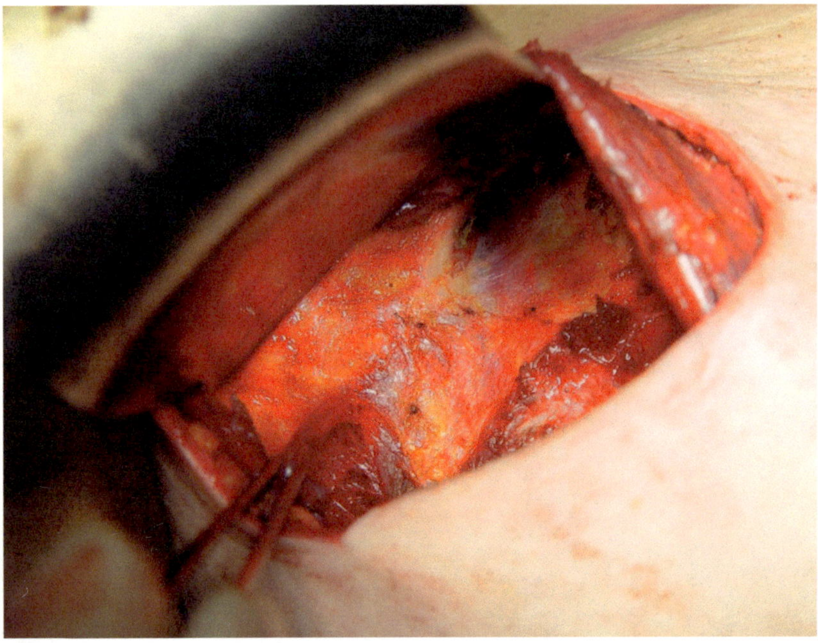

Figure 10. The deep fascia along the inframammary fold observed behind the section of the muscle fibers

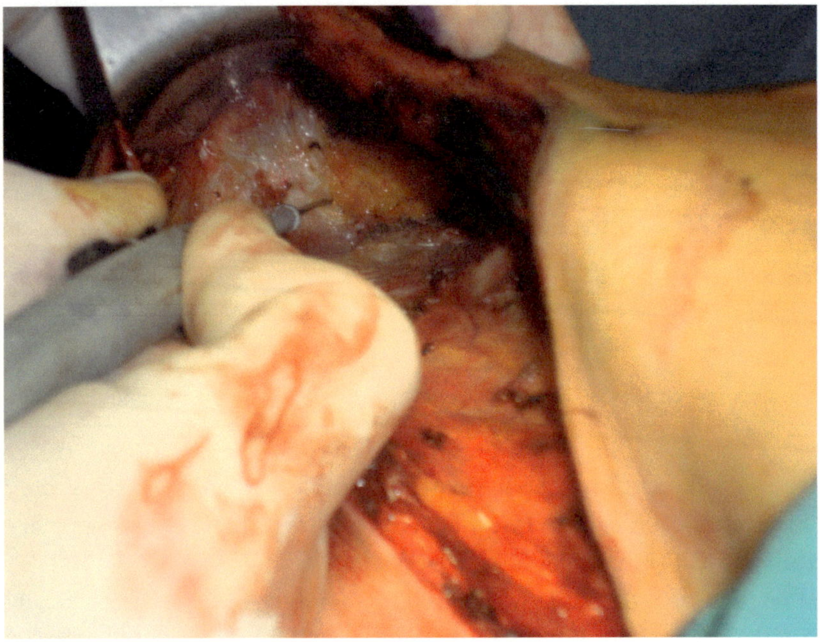

Figure 11. Total release of the deep fascia and deep retinacula cutis along the inframammary fold

4.2. Subcutaneous/subfascial preparation of the pocket: Part II — The dual-plane reconstruction

Summarizing the first part, the submuscular pocket results:

- partially scored medially, close to the sternal border, from the 4th rib down to the inframammary level;
- completely scored, including the whole musculo-fascial plane, along all the inframammary fold under the pectoralis maior and serratus anterior as far as the most lateral portion of the submuscular pocket. The final maneuver gives access to the deep adipose layer infero-laterally where fat is generally thicker.

Dissection allows to achieve a vertical enlargement of the lower pocket about 2-3 cm, seldom wider after scoring the deep retinacula cutis. This is that for more than a decade the Authors have been used to perform in the one-stage IBR with permanent implants, even some series of patients were recently published by other authors. [35] Expandable devices, Becker's or other types, were never used in these patients. Devices were tear-drop shaped and pre-filled with silicone gel highly cohesive. The patients were few compared with the patients with 2-stage reconstruction. Breast size was small to medium and weight lower than 300 grams. Because the possible results were not so satisfactory and the demand for sparing mastectomy was growing up, since 2008 the possibilities of transposing the former knowledge upon the inframammary reconstruction (Nava et al., 1998) were taken into account, in order to define the details of a proper technique for IBR in over 130 cases (Riggio et al., 2012). [27, 31]

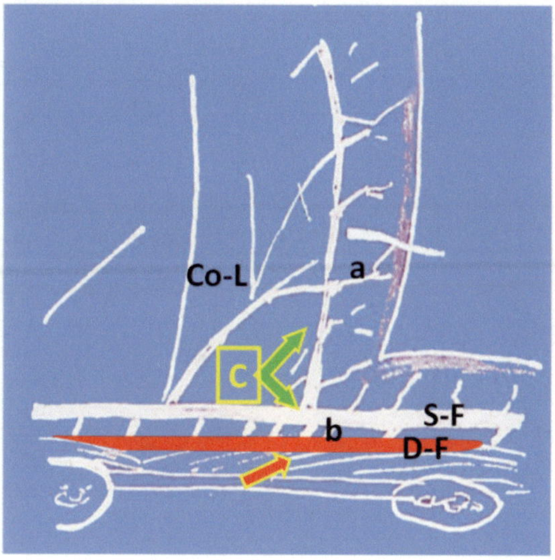

Figure 12. The surgical anatomy of the inframammary fascial system of connective tissue: a, superficial retinacula cutis; b, deep retinacula cutis; Co-L, Cooper's Ligaments; S-F, superficial fascia (horizontal white line); D-F, deep fascia overlying the muscles (horizontal red line); C, the levels of the electrosurgical scores in the dual-plane technique: green arrows into the superficial fascial plane and red arrow into the deep plane. It is possible to release the deep fascia a few millimeters beneath the fold, whereas the superficial fascia must be scored a few millimeters above.

The modified technique improves the enlargement of the lower breast substantially through the total release of the superficial fascia together with the superficial retinacula cutis above the whole inframammary line (Fig.12). It is fundamental that every surgeon may notionally understand, practically recognize, and surgically respect the fine anatomy of the submammary fold.

The multiple scores can obtain a better enlargement of the lower breast compared to the same manoeuvre performed in the second stage of reconstruction after expander because soft tissues can here contain some grade of fibrosis and the pre-existing connective frame be distorted. The scores must be performed behind the skin plane perpendicularly, avoiding any dermal bruising, and just above the corresponding external submammary line, a few millimeters, so as to avoid the bottoming-out of the pocket (Fig. 13, 14, 15, 16)

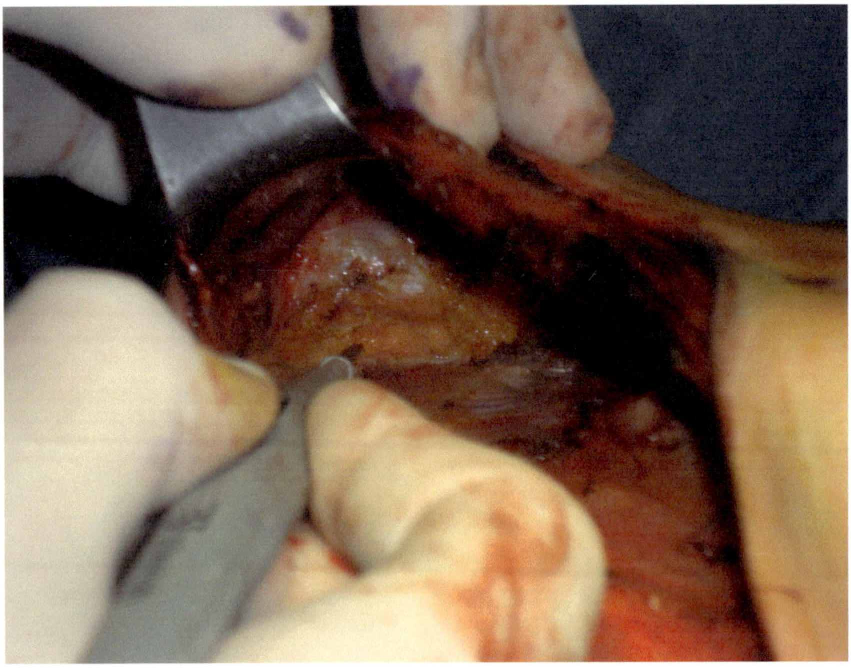

Figure 13. The vertical scoring of the superficial fascia through the previous deep fasciotomy and access to the deep subcutaneous layer, along the inframammary fold. The upper and lower free borders are part of the deep fascia already scored.

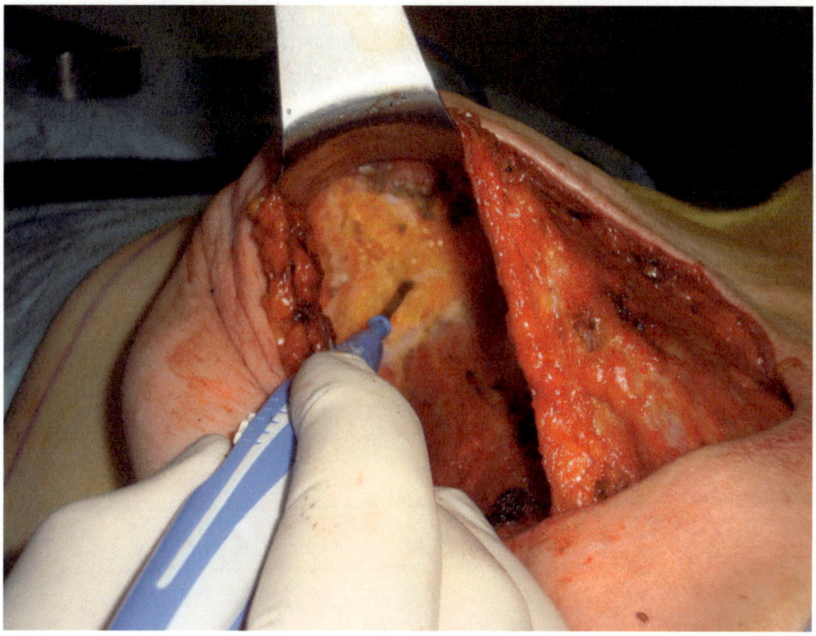

Figure 14. The tip of the electrical scalpel indicates where the superficial fascia layer is placed, above the inframammary fold, and the advancement of the pocket enlargement.

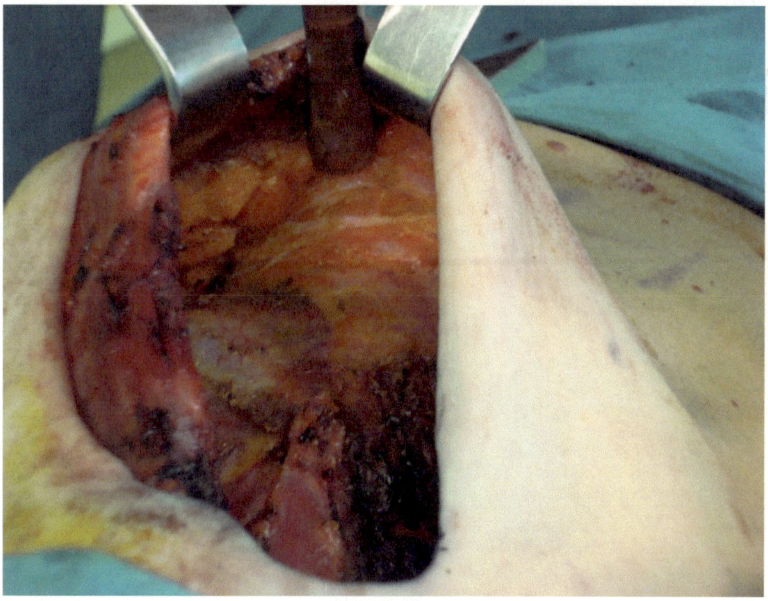

Figure 15. The submammary pocket after superficial fasciotomy, a few millimeters above the inframammary fold. The scored borders of the superficial fascia are visible below the middle retractor.

The dual-plane technique is able to add further 3-4 cm of height in the lower pocket, made of soft and vascularized tissue (Fig.16), totally integrated to the upper coverage made of muscular tissue (pectoralis maior and serratus anterior muscles). The total release of the connective inframammary frame can reach the 7 cms including the previous deep-fascial. It lets free skin and adipofascial layer spontaneously to reach the top of extensibility. This extension is to be compared with a rapid expansion. In the meantime, muscles are free to move upwards and so accomplishing the ultimate dual-plane costruction of an implant coverage that is totally and continuosly vascularized: the lower third of pliable soft tissue and the upper two thirds of firmer muscular tissue (Fig.17, 18).

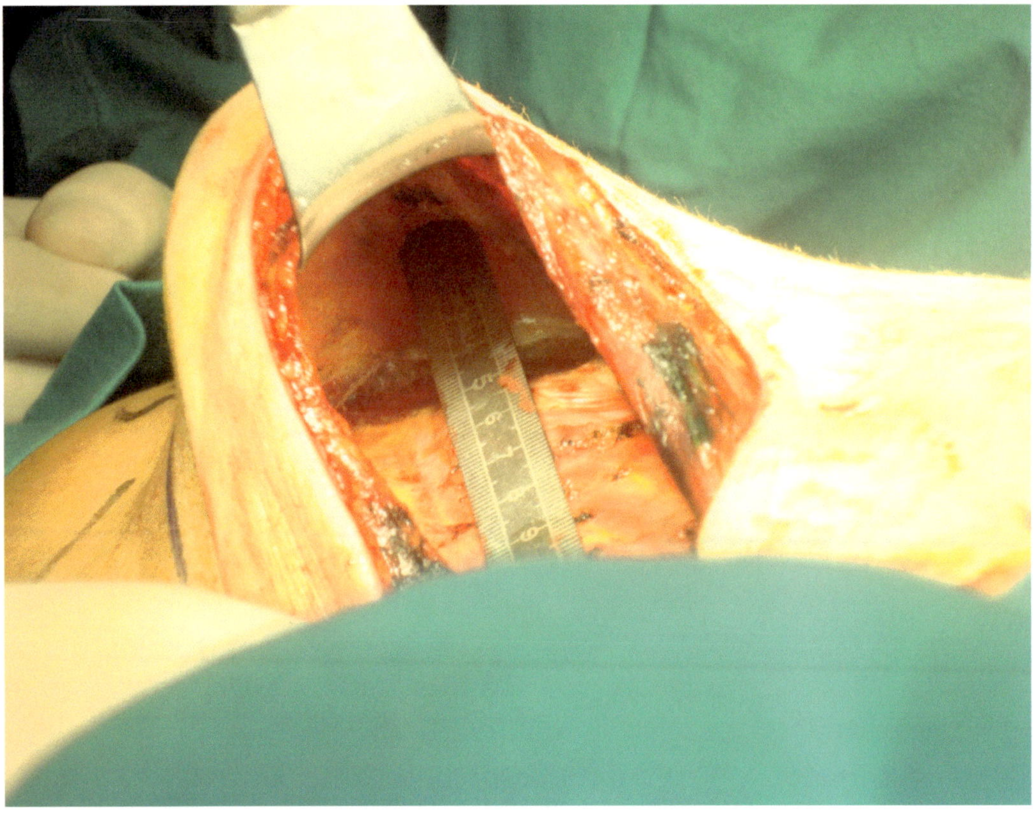

Figure 16. The autologous composite pocket is completing.

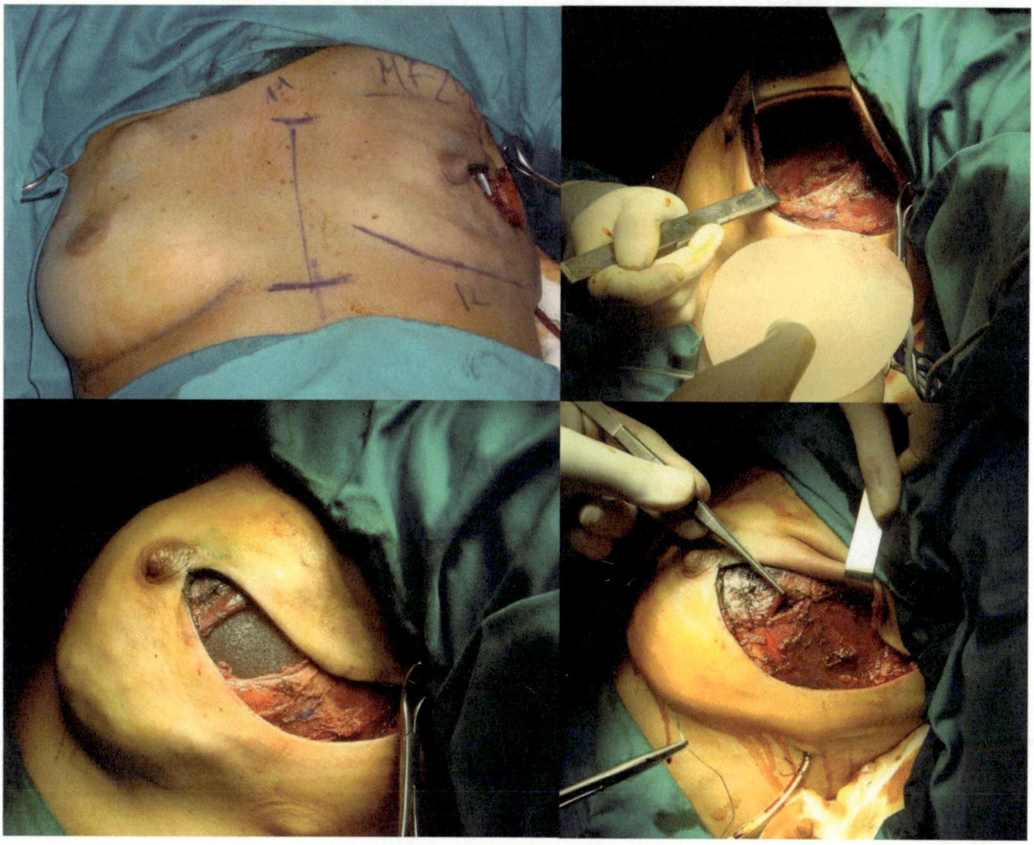

Figure 17. The insertion of the permanent anatomical implant behind the dual-plane coverage. This pocket is totally isolated by the subcutaneous pocket of the removed parenchyma. A drain is inserted under the implant and another between the axillary and subcutaneous compartments. The closure of the pocket is carried out between the free border of the pectoralis maior and the surgical edge of the serratus anterior, using several figure-to-eight stitches of vicryl 2.0.

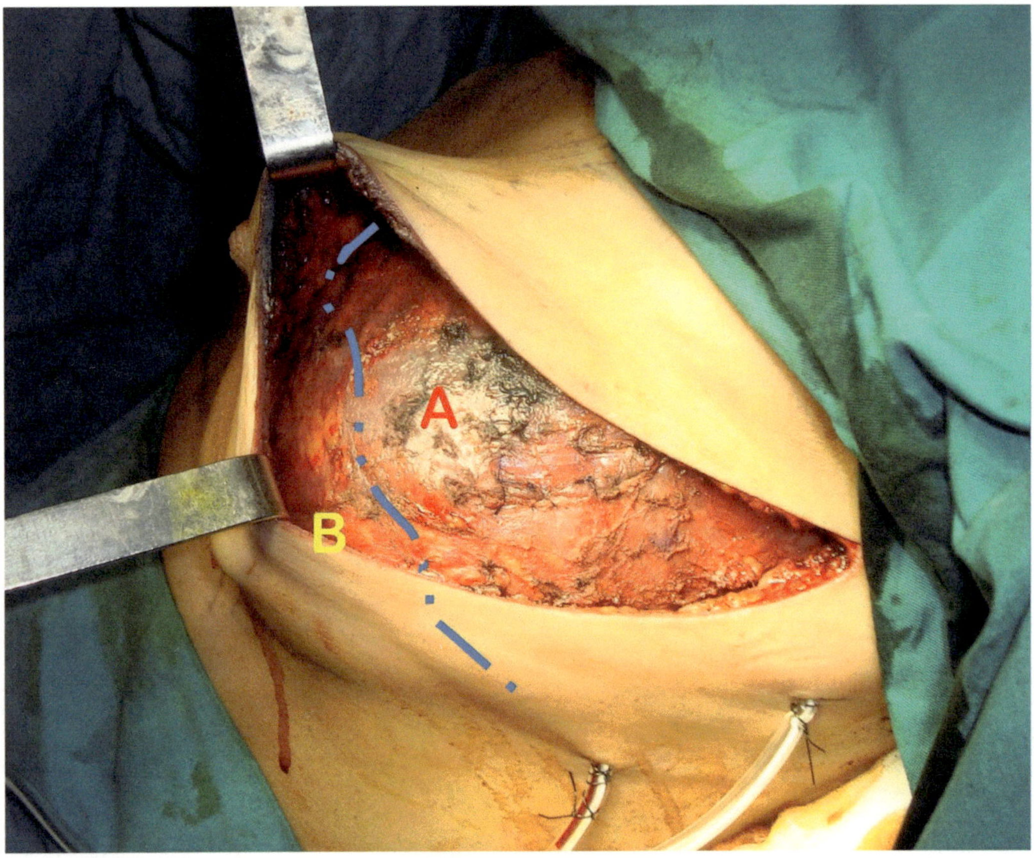

Figure 18. The composite coverage, skin-adipo-fascial tissue downwards and muscular upwards is nourished by a continuous vascular network, preventing complications related to reduced vascular supply and to biomatrix. The blue line illustrates the implant envelope divided in muscular *(A)* and subcutaneous-subfascial coverage *(B)*.

Of course, the breast shape will be given by the anatomical implant but only the high-cohesiveness of the silicone gel can maintain and hence stretch the pocket in the following weeks (Fig.19). A saline implant or expander does not retain any true form; even if totally inflated it will never be the same of a "gummy-bear" implant. The different bio-mechanical effect also helps in re-establishing the true projection of implant that initially appears to be constricted by the tension of the muscular coverage.

http://dx.doi.org/10.5772/56466

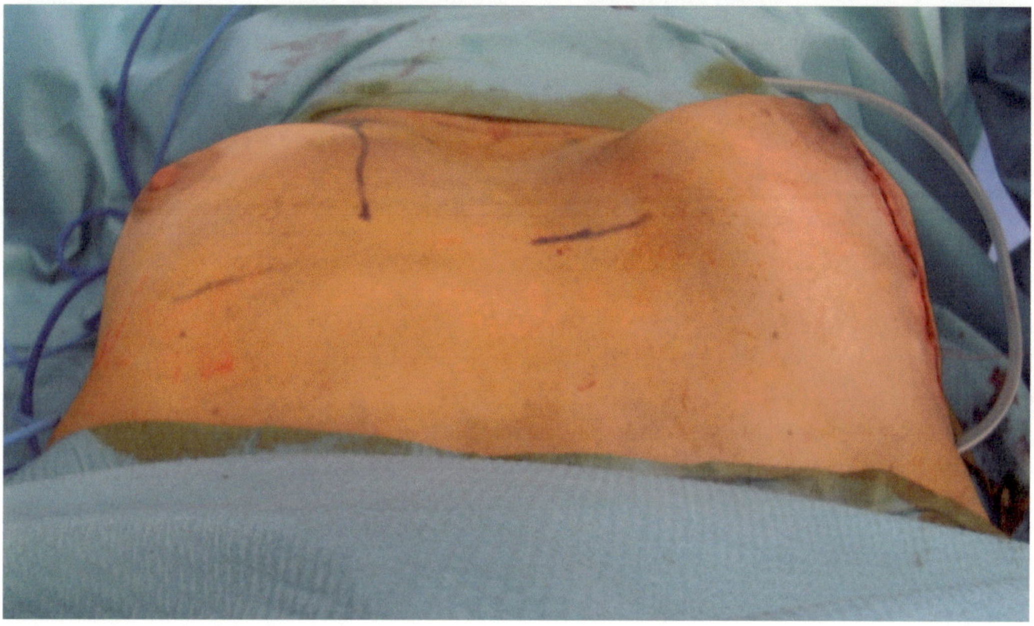

Figure 19. The one-stage immediate reconstruction of a nipple-sparing mastectomy using a permanent silicone implant (Natrelle 410MX 370-grams by Allergan Inc.) in dual-plane autologous pocket. No ADM or synthetic mesh was used. High profile and fullness of this implant-based reconstruction are already visibile after skin closure compared with the healthy breast. *Intra-operative bird's-eye view, patient in supine position.*

4.3. Tips and tricks

The fixation of the central inframammary fold. After scoring the superficial fascia above the inframammary fold, even if the symmetry was totally respected, the level inside appears to be bottomed out inside in some patient. It ought to be due to the abdominal superficial tension which pulls down the lower edge of the fascia already resected. The following procedure can solve the defect according to the former technique of inframammary redefinition already introduced by the same Author Nava. One or two stitches of absorbable material, usually vicryl 0, fix the lower edge of the superficial fascia already scored at the midpoint of the inframammary line into the residual deep fascia or deeper fibers of the serratus anterior or, if necessary, the intercostal fascia (Fig.20). Sometimes, when mastectomy is unilateral, the same procedure is performed for major definition of the central fold as to create a minimal folding to the inframammary line at the aim of a better symmetry with the contralateral breast or only to avoid even minimal descent of the implant.

The external partial myotomies. This is a technical detail introduced by the first Author Riggio, and specifically used in the new one-stage dual-plane IBR for those cases where the central strain strength of the pectoralis maior muscle is higher than usual. The muscle scoring must be carried out after the closure of the device pocket and after estimating the grade of compression produced by the muscle force against the implant. By this way two effects come out: 1) reducing the tension along the suture line of the device pocket, 2) decompressing the

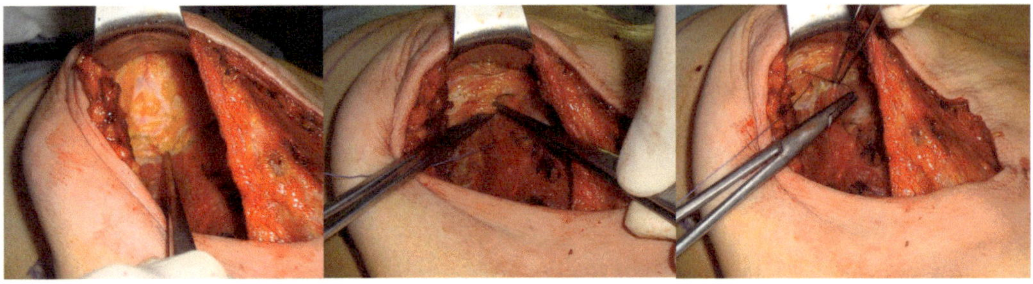

Figure 20. The lower edge of the superficial fascia is identified corresponding to the central point of the inframammary line and then pinched and fixed to the muscular fascia using a single stitch of vicryl 0, after Nava et al..

lower pole of the high-cohesive implant and improving the immediate profile of the lower breast. The correct placement, length, and direction of the partial sections are illustrated in the following Fig.21 and 22. The scores includes fascia and superficial fibers of the pectoralis maior muscle, close to the central part of the coverage.

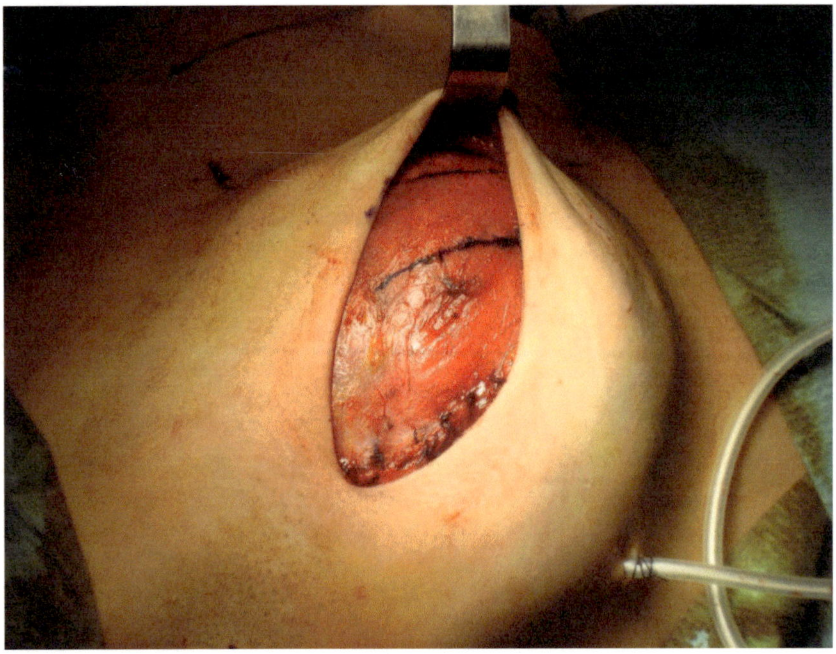

Figure 21. One or two lines of incision are drawn with blue 4 cm far from the suture of the pocket, in this figure visible near the lateral skin border. They are parallel to the suture line but usually crossing the oblique orientation of the muscle fibers.

http://dx.doi.org/10.5772/56466

The internal lateral myotomies. Similar incisions (one-two scores) can be carried out along the inner surface of the harvested serratus anterior muscle, that means inside the pocket laterally, before the implant insertion. The scoring must be vertical and is useful to release and lengthen the inferior-lateral pocket much better. They can be partial or total depending on the stiffness more than the thickness of the serratus fibers.

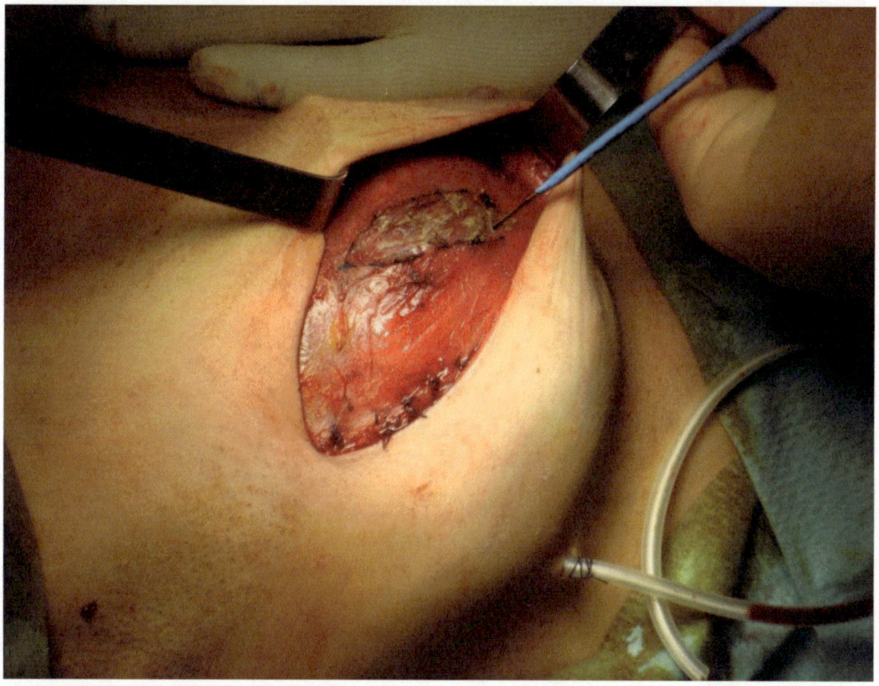

Figure 22. Scoring the fascia and the most superficial fibers of the mid-lower portion of the pectoralis maior muscle corresponding to the central part of the dual-plane pocket. This fine procedure was named by Riggio as external partial myotomy for the tension discharge.

5. Conclusions

The dual-plane technique can be indicated for a selected group of patients, the others follow different guidelines for reconstruction (Fig.23, 24).

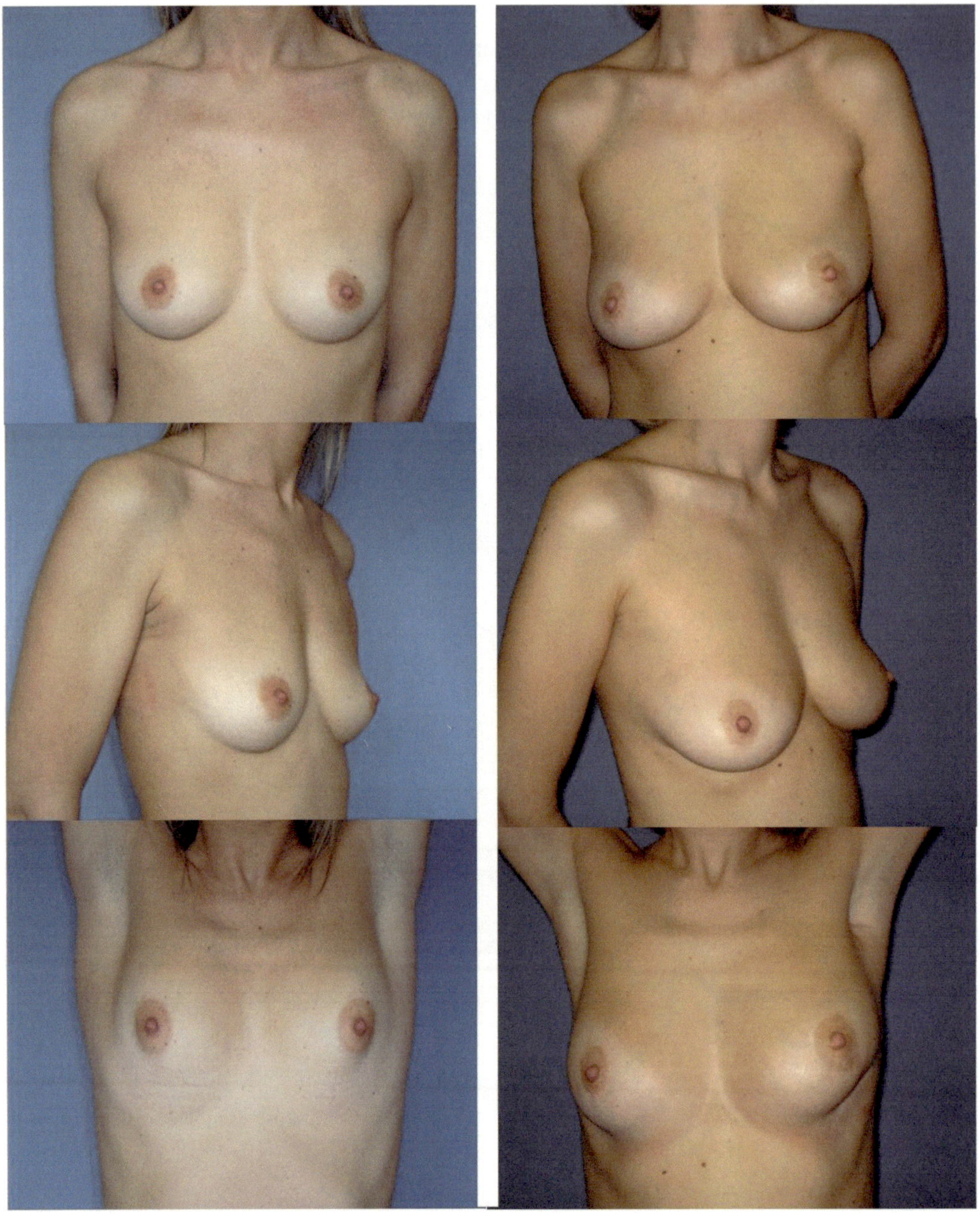

Figure 23. Here are the cases of two sisters affected by BRCA2, 35-year-old and 37-year-old respectively, with similar breast but different cancer history, pre-op views. The first underwent bilateral risk-reducing without sparing the nipple bilaterally, no prior cancer *(left column)*. In the meantime, also the second sister underwent risk-reducing mastectomy but the prior conservative cancer treatment (quadrantectomy + radiation therapy + chemotherapy) changed the reconstructive perspectives in the left breast *(right column)*.

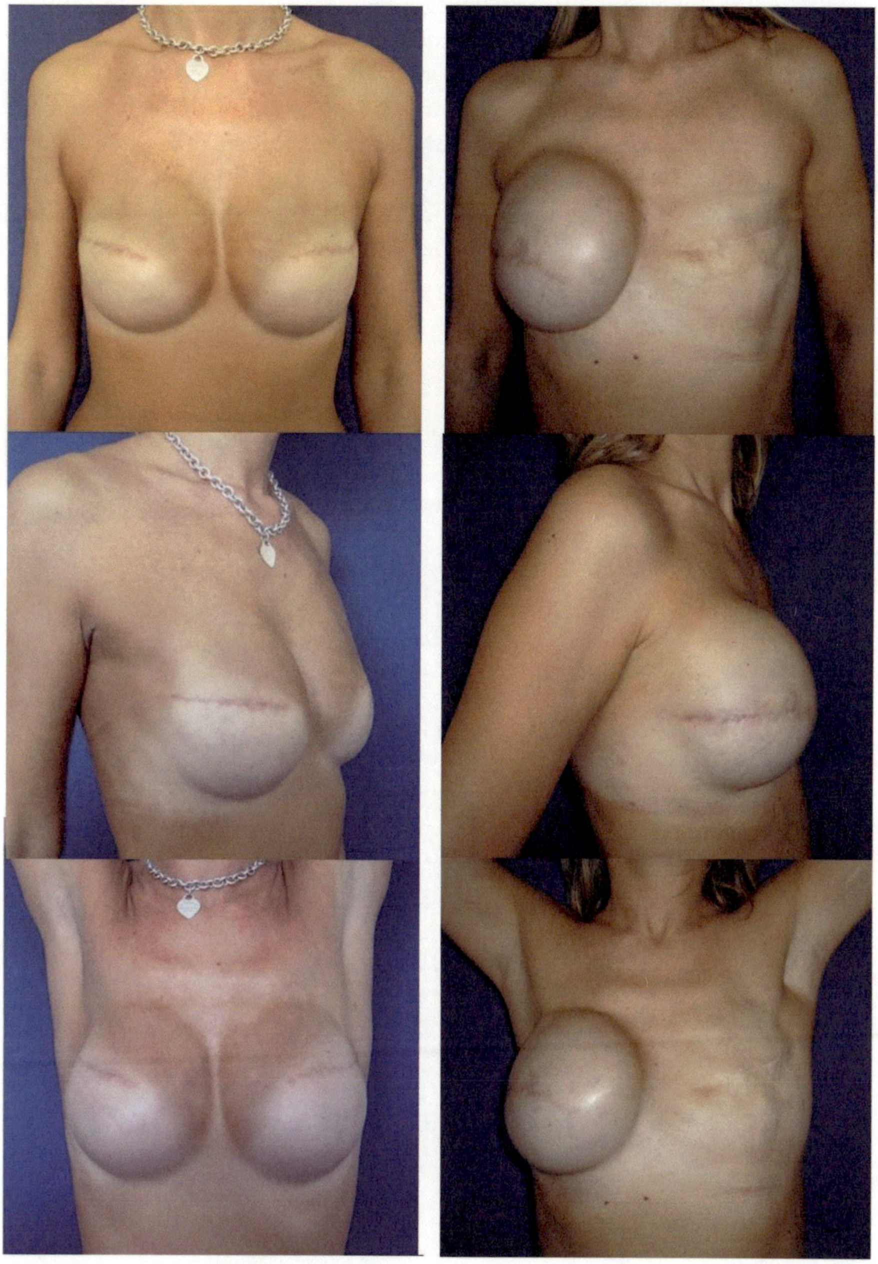

Figure 24. The same two patients, post-op views. The first sister received one-stage IBR with full-height/full-projection implants, Allergan Natrelle 410FF 375g, result after five months *(left column)*. The second received IBR with expander insertion on the right whilst the left reconstruction was posposed because of previous radiotherapy and the refusal for DIEP flap *(right column)*; she preferred to be treated with serial lipofilling and then expander. Pocket preparation and following outcome are different if used the dual-plane composite pocket for stable implant instead of a standard submuscular pocket for saline expander. Expander in the right breast inflated about 400cc, after the first lipofilling in the left side, nine months after mastectomy.

The presence of the following features bring together to perform a safe IBR with the technique described in the chapter: a) low to medium size; b) absent to poor ptosis; c) intra-operative careful respect for the deep fascia along the lateral borders of pectoralis maior and serratus anterior muscles; d) intra-operative preservation of the submammary fascial system Both risk-reducing and oncological sparing mastectomies can be equally reconstructed with the technique. Nipple-sparing and/or bilateral mastectomies can achieve better results (Fig.25). As well the unilateral mastectomy combined to contralateral augmentation. More than the 30% of IBR involves either immediate (Fig.26) or delayed augmentation of the healthy breast (Fig.27).

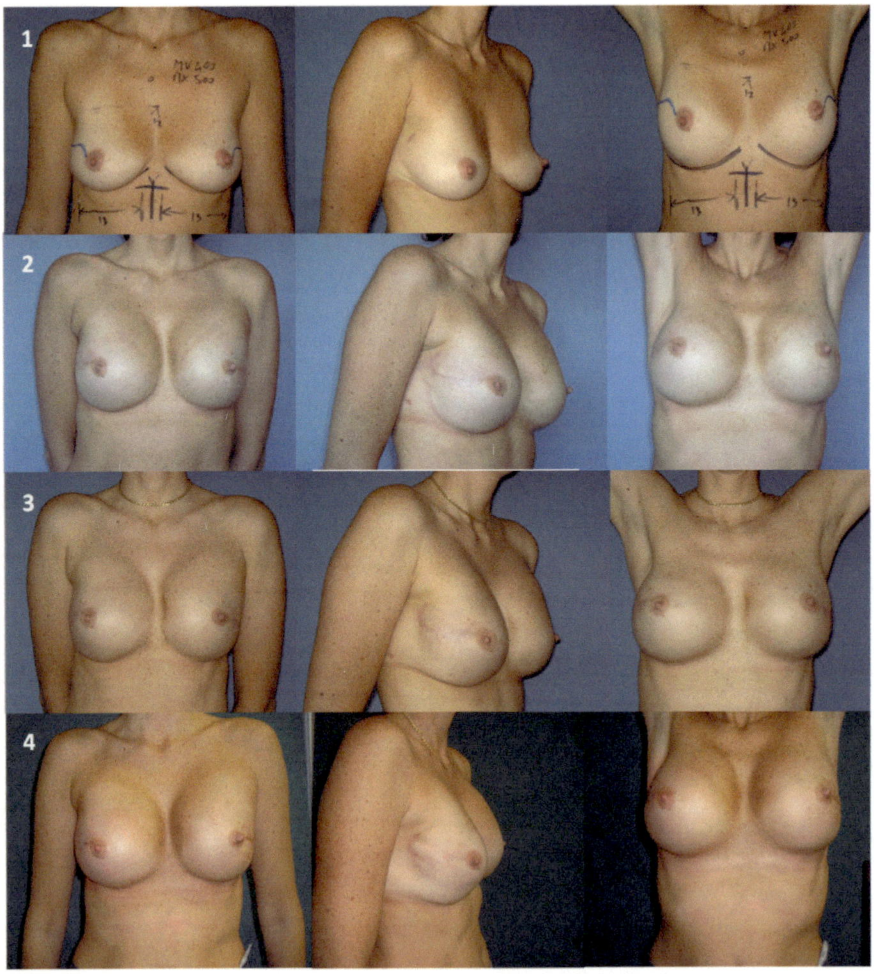

Figure 25. A 38-year-old patient with small breast, no ptosis, affectd by right breast cancer in BRCA1. Right nipple-sparing total mastectomy + left risk-reducing bilateral mastectomy and one-stage IBR with Allergan Natrelle implants 410FX 495g. The breast was largely augmentated. Preop *(line 1)*, post-op views after 3.5 months *(line 2)*, post-op views after 8 months *(line 3)*, post-op views after 3 years and 9 months *(line 4)*. The Baker's grade of capsular contracture was consistently 2 in both sides.

http://dx.doi.org/10.5772/56466

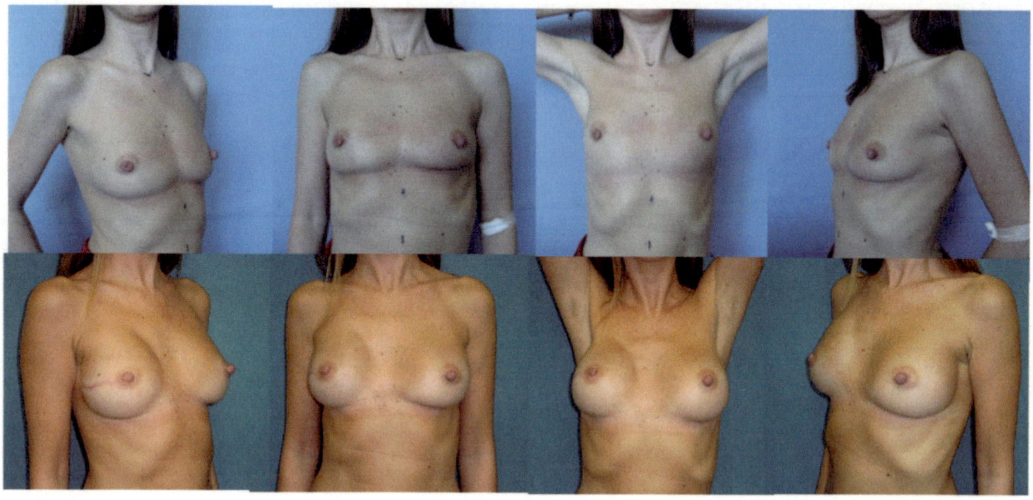

Figure 26. A 37-year-old patient with right breast cancer. Nipple-sparing mastectomy and one-stage IBR with Allergan Natrelle 410MX 290g + breast submuscular augmentation with 410MF 195g. Pre-op and post-op views after 7 months.

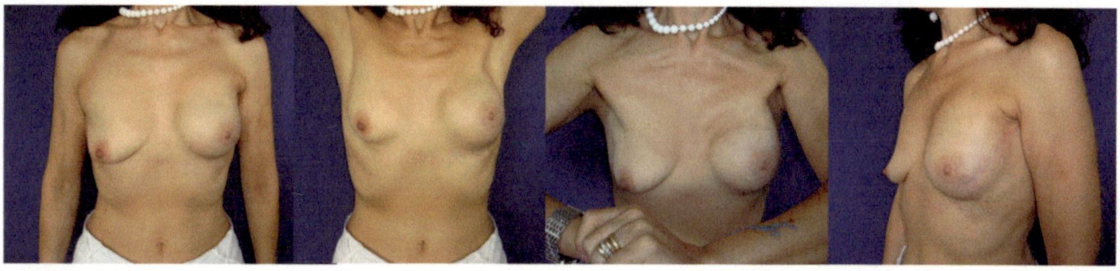

Figure 27. A 49-year-old patient with leftt breast cancer. Nipple-sparing mastectomy and one-stage IBR with Allergan Natrelle full-height/full projection 410FX 315g. The contralateral augmentation was postponed because contemporary correction of the healthy breast in presence of both moderate ptosis and lower constricted pole was evaluated to have few chances of achieving symmetrization safely in a single stage.

Although some surgeon disagrees, no tension spreads on the skin cover using the dual-plane technique. Fast reaching of the definite volume and related major pressure of the device top do not represent a distinct risk for skin necrosis. The technique was safely used in moderate smokers. This is possible because the device volume discharges pressure along the muscular cover at the first moment and, only after some weeks, the muscle is stretching. However skin cover is never tightened by the cohesive implant because skin surface after mastectomy is generally loose and larger than the parenchyma volume, especially in the lower half. Therefore the mammary skin could envelop a bigger prosthesis with poor tension. The largest implant was of 580g. Immediate increase of the previous breast size carry advantages as the overfilling of the breast boundaries, reduction of skin folding, and minor areola-nipple displacement because better stabilizes its position. The volume correction of minor differences were deliberately postponed after complete healing, i.e. at least six months later, and concerned 10% as minimal. The choice for a delayed operation of the healthy breast was prudently dictated by the most predictable evaluation of breast symmetry and shape. This became mandatory if the contralateral breast had need for some mastopexy with augmentation or alone.

Author details

Egidio Riggio* and Maurizio B. Nava

Plastic Reconstructive Surgery Unit, Fondazione IRCCS Istituto Nazionale dei Tumori, Milano, Italy

References

[1] Toth, B. A, & Lappert, P. Modified skin incisions for mastectomy: the need for plastic surgical input in preoperative planning. Plast Reconstr Surg (1991)., 87, 1048-53.

[2] Wellisch, DK, & Schain, ., Little JWIII. The psychological contribution of nipple addition in breast reconstruction. Plast Reconstr Surg 1987;80:699-704.

[3] Nava, M. B, Cortinovis, U, Ottolenghi, J, Riggio, E, Pennati, A, Catanuto, G, Greco, M, & Rovere, G. Q. Skin-reducing mastectomy. Plast Reconstr Surg (2006). discussion 611-13., 118(3), 603-10.

[4] Rusby, J. E, Smith, B. L, & Gui, G. P. Nipple-sparing mastectomy. Br J Surg (2010)., 97(3), 305-16.

[5] Metcalfe, K. A, Semple, J. L, & Narod, S. A. Time to reconsider subcutaneous mastectomy for breast-cancer prevention? Lancet Oncol (2005)., 6, 431-34.

[6] Garcia-etienne, C. A, & Borgen, P. I. Update on the indications for nipple-sparing mastectomy. J Support Oncol (2006)., 4, 225-330.

[7] Ashikari, R. H, Ashikari, A. Y, Kelemen, P. R, & Salzberg, C. A. Subcutaneous mastectomy and immediate reconstruction for prevention of breast cancer for high-risk patients. Breast Cancer (2008)., 15, 185-91.

[8] Laronga, C, Kemp, B, Johnston, D, Robb, G. L, & Singletary, S. E. The incidence of occult nipple-areola complex involvement in breast cancer patients receiving a skin-sparing mastectomy. Ann Surg Oncol (1999)., 6, 609-613.

[9] Sacchini, V, Pinotti, J. A, Barros, A. C, Luini, A, Pluchinotta, A, Pinotti, M, et al. Nipple-sparing mastectomy for breast cancer and risk reduction: oncologic or technical problem? J Am Coll Surg (2006)., 203, 704-714.

[10] Crowe, J. P, Patrick, R. J, Yetman, R. J, & Djohan, R. Nipple-sparing mastectomy update: one hundred forty-nine procedures and clinical outcomes. Arch Surg (2008). , 143, 1106-10.

[11] Gerber, B, Krause, A, Dieterich, M, Kundt, G, & Reimer, T. The oncological safety of skin sparing mastectomy with conservation of the nipple-areola complex and autologous reconstruction: an extended follow-up study. Ann Surg (2009). , 249, 461-468.

[12] Kroll, S. S, & Baldwin, B. A comparison of outcomes using three different methods of breast reconstruction. Plast Reconstr Surg (1992). , 90, 455-62.

[13] William O'BrienPer-Olof Hasselgren, Robert P. Hummel, Robert Coith, David Hyams, Lawrence Kurtzman, Henry W. Neale. Comparison of postoperative wound complications and early cancer recurrence between patients undergoing mastectomy with or without immediate breast reconstruction. The American Journal of Surgery, July (1993). , 166(1), 1-5.

[14] Spear, S. L, & Majidian, A. Immediate breast reconstruction in two stages using textured, integrated-valve tissue expanders and breast implants: A retrospective review of 171 consecutive breast reconstructions from 1989 to 1996. Plast Reconstr Surg (1998). , 101, 53-63.

[15] Gui, G. P, Tan, S. M, Faliakou, E. C, Choy, C, Hern, A, & Ward, R. A. Immediate breast reconstruction using biodimensional anatomical permanent expander implants: a prospective analysis of outcome and patient satisfaction. Plast Reconstr Surg (2003). , 111(1), 125-38.

[16] Ho, G, Nguyen, T. J, Shahabi, A, Hwang, B. H, Chan, L. S, & Wong, A. K. A systemic review and meta-analysis of complications associated with acellular dermal matrix-assisted breast reconstruction. Ann Plast Surg. (2012). , 68, 345-56.

[17] Cassileth, L, Kohanzadeh, S, & Amersi, F. One-Stage immediate breast reconstruction with implants: A new option for immediate reconstruction. Ann Plast Surg. (2011). Jul 5 [Epub ahead of print].

[18] Spillane, C. A, Ashikari, A. Y, Koch, R. M, & Chabner-thompson, E. An 8-Year experience of direct-to-Implant Immediate Breast reconstruction using Human acellular dermal matrix (Alloderm). Breast. (2010). , 127, 514-23.

[19] Singh, N, Reaven, N. J, & Funk, S. E. Immediate 1-stage vs. tissue expander postmastectomy implant breast reconstructions: A retrospective real-world comparison over 18 months. J Plast Reconstr Aesthet Surg. (2012). , 65, 917-23.

[20] Connor, J, et al. Retention of structural and biochemical integrity in a biologic mesh supports tissue remodeling in a primate abdominal wall model. Regen Med. (2009). , 4(2), 185-95.

[21] Hoganson, D. M, Owens, G. E, Doherty, O, Bowley, E. M, Goldman, C. M, Harilal, S. M, Neville, D. O, Kronengold, C. M, & Vacanti, R. T. JP.Preserved extracellular ma-

trix components and retained biological activity in decellularized porcine mesothelium. Biomaterials. (2010). Sep;, 31(27), 6934-40.

[22] Products TiLOOP® Bra: http://wwwpfmmedical.com/en/productcatalogue/pfm-medical/mesh_implants_breast_surgery/tiloopR_bra/index.html

[23] Riggio, E. and Valentina Visintini Cividin V. Breast Reconstruction Approach to Conservative Surgery. ((2012). in Breast Reconstruction- Current Techniques, Marzia Salgarello (Ed.), 978-9-53307-982-0InTech, 243-278.

[24] Pomahac, B, Recht, A, May, J. W, Hergrueter, C. A, & Slavin, S. A. New trends in breast cancer management: is the era of immediate breast reconstruction changing? Ann Surg. (2006). Aug;, 244(2), 282-8.

[25] Rozen, W. M, Ashton, M. W, & Taylor, G. I. Defining the role for autologous breast reconstruction After mastectomy: social and oncologic implications. Clinical Breast Cancer, (2008)., 8(2)

[26] Maxwell, G. P, Storm-dickerson, T, Whitworth, P, Rubano, C, & Gabriel, A. Advances in nipple-sparing mastectomy: oncological safety and incision selection. Aesth Surg J (2011)., 31(3), 310-9.

[27] Riggio, E, Ottolenghi, J, & Nava, M. Breast operative technique for single-stage reconstruction after conservative skin sparing mastectomies: a preliminary study. Surg Tech Development. (2012)., 2, 4-9.

[28] Garwood, E. R, Moore, D, Ewing, C, Hwang, E. S, Alvarado, M, Foster, R. D, & Esserman, L. J. Total skin-sparing mastectomy: complications and local recurrence rates in 2 cohorts of patients. Ann Surg (2009)., 249(1), 26-32.

[29] Riggio, E, Quattrone, P, & Nava, M. Anatomical study of the breast superficial fascial system: the inframammary fold unit. Eur J Plast Surg (2000)., 23, 310-315.

[30] Lockwood, T. E. Superficial fascial system (SFS) of the trunk and extremities: a new concept. Plast Reconstr Surg (1991)., 87, 1009-1018.

[31] Nava, M, Quattrone, P, & Riggio, E. Focus on the breast fascial system: a new approach for inframammary fold reconstruction. Plast Reconstr Surg (1998). , 102, 1034-1045.

[32] Vallejo da Silva ARodriguez FR, Loures CM, Gloria Silami Lopes V. Mastectomy in the era of implant-based reconstruction: Should we be removing the pectoralis fascia? Breast. (2012). Jul 22. [Epub ahead of print]

[33] Gefen, A, & Dilmoney, B. Mechanics of the normal woman's breast. Technol Health Care ((2007))., 15 (4), 259-71

[34] Riggio, E. Breast Augmentation with Extra-projected and High-Cohesive Dual-Gel Prosthesis 510: A Prospective Study of 75 Consecutive Cases for a New Method (the Zenith System). Aesthetic Plast Surg (2012)., 36(4), 866-78.

http://dx.doi.org/10.5772/56466

[35] Salgarello, M, & Farallo, E. Immediate breast reconstruction with definitive anatomical implants after skin-sparing mastectomy. Br J Plast Surg (2005). , 58(2), 216-22.

Chapter 4

Prosthetic Breast Reconstruction with Acellular Dermal Matrix

Katie Weichman and Joseph Disa

Additional information is available at the end of the chapter

http://dx.doi.org/10.5772/56331

1. Introduction

The use of prosthetic devices for breast reconstruction began in the early 1960's with silicone-gel filled implants. Currently, traditional two-stage tissue expander to implant prosthetic breast reconstruction remains the most common type of breast reconstruction performed in the United States. Most recent ASPS statistics estimate greater than 70% of reconstructions are implant based.[1]

Over the years, implant technology and surgical techniques have evolved, resulting in the improved outcomes in breast reconstruction. National trends have moved away from total submuscular coverage toward "dual-plane" positioning of implants. Dual-plane placement provides multiple advantages including decreased chest wall morbidity and increased patient comfort. However, limitations of dual-plane positioning include lack secure coverage of the inferior pole of the implant, less control over the position of the inframammary fold (IMF), and a tendency towards superior migration of the pectoralis major muscle and expander during expansion. [2]-[4] Additional limitations of traditional tissue expander reconstruction remains the time required to reach maximal expansion and difficulty in inferior pole expansion. [5]

Acellular dermal matrix (ADM), was initially employed in breast surgery for revision breast augmentation to prevent rippling and contour abnormalities. It is currently being utilized to address the limitations associated with the dual plane and total submuscular techniques.[6] Its use in immediate implant based breast reconstruction became popular in 2005 after Brueing et al. published a case series describing its use as a sling to cover the inferior-lateral pole in immediate permanent implant reconstruction.[5],[4]Subsequently several case series were published to further support this technique and expand its use to two-stage tissue expander reconstruction. [3],[7]-[11]Proponents of this technique advocate two main advantages: inferior-lateral pole coverage of the implant where the pectoralis muscle is absent and greater initial tissue expansion. [7],[11]-[14][16]-[18]Other proposed advantages include decreased postoperative pain, decreased donor site morbidity, and improved aesthetic outcomes. Several disadvantages have been proposed in the literature including increased postoperative infectious complications, seroma, and explantation.[13],[19]-[21] (Figure 1)

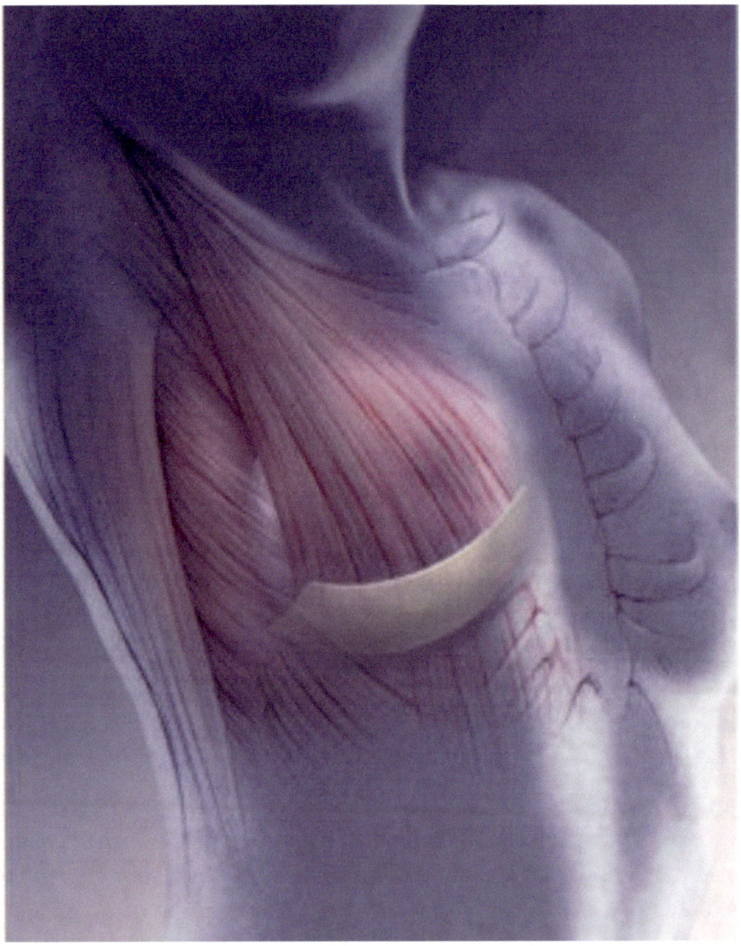

Figure 1. Placement of Accellular Dermal Matrix

2. Types of acellular dermal matrix

While the majority of breast reconstruction with acellular dermal matrix has been described with the use of human matricies, porcine and bovine products are available and have been described for use. Human acellular dermal matricies published in the literature for use in breast reconstruction include; Alloderm (LifeCell, Branchburg, NJ), Flex HD (Ethicon, Sommerville, NJ), Neoform (Mentor, Santa Barbara, CA), DermaMatrix (Synthes, West Chester, PA). Porcine derived matrices include; Strattice (LifeCell, Branchburg, NJ) and Permacol (Covidien, Boulder, CO). Currently there is only one bovine dermal matrix on the market, Surgimend (TEI Biosciences, Boston, MA).

3. Timing

Prosthetic breast reconstruction with acellular dermal matrix can be accomplished either in the immediate or delayed fashion. The advantage of immediate reconstruction is that the first step of breast reconstruction is accomplished at the time of the mastectomy under the same general anesthesia. In this setting, maximum amount so breast skin can be preserved as the prosthetic device will occupy some of the mastectomy space. In the setting of single stage breast reconstruction using a permanent implant, immediate reconstruction allows for the placement of an optimally sized device.

Delayed breast reconstruction using this technique is also possible, however, significantly more tissue expansion is generally necessary. In this method, the mastectomy skin flaps are re-elevated and expanded postoperatively to re-create a pocket for the ultimate placement of a permanent breast implant. Although delayed breast reconstruction with a tissue expander requires an intraoperative procedure, it benefits from simplification of the initial phase of patient management. In the setting of high-risk disease and patients who may require chemotherapy and radiation therapy, delayed reconstruction will not result in a delay of initiation of the adjuvant treatments.

4. Patient selection

While the majority of patients are candidates for prosthetic breast reconstruction and additionally prosthetic reconstruction with acellular dermal matrix. There are several limitations with the overall shape of the permanent implants that dictate the quality of the final result. Factors to consider include need for bilateral or unilateral reconstruction, the patients overall body habitus including body mass index (BMI) and chest width, comorbidities, and patients psychological profile. The ideal candidates for prosthetic reconstruction with acellular dermal matrix are thin patients undergoing bilateral breast reconstruction with adequate mastectomy skin flaps and thin patients with a non-ptotic breast undergoing unilateral reconstruction with adequate mastectomy skin flaps. In these situations, achieving reasonable symmetry is typically achievable.

However, as both breast size and degree of ptosis increases, symmetry in unilateral prosthetic breast reconstruction becomes more difficult to achieve. In this setting, patients may be candidates for contralateral symmetry procedures such as mastopexy or reduction mammoplasty. While the ultimate goal is to provide exact symmetry, patients should be aware that symmetry may only be accomplished in brassiere and clothing.

While there are no defined absolute contraindications for use of Acellular dermal matrix in prosthetic breast reconstruction, obesity, smoking history, and breast size >600grams have been shown to be associated with increased rates of postoperative complications. [19]-[21]

5. Technique

The primary goal of prosthetic breast reconstruction is to achieve a breast mound that is symmetric with either the normal contralateral breast or the contralateral reconstruction. Clear communication between the ablative and reconstructive surgeons is necessary to achieve superior results. Mastectomy incisions are planned and marked together and the inframammary fold should additionally be marked and preserved when possible. Additionally, mastectomy skin flaps should be of adequate thickness to maintain blood supply to the skin and prevent mastectomy skin flap loss.

After mastectomy, careful hemostasis should be obtained within the mastectomy pockets. Then the inferolateral origin of the pectoralis major muscle, along with the investing fascia, is elevated off the anterior chest wall. Using electrocautery dissection, a subpectoral pocket is developed to the extent of the previously marked perimeter of the breasts. After the pocket has been successfully developed, an appropriately sized, usually 4-8cm x 14-16cm, sheet of acellular dermal matrix is prepared according to the manufacturer's recommendations. The ADM is then sutured to chest wall to recreated the inferior and lateral mammary folds. Most surgeons prefer the use of an absorbable suture including either 2-0 polydioxanone (PDS) (Ethicon, Somerville, NJ) or 2-0 Vicryl (Ethicon, Sommerville, NJ) suture. The inframammary ADM is curved laterally and cephalad along the lateral border of the breast perimeter to recreate the natural curvilinear origins of the inferolateral aspect of the detached pectoralis muscle and breast mound unit. Once the ADM has been secured to the inframammary fold, the width of the pocket is measured and tissue expander size is chosen based on the base width. Hemostasis in the pocket is then meticulously achieved. The tissue expander is then prepared in the standard sterile fashion on the back table and then placed in the pocket. The superior border of the ADM is sutured to the inferior and lateral border of the pectoralis muscle thus creating and inferolateral sling of ADM. (Figure 2 and Figure 3)

This tissue expander can be inflated intraoperatively to a volume determined appropriate by surgeon judgment. Care is taken to obliterate dead space but to not impart excessive pressure on the mastectomy skin flaps. One or two closed suction drains are utilized to drain the

http://dx.doi.org/10.5772/56331

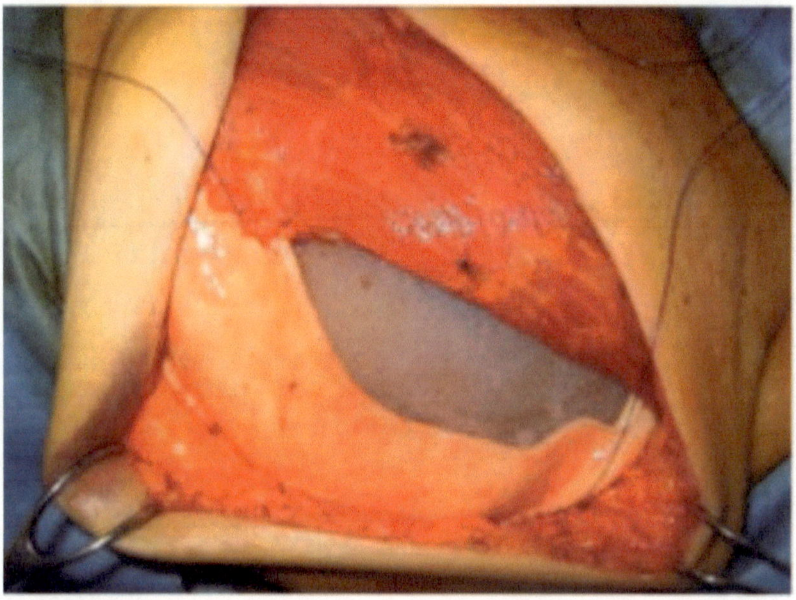

Figure 2. Intraoperative illustration of tissue expander placement into the pectoralis major and acellular dermal matrix pocket

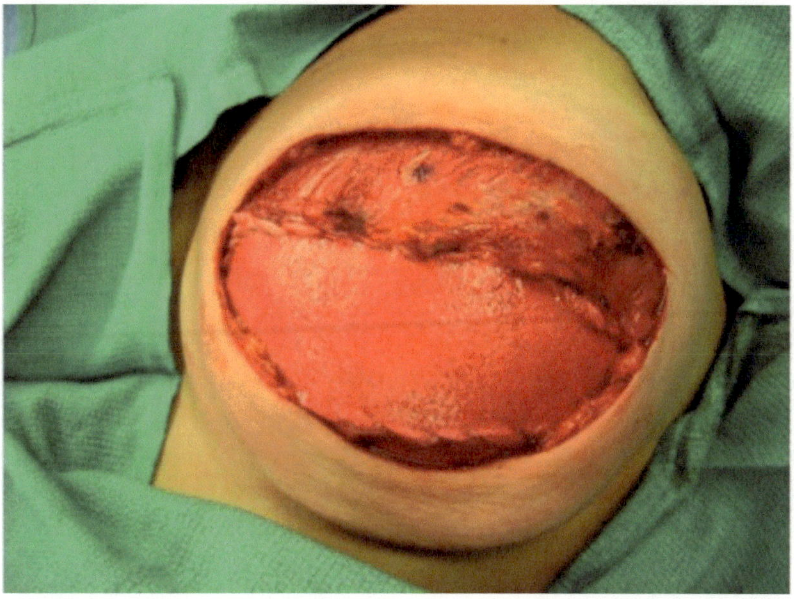

Figure 3. Intraoperative closure of pectoralis major and acellular dermal matrix over the tissue expander

mastectomy space. The mastectomy skin flaps can be tailored to remove excess or non-viable skin prior to final closure. (Figure 4)

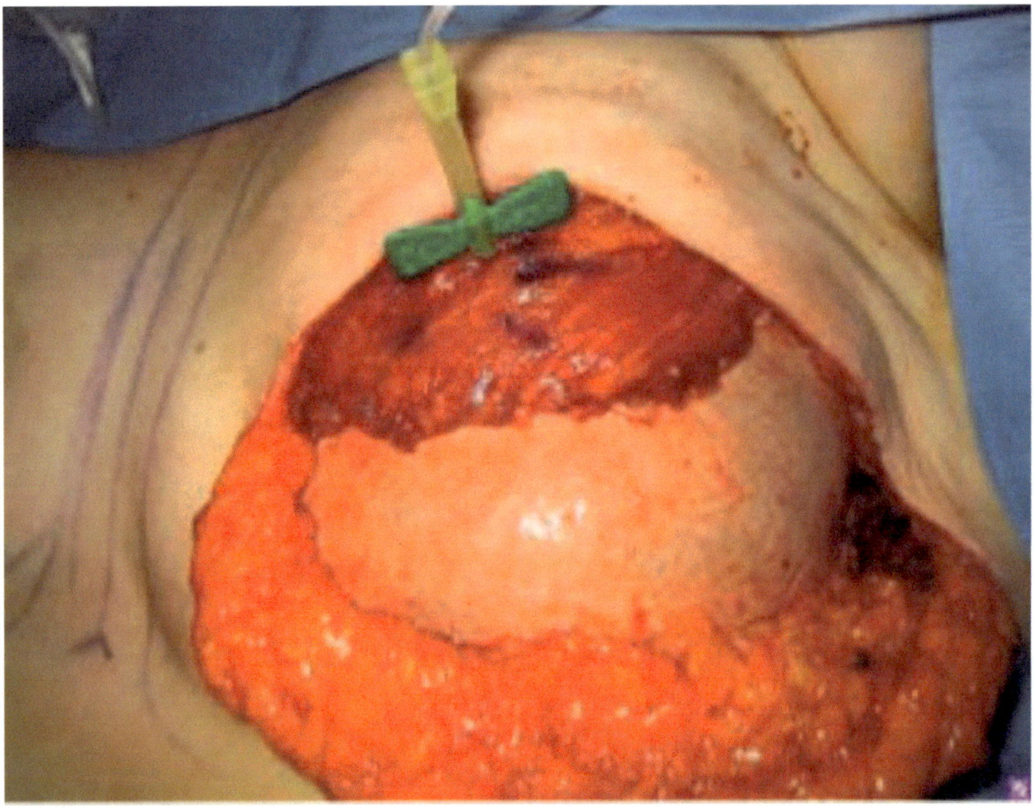

Figure 4. Intraoperative tissue expansion

6. Expansion

Tissue expansion begins in the office approximately 10-14 days after surgery when wound healing is stable and patient no longer has pain. Tissue expansion ensues in the standard fashion using the magnetic expander port finding device to find the site of the valve. The area is then cleansed with antiseptic solution and butterfly needle is used to gain access to the tissue expander. Approximately 30-120mL of saline is injected into the expander during each expansion session. Expansions typically occur at weekly to monthly intervals. The final goal of expansion is guided by desired reconstruction breast size and/or achieving maximum symmetry with contralateral breast. Overexpansion (greater than tissue expander volume) helps to create ptosis in the secondary exchange procedure. In general, soft tissues are allowed to rest for at least one month between the time of last expansion and the implant exchange procedure. [22] (Figure 5)

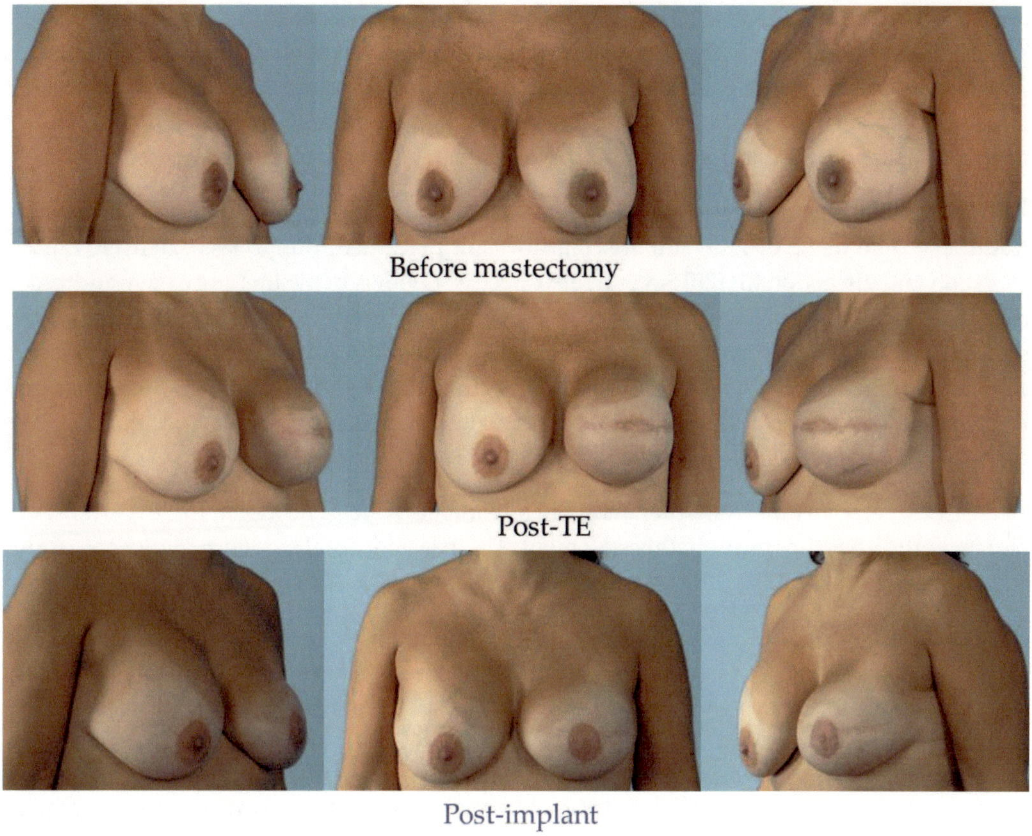

Figure 5. 49 year old female with left breast cancer who underwent left mastectomy with acellular dermal matrix and tissue expander followed by exchange for permanent implant.

7. Proposed advantages

ADM was initially described for use in single stage immediate permanent implant reconstruction and one proposed advantage of the use of ADM is to decrease or eliminate the use of tissue expanders. In the initial report by Breuing, and five subsequent retrospective studies, the efficacy and success of one stage reconstruction has been shown. [7],[9],[12],[14],[15],[23] In these retrospective reviews the overall complication rate is found to be between 6.9% and 25%. [24] Breuing reports a 6.9% (2/30) complication rate in single state reconstructions and Zienowicz's et al. shows a complication rate of 25% (6/24) all of which were mastectomy skin flap necrosis, treated only with local wound care.[12],[25] The largest review of immediate one stage implant reconstructions by Colwell et al. describes an overall complication rate of 14.8% (49/331), including 9.1% (30/331) cases of mastectomy skin flap necrosis. Of the cases of mastectomy skin flap necrosis five implants (1.5%) required explantation. [9] These results demonstrate the successful use of ADM as an adjunct to immediate one stage permanent implant reconstruction. However, it is important to realize, one stage reconstruction is not always possible in patients undergoing prosthetic reconstruction. In order to achieve maximum success in direct to implant reconstruction, proper patient selection is paramount. Specifically, the heath and viability of mastectomy skin flaps needs to be excellent and although it may be possible to make the reconstructed breast slightly larger than the native breast, ideal direct to implant candidates desire a similar or smaller sized reconstructed breast.[9]

Another proposed advantage of ADM is decreased postoperative pain associated with traditional dual plane or total submuscular implant placement due to less extensive muscle elevation and dissection.[5],[26] Several retrospective reviews in the literature have addressed this issue and while subjectively pain was shown to be diminished in patients being reconstructed with ADM. There are no studies that demonstrate objective data with statistical significance to support this claim. [10],[11],[15] However, a recent prospective randomized trial revealed no difference in postoperative pain when comparing total submuscular coverage to the patients undergoing reconstruction with ADM sling. [27]

Decreased operative time is another heralded advantage of ADM however, there is an absence of data in the literature proving this statement. There is anecdotal evidence in two case series suggesting this benefit. [5],[14]

Increased initial TE fill is a seemingly logical benefit to the use of acellular dermal matrix. The sling allows greater size of implant pocket and easier expansion within the pocket with less muscular recoil. This has been proven in many retrospective investigations with differences in initial tissue expander volumes as high as 300mL. [8],[12],[15]-[17],[19]-[21],[24] Two studies thwart this evidence, Preminger et al. comment that there is no statistically significant difference in expansion of the ADM cohort when compared to the non-ADM cohort at 224 mL versus 201 mL ($p=0.180$). [28] However, this approaches significance and sample size alone may prove the limitation of this particular value. Additionally, Vardanian et al. saw a similar fill in the ADM cohort at 150 ± 76mL as compared to 100 ± 69 mL in the non-ADM cohort.[29] However, it is important to realize that the factors contributing to increased tissue expander fill including body habitus, mastectomy skin flap condition, type of mastectomy performed (skin sparring, nipple areolar sparing), and surgeon judgment play roles in determining amount of tissue expander fill.

In addition to initial greater tissue expander fill, fewer number of overall expansions is another seemingly logical extension of the use of the ADM sling. Several studies have addressed this issue, however, the data is not as convincing. Four studies show that a statistically significant fewer numbers of expansions is required with the addition of ADM. [3,7,8,30] Sbitany shows a decreased total number of fills in the ADM group at 1.7 when compared to the non-ADM group at 4.3. [8] Similarly, Nahabedian reports a mean number of expansions in the ADM group at 3 as compared to the non-ADM group at 5.5. [7] On the other hand four studies have shown no difference in the number of expansions when comparing each cohort. [10],[17],[27],[28] Seth demonstrates an average number of expansions in the ADM group of 4.8 ± 2.4 as compared to the non-ADM group of 5.3 ± 2.4 ($p=0.02$).[17] Similarly, McCarthy in a prospective randomized trial shows no difference in time to completion of expansion at 5.6 months in the ADM cohort when compared 4.6 months in the non-ADM cohort ($p=0.93$). [27]

Several theories can explain the striking schism in the data regarding time to expansion, major factors accounting for these equivocal findings include surgeon technique and patients physical limitations. Some surgeons and institutions are more aggressive with tissue expansion volumes and time between expansions. Additionally, patients' ability to tolerate expansions is extremely variable. Given, this information, this proposed advantage is not likely clinically relevant.

Acellular dermal matrix was initially described for use in revision breast augmentation to treat capsular contractures. A natural translation would be to prevent capsular contractures in those undergoing breast reconstruction. Capsular contracture has been reported in rates as high as 14.1% in patients undergoing reconstruction without ADM.[31] Several authors have touted an absence of capsular contracture with ADM with follow up times ranging from 6.5 to 52 months. [5],[6],[11],[15],[23],[32] Vardanian et al. showed in a recent retrospective review that capsular contracture severity, as graded by modified Baker capsular contracture grading system, was significantly lessened in patient undergoing reconstruction with the addition of ADM.[29] Additionally, studies have not shown Baker capsular contracture grades greater than grade I or II.[10],[12] In a primate model Stump et al. evaluated the effect of ADM on capsule formation and found at 10 weeks there was no definable capsule in around the implants reconstructed with ADM compared to the implants without which had a definable capsule. To date, there is no long term data to support a protective effect of ADM to in reducing the incidence of capsular contracture.

Improved aesthetic outcomes of reconstructed breasts are the ultimate goal of plastic surgeons. However, evaluation of this outcome is very subjective and surgeon dependent. Many authors have argued that ADM provides better aesthetic outcomes but there is sparse data to support these claims. Two studies have objectively evaluated the aesthetic outcomes of breast reconstruction with ADM. Spear et al. defined a five-point scale and compared ADM reconstructed breast to contralateral non-reconstructed breasts. They found that scores for breast reconstructed with ADM did not significantly differ from the contralateral unreconstructed breast at 3.68 versus 3.98 (p =0.3). [3] Additionally, Vardanian et al. showed that overall aesthetic outcomes, graded by four independent observers on a scale of 1-4, was statistically significantly greater in the ADM group at 3.26 when compared to the non-ADM group at 2.87. Additionally, the inframammary fold was found to be in better position in the ADM group at 3.35 as compared to the non-ADM group at 2.94. [29]

8. Complications

Complications associated with prosthetic breast reconstruction with acellular dermal matrix are similar to those reconstructed without acellular dermal matrix and should be divided into early and late complications. Early complications include; hematoma, seroma, mastectomy skin flap necrosis, infection, and need for explantation. Late complications include: asymmetry, implant wrinkling, malposition, capsular contracture, and late infection.

The incidence of hematoma is generally accepted as less than 5%. The treatment and consequences are similar with all breast reconstruction. This involves identification of hematoma and rapid evacuation to prevent sequelae, which includes mastectomy skin flap compromise, infection, and capsular contracture.

Seroma, unlike hematoma, is fraught with much controversy in the face of acellular dermal matrix. ADM is hypothesized to increase the risk of seroma and two studies show statistically significantly higher incidences of seroma. [13],[16] Chun shows seromas at an incidence of 14.1% in the ADM cohort when compared to non-ADM cohort at 2.7%. [13] Similarly, Parks shows an incidence of 29.9% in the ADM cohort when compared to 15.7% in the non-ADM cohort.[16] However, there are many studies that do not show a statistically significant difference in the incidence of seroma associated with ADM. [17],[19]-[21],[29],[33] Many of these studies including Liu at 7.1% in the ADM group versus 3.9% in the non-ADM group and Lanier at 13.4% in the ADM group versus 6.7% in the non-ADM group approach but fail to reach statistical significance. [19],[21] Given these findings it is important to take minimize the risk of seroma, including wide drainage with closed suction drains placed in the subcutaneous pocket plus or minus the expander/implant pocket and careful measurements of outputs to avoid premature drain removal.

Mastectomy skin flap necrosis is always a major concern in the setting of prosthetic breast reconstruction. Given the primary surgical intent of mastectomy is to treat breast cancer or remove all breast tissue to prevent cancer development, mastectomy skin flap thickness is often indeterminate. Additionally, other factors such as length of the mastectomy skin flap, medical comorbidities, smoking history, and surgical technique can often contribute to the development of mastectomy skin flap necrosis. Superficial or partial-thickness flap necrosis can be managed conservatively with local wound care. However, full thickness necrosis in the setting of an ADM assisted reconstruction should be managed with early excision with temporary deflation of expander to facilitated tension free closure and subsequent expansion.[34] Mastectomy skin flap necrosis associated with overt prosthetic exposure typically results in explantation. It is important to realize that ADM represents a second foreign body in addition to the expander/implant. Secondary infection of both the expander/implant and ADM is possible with the presence of mastectomy skin flap necrosis.

While there is no direct association between mastectomy skin flap necrosis and acellular dermal matrix, the incidence of mastectomy skin flap necrosis has been seen to be higher in patients undergoing reconstruction with ADM in two series. Weichman et al. reports a mastectomy skin flap necrosis rate of 8.3% in the ADM cohort as compared to 3.2% in the non-ADM cohort and Chun et al. similarly shows an incidence of 23.4% in the ADM cohort as compared to 8.9% in the non-ADM cohort. [13],[20] Both series also show greater initial tissue expansion volume, which is thought to contribute to this increased incidence. Therefore, it is important to both prevent mastectomy skin flap necrosis through surgical judgment and careful inflation of initial tissue expander. Additionally, it is paramount to identify full thickness necrosis and treat expeditiously with excision and closure to prevent further sequlae. Some authors support the use of indocyanine green angiography to assess the mastectomy skin flap viability. However, the data to support this technology available in the literature is inconclusive.

Infectious complications of prosthetic breast reconstructions are cited as high as 35.4%.[35],[36] Reconstruction with the addition of ADM poses a second foreign body and therefore infectious complications could be more likely. The literature displays divergent evidence with regards to infectious complications in the presence of ADM. There are a multitude of reports showing equivalent infectious complications when comparing ADM to non-ADM breast reconstructions. [3],[7-9],[15]-[18],[29],[37],[38]Conversely there are many reports showing increased infectious complications in patients with ADM reconstruction. [13],[19]-[21],[33] It is important to recognize infectious complications and treat expeditiously with either oral or intravenous antibiotics as per surgeon judgment.

9. Conclusions

Acellular dermal matrix is an influential addition to the plastic surgical armamentarium for breast reconstruction. Superior aesthetic results have been seen in patients undergoing both immediate one-stage implant reconstructions and two-stage tissue expander reconstruction. Surgeons should realize, however, that ADM is another tool in prosthetic breast reconstruction and not necessarily a panacea. Surgeon judgment based upon experience and evidence based best practices should guide the use of ADM in prosthetic breast reconstruction.

Author details

Katie Weichman[1] and Joseph Disa[2]

1 New York University Medical Center, Institute of Reconstructive Plastic Surgery, New York, NY, USA

2 Memorial Sloan Kettering Cancer Center, New York, NY, USA

References

[1] Surgeons ASoP. American Society of Plastic Surgeons 2011 Statistics. 2011; http://www.plasticsurgery.org/News-and-Resources/2011-Statistics-.html

[2] Spear SL, Majidian A. Immediate breast reconstruction in two stages using textured, integrated-valve tissue expanders and breast implants: a retrospective review of 171 consecutive breast reconstructions from 1989 to 1996. *Plast Reconstr Surg.* Jan 1998;101(1):53-63.

[3] Spear SL, Parikh PM, Reisin E, Menon NG. Acellular dermis-assisted breast reconstruction. *Aesthetic Plast Surg.* May 2008;32(3):418-425.

[4] Spear SL, Pelletiere CV. Immediate breast reconstruction in two stages using textured, integrated-valve tissue expanders and breast implants. *Plast Reconstr Surg.* Jun 2004;113(7):2098-2103.

[5] Breuing KH, Warren SM. Immediate bilateral breast reconstruction with implants and inferolateral AlloDerm slings. *Ann Plast Surg.* Sep 2005;55(3):232-239.

[6] Baxter RA. Intracapsular allogenic dermal grafts for breast implant-related problems. *Plast Reconstr Surg.* Nov 2003;112(6):1692-1696; discussion 1697-1698.

[7] Nahabedian MY. AlloDerm performance in the setting of prosthetic breast surgery, infection, and irradiation. *Plast Reconstr Surg.* Dec 2009;124(6):1743-1753.

[8] Sbitany H, Sandeen SN, Amalfi AN, Davenport MS, Langstein HN. Acellular dermis-assisted prosthetic breast reconstruction versus complete submuscular coverage: a head-to-head comparison of outcomes. *Plast Reconstr Surg.* Dec 2009;124(6): 1735-1740.

[9] Colwell AS, Damjanovic B, Zahedi B, Medford-Davis L, Hertl C, Austen WG, Jr. Retrospective review of 331 consecutive immediate single-stage implant reconstructions with acellular dermal matrix: indications, complications, trends, and costs. *Plast Reconstr Surg.* Dec 2011;128(6):1170-1178.

[10] Namnoum JD. Expander/implant reconstruction with AlloDerm: recent experience. *Plast Reconstr Surg.* Aug 2009;124(2):387-394.

[11] Bindingnavele V, Gaon M, Ota KS, Kulber DA, Lee DJ. Use of acellular cadaveric dermis and tissue expansion in postmastectomy breast reconstruction. *J Plast Reconstr Aesthet Surg.* 2007;60(11):1214-1218.

[12] Zienowicz RJ, Karacaoglu E. Implant-based breast reconstruction with allograft. *Plast Reconstr Surg.* Aug 2007;120(2):373-381.

[13] Chun YS, Verma K, Rosen H, et al. Implant-based breast reconstruction using acellular dermal matrix and the risk of postoperative complications. *Plast Reconstr Surg.* Feb;125(2):429-436.

[14] Gamboa-Bobadilla GM. Implant breast reconstruction using acellular dermal matrix. *Ann Plast Surg.* Jan 2006;56(1):22-25.

[15] Salzberg CA. Nonexpansive immediate breast reconstruction using human acellular tissue matrix graft (AlloDerm). *Ann Plast Surg.* Jul 2006;57(1):1-5.

[16] Parks JR, Hammond SE, Walsh WW, Adams RL, Chandler RG, Luce EA. Human Acellular Dermis (ACD) vs. No-ACD in Tissue Expansion Breast Reconstruction. *Plast Reconstr Surg.* Jun 8 2012.

[17] Seth AK, Hirsch EM, Fine NA, Kim JY. Utility of acellular dermis-assisted breast reconstruction in the setting of radiation: a comparative analysis. *Plast Reconstr Surg.* Oct 2012;130(4):750-758.

[18] Glasberg SB, Light D. AlloDerm and Strattice in breast reconstruction: a comparison and techniques for optimizing outcomes. *Plast Reconstr Surg.* Jun 2012;129(6): 1223-1233.

[19] Lanier ST, Wang ED, Chen JJ, et al. The effect of acellular dermal matrix use on complication rates in tissue expander/implant breast reconstruction. *Ann Plast Surg.* May; 64(5):674-678.

[20] Weichman KE, Wilson SC, Weinstein AL, et al. The use of acellular dermal matrix in immediate two-stage tissue expander breast reconstruction. *Plast Reconstr Surg.* May 2012;129(5):1049-1058.

[21] Liu AS, Kao HK, Reish RG, Hergrueter CA, May JW, Jr., Guo L. Postoperative complications in prosthesis-based breast reconstruction using acellular dermal matrix. *Plast Reconstr Surg.* May;127(5):1755-1762.

[22] Disa JJ, Ad-El DD, Cohen SM, Cordeiro PG, Hidalgo DA. The premature removal of tissue expanders in breast reconstruction. *Plast Reconstr Surg.* Nov 1999;104(6): 1662-1665.

[23] Breuing KH, Colwell AS. Inferolateral AlloDerm hammock for implant coverage in breast reconstruction. *Ann Plast Surg.* Sep 2007;59(3):250-255.

[24] JoAnna Nguyen T, Carey JN, Wong AK. Use of human acellular dermal matrix in implant- based breast reconstruction: evaluating the evidence. *J Plast Reconstr Aesthet Surg.* Dec 2011;64(12):1553-1561.

[25] Breuing KH, Colwell AS. Immediate breast tissue expander-implant reconstruction with inferolateral AlloDerm hammock and postoperative radiation: a preliminary report. *Eplasty.* 2009;9:e16.

[26] Topol BM, Dalton EF, Ponn T, Campbell CJ. Immediate single-stage breast reconstruction using implants and human acellular dermal tissue matrix with adjustment of the lower pole of the breast to reduce unwanted lift. *Ann Plast Surg.* Nov 2008;61(5):494-499.

[27] McCarthy CM, Lee CN, Halvorson EG, et al. The use of acellular dermal matrices in two-stage expander/implant reconstruction: a multicenter, blinded, randomized controlled trial. *Plast Reconstr Surg.* Nov 2012;130(5 Suppl 2):57S-66S.

[28] Preminger BA, McCarthy CM, Hu QY, Mehrara BJ, Disa JJ. The influence of AlloDerm on expander dynamics and complications in the setting of immediate tissue expander/implant reconstruction: a matched-cohort study. *Ann Plast Surg.* May 2008;60(5):510-513.

[29] Vardanian AJ, Clayton JL, Roostaeian J, et al. Comparison of implant-based immediate breast reconstruction with and without acellular dermal matrix. *Plast Reconstr Surg.* Nov 2011;128(5):403e-410e.

[30] Parks JW, Hammond SE, Walsh WA, Adams RL, Chandler RG, Luce EA. Human Acellular Dermis versus No Acellular Dermis in Tissue Expansion Breast Reconstruction. *Plast Reconstr Surg.* Oct 2012;130(4):739-746.

[31] Spear SL, Newman MK, Bedford MS, Schwartz KA, Cohen M, Schwartz JS. A retrospective analysis of outcomes using three common methods for immediate breast reconstruction. *Plast Reconstr Surg.* Aug 2008;122(2):340-347.

[32] Becker S, Saint-Cyr M, Wong C, et al. AlloDerm versus DermaMatrix in immediate expander-based breast reconstruction: a preliminary comparison of complication profiles and material compliance. *Plast Reconstr Surg.* Jan 2009;123(1):1-6; discussion 107-108.

[33] Antony AK, McCarthy CM, Cordeiro PG, et al. Acellular human dermis implantation in 153 immediate two-stage tissue expander breast reconstructions: determining the incidence and significant predictors of complications. *Plast Reconstr Surg.* Jun;125(6): 1606-1614.

[34] Antony AK, Mehrara BM, McCarthy CM, et al. Salvage of tissue expander in the setting of mastectomy flap necrosis: a 13-year experience using timed excision with continued expansion. *Plast Reconstr Surg.* Aug 2009;124(2):356-363.

[35] Francis SH, Ruberg RL, Stevenson KB, et al. Independent risk factors for infection in tissue expander breast reconstruction. *Plast Reconstr Surg.* Dec 2009;124(6):1790-1796.

[36] Spear SL, Seruya M. Management of the infected or exposed breast prosthesis: a single surgeon's 15-year experience with 69 patients. *Plast Reconstr Surg.* Apr 2010;125(4):1074-1084.

[37] Ho G, Nguyen TJ, Shahabi A, Hwang BH, Chan LS, Wong AK. A systematic review and meta-analysis of complications associated with acellular dermal matrix-assisted breast reconstruction. *Ann Plast Surg.* Apr 2012;68(4):346-356.

[38] Kim JY, Davila AA, Persing S, et al. A meta-analysis of human acellular dermis and submuscular tissue expander breast reconstruction. *Plast Reconstr Surg.* Jan 2012;129(1):28-41.

Chapter 5

Fat Grafting in Breast Reconstruction with Expanders and Prostheses in Patients Who Have Received Radiotherapy

Jose Ma Serra-Renom, Jose Ma Serra-Mestre and Francesco D'Andrea

Additional information is available at the end of the chapter

http://dx.doi.org/10.5772/56073

1. Introduction

Around 70% of breast reconstruction interventions currently incorporate tissue expansion and prostheses (Plastic Surgery Statistics Report, 2010). The popularity of the technique is due in part to its apparent simplicity. However, to ensure satisfactory results and to avoid long-term complications a long learning curve is required, and certain modifications should be made to the conventional techniques.

Breast reconstruction incorporating tissue expansion and prostheses presents a series of clear advantages. The most significant are its less invasive nature and its shorter recovery times – both highly important issues in patients who have already suffered major physical and psychological distress. It is also particularly beneficial in bilateral cases, in which achieving symmetry is a key objective, and in thin patients with small breasts. The technique obtains good results without increasing the morbidity of donor sites or causing the formation of new scars, as it uses the surrounding tissue which has the same color, texture and sensitivity.

At the same time, however, the technique has certain limitations, which we will discuss below. A high percentage of patients undergo radiotherapy, thereby increasing tissue fibrosis and the formation of capsular contracture and negatively affecting surgical outcomes. The use of textured implants, and above all the performance of fat grafting has significantly reduced the effect of this complication by providing thicker subcutaneous tissue [1,2] and improving the quality of the irradiated tissue [3].

2. Fat grafting in the breast

Fat injection is widely accepted as a useful technique for handling defects and asymmetries in breast surgery [4-6]. The availability of sufficient donor tissue, the low morbidity of the liposuctioned area, the benefit of the liposuction to the patient, and the ease of application have been decisive factors in its recent expansion. Today, however, fat is seen not only as an autologous filler, but also as a regenerator of the injected tissue thanks to the preadipocytes it contains. This regenerative capacity is of particular interest in breast surgery due to the tissue damage caused by radiotherapy.

Rigotti [3] demonstrated the improvement in irradiated tissues after serial injection of fat, reporting values on the LENT-SOMA scale (which provides an objective assessment of post-radiation skin changes) from 3-4 to 0-1. Along the same lines, our research group demonstrated the formation of a new subcutaneous plane in the post-mastectomized breast after radiation therapy, reducing the formation of the capsule around the prosthesis and improving tissue quality [1]. These results have since been corroborated by other authors [7-10].

The use of fat grafts has been a matter of controversy since the 1980s. It has been suggested that fat injection modifies radiological images in both mammography and magnetic resonance imaging (MRI), which may hinder the radiological control after surgery and may interfere with the early detection of breast cancer. In our view, however, the radiological findings after fat injection are not pathognomonic for tumor growth, but in fact are clearly differentiated images which radiologists in the twenty-first century should be able to recognize – just as they have had to learn to distinguish the changes appearing in other conventional breast surgery (reduction, augmentation, mastopexy, and so on) which are commonly accepted today.

When performing breast reconstruction, the breast already presents scars and calcifications as a result of tumor removal. In its 2009 publication, the ASPS Fat Graft Task Force updated its recommendation on the use of fat injection [11].

So far, no increase in local recurrence of breast cancer has been found in association with fat injection, nor any increase in the risk of new cancers. In fact, breast augmentation surgery raises aromatase activity 20 times more than fat grafting.

2.1. Volume maintenance and fat graft viability

It is important to identify the variables that may affect the adipocytes and adipose-derived stem cells (ASC) during the processing of fat tissue from its extraction to its injection into the recipient site. Numerous studies have been performed, but certain aspects remain unresolved. It is not the aim of this chapter to discuss the physiology of fat tissue in great technical detail; below is a brief summary of some of the procedures for optimizing outcome in terms of cell viability and, as a result, greater volume maintenance.

Fat harvesting

As far as the choice of donor site is concerned, we advocate obtaining the fat from the peri-umbilical area due to the ease of preparing a single surgical field comprising the donor, the

http://dx.doi.org/10.5772/56073

abdomen, and the recipient, the breast. The abdomen usually has enough fat to allow removal and to hide the incisions made in the navel and the pubis. This also enables us to extract the fat in a criss-cross pattern and avoids leaving visible scars and irregularities, even if they are minimal.

In the literature there is no consensus regarding the best donor site. One study favors the lower abdomen, where it is believed that there is a higher concentration of stem cells (ASC) [12]; however the results were obtained on the basis of c-kit expression, which measures not just the stem cells but lymphocytes as well. For Fraser et al [13], the hips are the best area, while other authors see no particular advantages between different areas of extraction.

Local anesthesia (especially lidocaine and epinephrine) has been reported to impair adipocyte metabolism, reducing glucose transport and the viability of the ASC [14]. However, that study was performed in vitro and did not take into account the actual concentration of anesthetic in the fluid being infiltrated. The authors note that the time between infiltration and aspiration may be relevant in prolonging contact between cells and the anesthetic [14].

Another important variable in the cell viability of the stromal fraction is the aspiration pressure. Today it is accepted that the lower the pressure, the higher the survival [15], so we favor the use of a 10 cc syringe with the plunger withdrawn 2 cc (0.37 at) for the extraction of small volumes, or a fat aspirator at 0.5 at for larger volumes.

The choice of cannula does not seem to be a problem, although there is a relationship between the diameter of the cannula and the aspiration pressure.

Fat Processing

Some studies report that washing achieves higher cell viability and survival than Coleman's centrifugation method (3000 rpm x 3 min) [16], although the results obtained with the two techniques are similar and both can be considered valid. Numerous studies have assessed the effects of centrifugation on fat aspirates to optimize the centrifugal force for fat transplantation and to obtain a high number of intact ASC [17, 18]. A centrifugal force of 1200 g is recommended.

Other decisive factors in cell viability are the time the fat tissue is extracted and the temperature to which it is exposed. Matsumo et al [19] studied the oil ratio, the presence of glycerol-3-phosphate dehydrogenase and adipose stem cells in different samples at different temperatures and times of preservation. They concluded that ASC persisted at room temperature practically for four hours, with a progressive destruction up to 24 hours. Carvalho et al. [20] reported that acceptable fat tissue viability can be maintained at room temperature until 24 hours after extraction. For longer periods, adipose tissue preservation banks have recently been designed.

Fat Grafting

The key factor is to achieve the correct three-dimensional distribution of fat in different planes from the depth to surface, creating a criss-cross pattern and avoiding the accumulation of large quantities of fat. The diameter of the hole of the cannula used to make the injection should be the same as the one used to extract the fat, in order to keep mechanical damage to the adipocytes to a minimum.

2.2. Procedure

Atraumatic procurement of adipose tissue

When surgery is performed under general anesthesia or sedation, we create the tumescence of the abdominal region using a multiperforated tumescent cannula with a luer lock connection measuring 1.6 mm x 9-15 cm, with a saline and adrenaline solution at a ratio of 500 cc saline, 1 mg of adrenaline and 20 cc of lidocaine 2%.

When surgery is performed under local anesthesia in a second operation to optimize the outcome, two hours prior to surgery the extraction area (previously indicated to the patient during a visit) is covered with a topical anesthetic cream (EMLA TM). A light massage is performed to ensure good penetration and the whole area is then covered with abundant cream and a plastic film. At the time of surgery the cream is removed and we infiltrate a small quantity of undiluted anesthetic at the two points where the incisions will be made. We then create the tumescence with a 30 cc solution of 2% lidocaine and 0.5 mg adrenaline. In both cases, we wait 20 minutes for the anesthetic to take effect.

Via the same incision used to make the tumescence, we introduce the 2 mm x 15 cm Coleman cannula connected to a 10 ml syringe with a luer lock tip, and maintain the plunger withdrawn about 2 ml with the dominant hand; with the other we make a pinch in the abdomen and make forward and backward movements at this level without losing the vacuum. In this way the syringe fills up with fat using a moderate vacuum pressure in order to keep trauma to a minimum. In cases in which greater quantities of fat are required and liposuction is performed, we use a 3 mm liposuction cannula and the liposuction device at a pressure of 0.5 atmospheres (FIG.1).

As it is very important not to leave irregularities in the abdomen, it is advisable to change the site and direction of the aspirations. To prevent irregularities it is also useful to make an incision in the pubis and to criss-cross the tunnels of the pubis and umbilicus.

Once the fat extraction is completed, we regularize the donor site using a flat liposuction cannula without aspiration. As we fill the syringes, we remove the plunger, cover the distal end and place them upright on a support rack. We now suture the incisions and apply a bandage to the abdomen for a week. After this period, abdominal massages are performed.

Adipose tissue processing

Centrifugation

When the necessary amount of fat has been extracted, it is centrifuged at 2000 rpm for two minutes.

After centrifuging, three levels can be observed in each of the syringes. The lower one contains blood and debris, water and components of the solution used for the tumescence; the middle layer consists of adipocytes and ASCs, and the top layer is formed by the oil resulting from

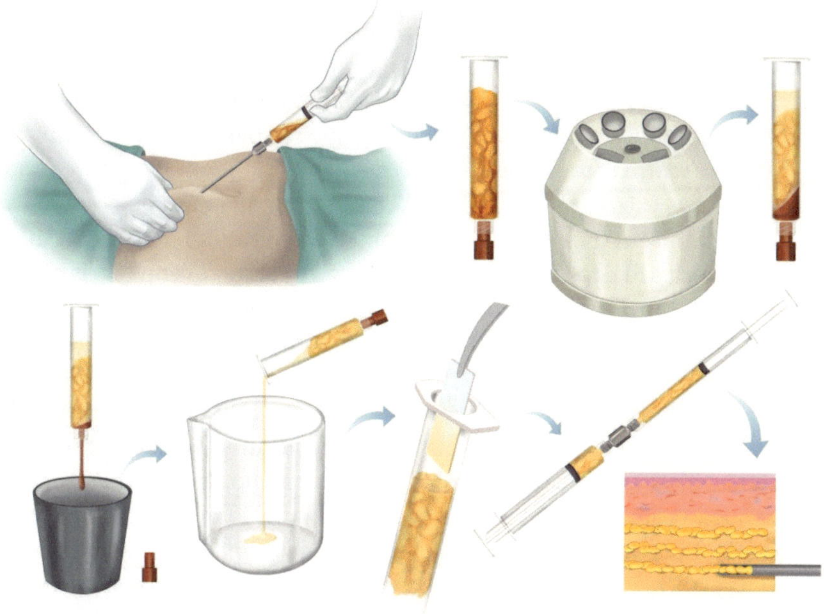

Figure 1. Harvest of fat grafts → Fat grafts are processed after centrifugation. The upper (oil) portion and the lower (red blood cells) portion should all be discarded. The fat is then injected creating several levels of injection.

the broken down fatty acids. This must be removed, as it has an acid pH and makes it difficult for the fat to "take" as a graft. To separate the hematic level we open the bottom plug and allow the blood to flow out into a tray. The broken down fatty acids in the top level can be removed by decantation, and if necessary the oil can be removed with the aid of a small lined gauze. Once the fat has been obtained, we connect the 10 ml syringe to the 1 ml syringes with a Luer Lock Transfer connector. This device is used to transfer fat by attaching a syringe to each end with a stopcock.

Washing

In this process we separate the tumescent liquid, anesthetics, lipids and broken down blood cells from the adipose tissue by washing and filtering the fat with saline solution or Ringer Lactate.

Once "purified" the fat is transferred to 10 ml syringes, and then, as with the method described above, it is transferred to the 1ml syringes via a Luer Lock Transfer connector, ready for injection.

Recently marketed systems such as Puregraft TM wash and filter the fat through membranes similar to those used in dialysis.

Injection of adipose tissue

To monitor the results as we inject the fat, we change the patient's position on the operating table and seat her. With a nº 11 scalpel we make the incisions needed, and with a blunt microinfiltration cannula (Coleman number 192729 or, if there is abundant fibrosis, the V7microinfiltration dissecting cannula), straight or convex, with a blunt tip and a 2 mm lateral orifice connected to a 1 ml syringe, we make the tunnels and inject the fat. Thus the injected fat enters in a single line and in small quantities [1ml), thereby enhancing graft survival and the integration of the adipose tissue implanted into the recipient site. This blunt cannula has a side hole in the tip, which is the same size as the holes of the cannula that we used to extract the fat, to avoid injury. These grafts should deposit very small amounts of fat in each tunnel, about 1 mm. First we introduce the cannula without infiltrating, and then infiltrate as we withdraw it. The effect is like the beads on a necklace; we create several levels of injection and it is essential to repeat the procedure several times at different levels so as to ensure that these micro-beads of fat "take" properly. It is also very important to introduce the fat in different areas creating a mesh or criss-cross pattern and making tunnels at all levels to prevent the accumulation of fat. The surrounding tissue revitalizes each lipoma, each small bead of fat tissue, and the body incorporates it as living tissue. In addition we should note that this fat contains preadipocytes, stem cells with a high capacity for angiogenesis. Therefore, by injecting this fat, we are not just adding volume but we are introducing mesenchymal stem cells with a great angiogenic capacity for the tissue repair of the implanted area. We finish with a 6/0 suture in each one of these holes and immobilize the area with hypoallergenic adhesive plasters to prevent the movement of the grafts.

2.3. Hotspots in fat injection with expanders and implants

From the cosmetic point of view, fat grafting overcomes the limitations of breast reconstruction with implants. To do so, along with the three-dimensional dispersion of the fat at various levels from the depth to the surface through the creation of the mesh or criss-cross pattern described above, the areas in which breast prostheses are not able to correct the defect require special attention. On the one hand, in the upper quadrants (especially in the upper outer quadrant) fat grafting provides the shape for the tail of the breast, something that the breast prosthesis does not do. In the upper-medial quadrant with the injection of fat we can reconstruct the cleavage. In the lower quadrants, fat grafting improves aesthetic appearance and adds thickness to the subcutaneous tissue, enhancing naturalness and creating a better-defined inframammary fold (FIG. 2).

3. Immediate breast reconstruction

3.1. Preoperative marking

Prior to surgery, we mark the reference lines with the patient in standing position.

First, the surgical oncologist draws the incision of the mastectomy to be performed. Then we draw the pocket we will create for insertion of the expander. To do this, we mark the midline from the sternal notch to the navel and delimit the width of the pocket, marking the anterior axillary line and a line 1.5 cm from the midline. We mark the current inframammary fold and an orientative point where we will place the new one, parallel to the current fold and at a

http://dx.doi.org/10.5772/56073

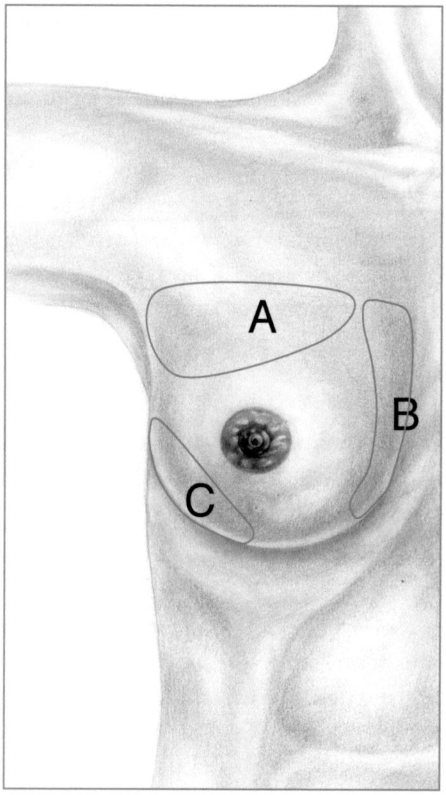

Figure 2. Areas in which breast prostheses are not able to correct the defect.

distance corresponding to half the result of the pinch test (the thickness of the skin and of subcutaneous fat panniculus), in most cases around 1-2 cm below. Note that these measures are approximate, and the new definitive fold will be placed using as a reference the healthy contralateral side, now reformed, 1 or 2 cm below the sixth rib.

In the contralateral healthy side, breast reduction, mastopexy or augmentation may be required. We prefer to perform symmetry surgery during this first stage since this gives us a second chance to correct the scars of the breast reduction or mastopexy when we replace the expander with the final prosthesis. In addition, if we have performed breast augmentation, being able to use the definitive contralateral breast as a reference helps us to calculate the size of the prosthesis needed on the mastectomized side during the second intervention.

3.2. Surgical technique

Approach to the contralateral breast

Among the main objectives of the reconstruction is to make the shape and volume of the two breasts as symmetrical as possible. In most patients, this requires cosmetic treatment of the healthy breast. We favor performing any cosmetic treatment necessary during the first stage. Better results are achieved if we perform the symmetrization with the expander and the fat grafting with the healthy, reformed side as our reference; this approach also allows us to make any alterations necessary in the second intervention.

If the healthy breast is small, we perform a breast augmentation. If a mastopexy is indicated, our technique of choice is the vertical scar technique [21]. If breast reduction is required, first we measure the distance from the sternal notch to the nipple. If it is less than 30 cm, we use our vertical scar technique [21]; if it is between 30 and 35 cm we use the "T" scar technique [22], and when it is above 35 cm we perform a free nipple implant and use the inferior pedicle to give projection to the breast, held in place by a band of the pectoralis major muscle [23].

First stage

At the same time as the aesthetic treatment of the healthy breast, and once the mastectomy is complete, we partially detach the pectoralis major muscle at the level of the fourth, fifth and sixth ribs (Fig.3A).

We begin this detachment with the free external edge of the muscle. It is important to perform this dissection above the pectoralis minor muscle; if carried out below this muscle, the dissection causes much more bleeding. It is very important to dissect the free edge of the pectoralis major muscle. Once identified, we introduce the index finger and with simple blunt dissection we identify the entire pocket without detaching any rib insertions, as this would cause bleeding. We place a retractor in the lateral edge and, using slight traction and taking care not to damage the muscle, we elevate the pectoralis major muscle like a tent. This simple maneuver allows us to detach the muscle from the sixth rib. We perform this detachment with the electric scalpel and with full vision. On reaching the sternon we detach the muscle up to the fourth rib.

We place the new inframammary fold 1 or 2 cm below the level of the sixth rib. Next, we suture the free lower edge of the pectoral muscle to the lower skin flap of the mastectomy, 2 cm from its free edge (Fig.3B).

It is important not to damage the muscle and to ensure that it does not tear when it is sutured to the subcutaneous tissue 2 cm from the lower edge of the mastectomy. Occasionally, if the subcutaneous tissue is thin we do not suture the muscle but place it 2 cm from the free edge, using transfixion stitches. We hold these stitches in place with steristrips.

Next we place the expander and fill it slightly with approximately 100cc of saline solution to prevent the formation of folds, but without creating tension in the skin, in order to avoid damage if the skin flaps are very thin. Finally we insert an aspiration drain and suture the skin.

Our technique [24] achieves an anatomical inclination in the upper quadrants as the expander is below the pectoral muscle, and the expansion of the lower quadrants is highly satisfactory since the muscle is detached and a curved shape is obtained, especially in the case of the lower external quadrant.

After two weeks, the expander is filled with 50 cc per week until the same size is achieved as the contralateral breast. Once the breasts are the same size, we perform a slight over-expan-

http://dx.doi.org/10.5772/56073

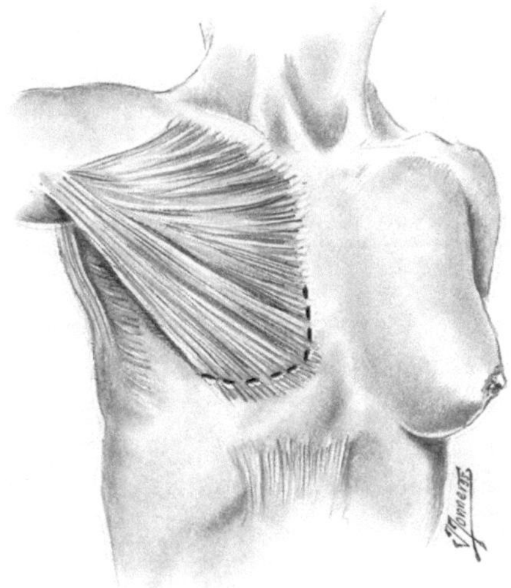

(A)

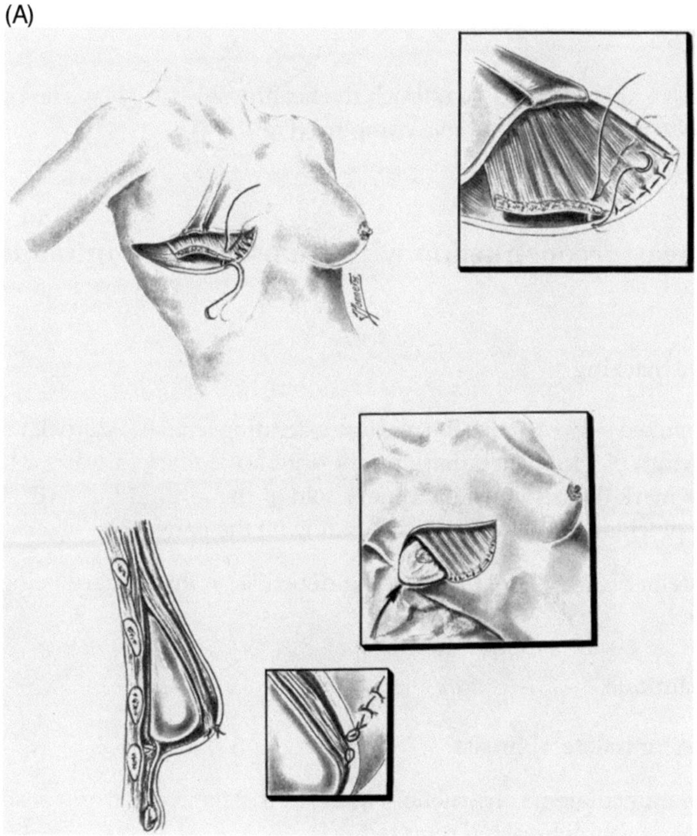

(B)

Figure 3. A: Partial detachment of the pectoralis major muscle from the fourth, fifth and sixth ribs. B: Suture of the lower free border of the pectoral major muscle to the lower skin flap of the mastectomy, 2 cm from the incision.

sion prior to the second intervention. If radiotherapy or chemotherapy is required, we follow the established protocol without any modifications.

Second stage

At 3 months after the first surgery, we replace the expander with the definitive prosthesis via a 4 cm incision in the lateral external third of the mastectomy scar and around the free edge of the pectoral muscle.

We use sizers to calculate the dimensions of the prosthesis required. After checking the correct volume, we insert the final prosthesis. We use anatomical prostheses with cohesive silicone. After inserting the prosthesis and suturing the skin, we perform fat grafting in the whole breast. In the upper quadrants we inject the fat in the subcutaneous plane between the muscle and skin, and also between the muscles, and in the lower quadrants between the capsule and the skin to achieve good reconstruction.

With this technique [1] we improve the quality of the tissue and reshape the breast to make it as symmetrical as possible to the contralateral breast, which if necessary will also receive fat grafting.

In this second stage, if necessary, we retouch the healthy side to achieve an optimal aesthetic result, and reconstruct the nipple-areola complex. (Fig.4 A-G).

4. Delayed breast reconstruction with endoscopy and intraoperative expansion

4.1. Preoperative marking

On the mastectomized side we mark the midline extending from the sternal notch to the navel. We define the width of the pocket, marking the anterior axillary line and a line 1.5 cm from the midline. We mark the new inframammary fold at the level of the sixth rib plus half the thickness of the pinching test (1 or 2 cm, depending on the patient).

On the contralateral healthy side, the marking depends on the surgery being performed, as explained above.

4.2. Surgical technique

Approach to the contralateral breast

As in the case of immediate reconstruction, in the first stage we perform aesthetic correction of the contralateral healthy breast, if required.

First stage

The expander is inserted by endoscopy through a 4 cm incision in the lateral external third of the mastectomy scar at the level of anterior axillary line, and with the aid of our endoscopic

http://dx.doi.org/10.5772/56073

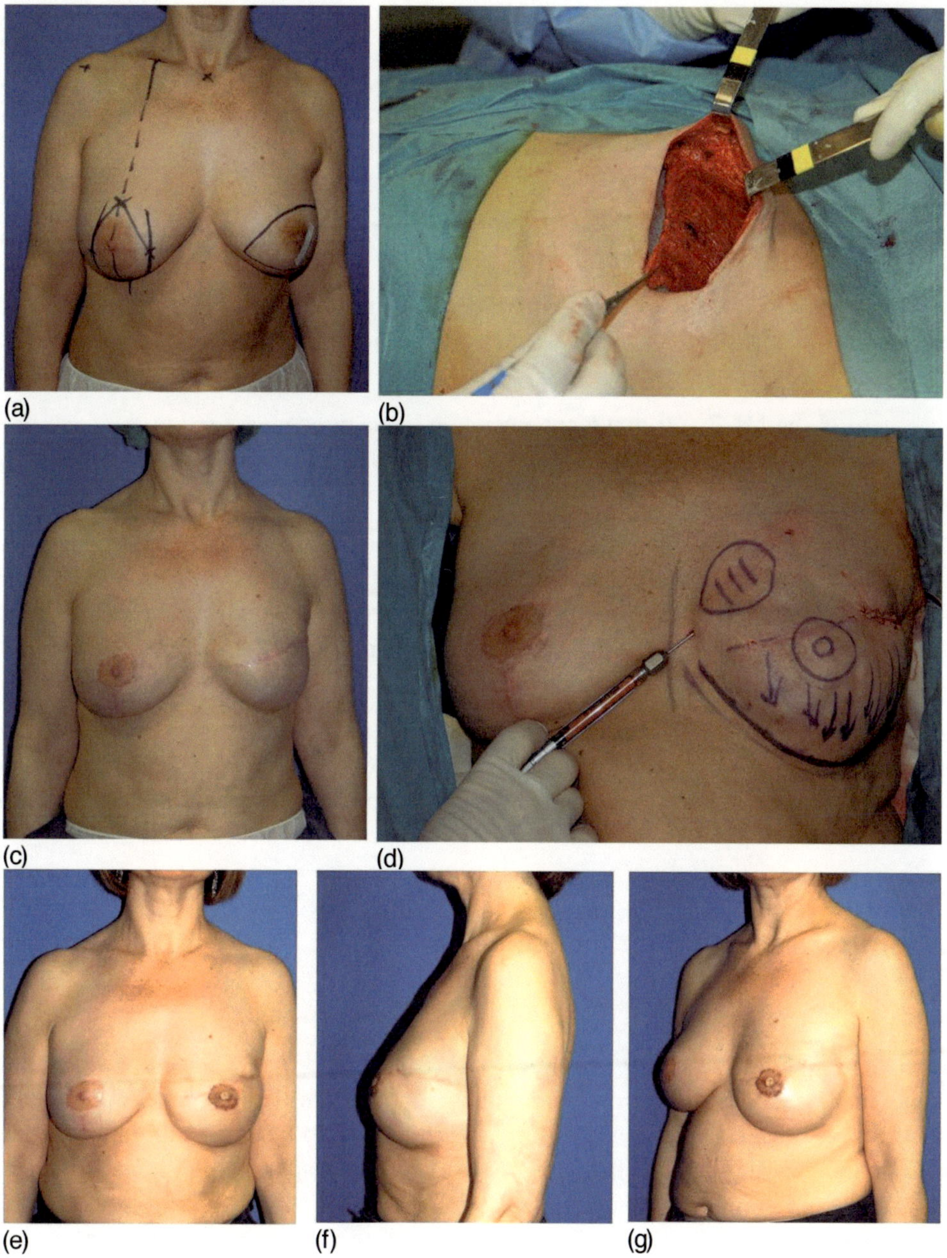

Figure 4. Patient aged 55 in whom a mastectomy was performed in the left breast, with immediate reconstruction with expander, prosthesis and fat grafting: (a) Preoperative frontal view. (b) Once the mastectomy is complete, we partially detach the pectoralis major muscle (c) Frontal view of the patient prior the second stage. (d) Fat grafting. (e) Frontal view 1 year after reconstruction. (f) Lateral view 1 year postoperatively. (g) Oblique view 1 year postoperatively.

retractor [25] we create the submuscular pocket in the upper quadrants and below the subcutaneous plane in the lower quadrants. We place the new fold at the same level as the contralateral breast. We then put the expander (with integral injection dome) in place and perform the volume increase required without causing damage to the skin. In up to 90% of cases, symmetrical volumes can be achieved between the two breasts in this first stage [26].

Simultaneously, a member of the team collects and prepares the fat. In this first stage we perform fat grafting only in the upper quadrants, injecting fat into the subcutaneous plane and the pectoral muscle.

Second stage

In this second stage, we replace the expander with the final prosthesis through the same incision as in the first stage and after calculating the dimensions of the prosthesis required using sizers.

We reconstruct the NAC and make any cosmetic corrections necessary in the contralateral breast (for example, to the scar formed by breast reduction if this operation has been performed).

In this second stage we inject fat between the capsule and the skin in the lower quadrants, and between skin and muscle and inside the muscle in the upper quadrants, in order to obtain good aesthetic results and to achieve symmetry between the two breasts. We also perform fat grafting of the contralateral breast if necessary: for example, to fill a small vacuum in the upper quadrants.

This injection of fat not only improves symmetry, but to a large extent avoids the formation of a hardened capsule and improves vascularization, skin quality and subcutaneous tissue neoformation after radiotherapy. It gives the reconstructed breast a very natural appearance and feel. (Fig. 5 A-G).

5. Complications and their management

Expanders and implants

The problems that may occur with the implant (extrusion and the formation of a capsule) are well known. Fortunately, extrusion or complete loss of the implant is rare. To prevent it, we always perform the incision in the lateral third of the mastectomy scar, in the anterior axillary line, so that the weakest point (the incision) does not correspond to the area in which the prosthesis exerts maximum pressure. In addition, the position of the muscle between the scar and the expander and the suture 2 cm from the free edge of the lower mastectomy flap keep the probability of this complication to a minimum. As for the formation of a periprosthetic capsule in the long term, Cordeiro [27] reports a rate of capsule grade III-IV formation of 18% and Alderman [28] a rate of 15%. Similar rates have been reported in other series.

While chemotherapy does not appear to alter the results, radiotherapy is a predisposing factor for the formation of a symptomatic periprosthetic capsule. The use of textured implants and especially the performance of fat grafting reduces this complication even in irradiated patients [1, 3, 8].

http://dx.doi.org/10.5772/56073

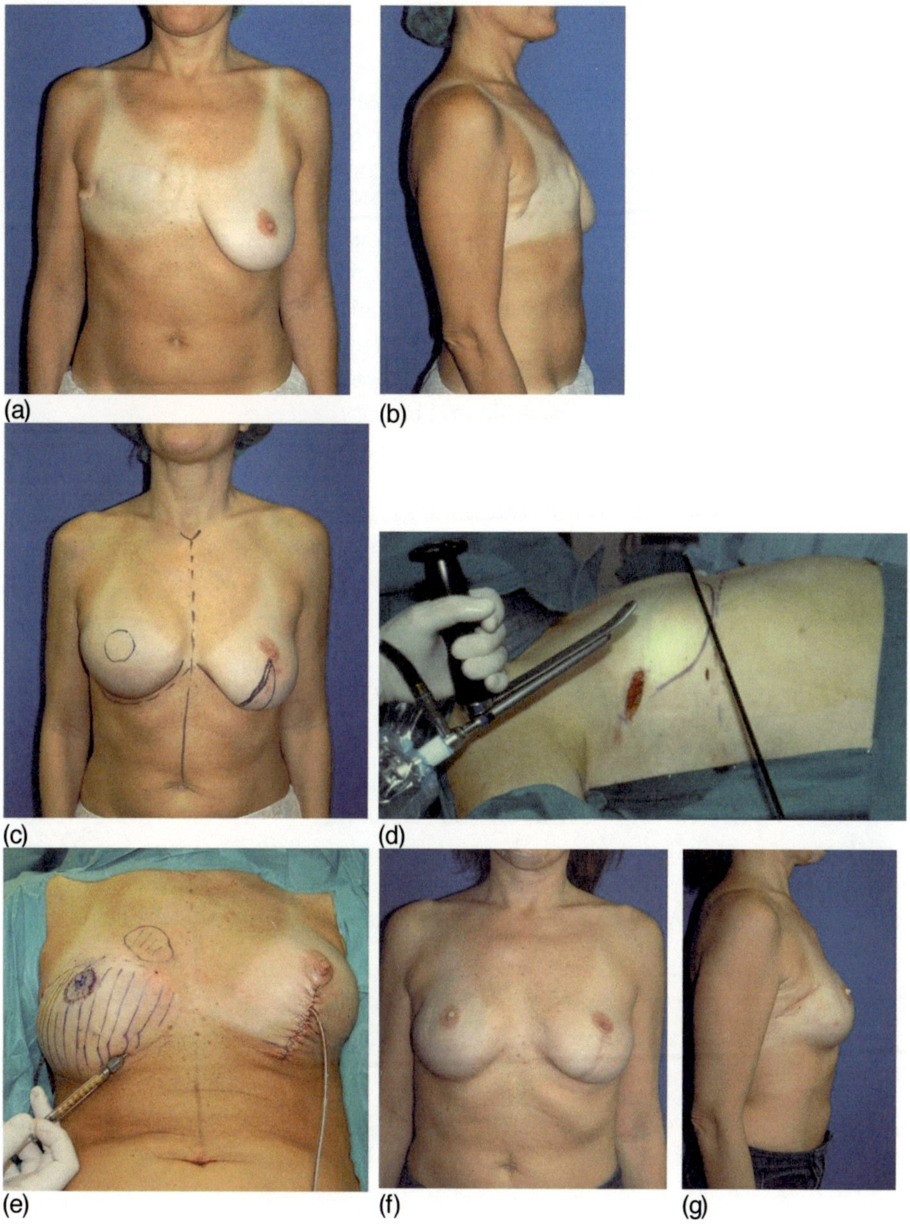

Figure 5. Patient aged 35 in whom a mastectomy was performed in the right breast, with delayed reconstruction with expander, prosthesis and fat grafting. (a) Preoperative frontal view. (b) Lateral view of the mastectomized side. (c) Frontal view of the patient prior the second stage. (d) The expander is inserted by endoscopy through a 4 cm incision in the lateral external third of the mastectomy scar at the level of anterior axillary line. (e) Fat grafting. (f) Frontal view at 1 year after reconstruction. (g) Lateral view of the mastectomized side.

Another possible complication is infection, which has an incidence of between 2% and 9%. In severe cases surgical cleaning, proper antibiotic coverage and implant removal are required.

It is also important to avoid damage to the mastectomy skin flaps, as this may lead to ischemia and partial necrosis of the skin.

Some authors hold that good results in terms of symmetry and naturalness cannot be achieved in unilateral cases. Our experience shows that with the changes we have made to the conventional technique [1, 24, 26] we obtain results that are consistent with the range of satisfaction rates reported by other authors, between 85% and 90%. The detachment of the pectoralis muscle allows proper expansion of the lower quadrants, while in the upper quadrants it produces a very natural inclination. Fat grafting improves the quality of the tissue, thickens the subcutaneous tissue and completes the symmetrization of the two sides. It also enables us to define the cleavage in the upper medial quadrants and the tail of the breast in the lateral quadrants. However, the key to achieving good results in unilateral cases is the correct choice of cosmetic treatment of the healthy contralateral breast.

Fat grafting

The injection of fat in breast surgery is a widely used method with very low complication rates. This is because fat is an autologous material, completely biocompatible, non-migratory and non-teratogenic; the tissue lost is replaced with similar tissue, applying the principle of "replace like with like".

In spite of the low rate of complications, the surgeon's experience and familiarity with the technique for obtaining, processing and injecting the fat are key elements for achieving good results.

It should be borne in mind that the fat is handled prior to its implantation and also that the adipose tissue is deprived of vascularization from the moment of extraction until its integration in the receptor tissue, with the result that there is a risk of infection. For this reason, maintaining maximum sterility during the procedure, ensuring asepsis of the area, and subsequent vigilance are all essential. Antibiotic prophylaxis immediately prior to surgery is very useful.

Another possible complication is damage to neighboring structures such as vessels or nerves. For this reason we use blunt cannulas and always before injecting the fat we perform a slight aspiration to ensure that we are not injecting the fat into vessels to avoid the risk of fat embolization.

As surgeons gain experience with these techniques, irregularities or the problems of hypo- and hypercorrection of the defects become less frequent. However, hypocorrection of defects is preferable to hypercorrection, because it can be resolved by further injections.

As in any surgical technique, inflammation or small hematomas will be present in the days immediately after the intervention. In these cases the use of anti-inflammatory drugs, cold therapy or even homeopathy may be helpful.

In the medium to long term calcifications may appear, but they bear no resemblance to the ones produced by tumor growth and are easy to recognize; there may also be oil droplets or fat cysts. If the fat has been injected incorrectly, in large accumulations, areas of necrosis or hardening may appear due to the encapsulation of this ischemic fat. This may cause patients serious concern because, understandably, they attribute it to the tumor.

As regards the area of extraction, it is very important to avoid irregularities. While obtaining the fat the direction of the tunnels should be varied and during the postoperative period drainage and massage should be provided, as after liposuction.

6. Conclusion

Major advances have recently been made in microsurgical reconstruction techniques and in the development of biomaterials for texturized breast implants. The search for improved results requires complementing conventional reconstruction techniques with other procedures. The injection of correctly treated fat helps to overcome the limitations of the various breast reconstruction techniques and achieves a very low complication rate.

By creating an appropriate pocket for the tissue expansion, achieving symmetry in the contralateral breast and injecting fat to palliate the sequelae of the radiotherapy, tissue reconstruction with expanders, prosthesis and fat grafting is a safe method that obtains satisfactory results.

Author details

Jose Ma Serra-Renom[1], Jose Ma Serra-Mestre[2*] and Francesco D'Andrea[3]

*Address all correspondence to: jmserramestre@gmail.com

1 Institute of Aesthetic and Plastic Surgery Dr. Serra-Renom Hospital Quiron Barcelona. Universitat Internacional de Catalunya, Spain

2 Department of Plastic Reconstructive and Aesthetic Surgery Second University of Naples, Italy

3 Department of Plastic Reconstructive and Aesthetic Surgery Second University of Naples, Italy

References

[1] Serra-Renom, J. M, Muñoz-Olmo, J. L, & Serra-Mestre, J. M. Fat grafting in postmastectomy breast reconstruction with expanders and prostheses in patients who have received radiotherapy: formation of new subcutaneous tissue. Plast Reconstr Surg. 2010 Jan; 125(1):12-8.

[2] Serra-Renom, J. M, Muñoz-Olmo, J. L, & Serra-Mestre, J. M. Breast reconstruction with fat grafting alone. Ann Plast Surg. 2011 Jun; 66(6):598-601.

[3] Rigotti G, Marchi A, Galie M, et al. Clinical treatment of radiotherapy tissue damage by lipoaspirate transplant: a healing process mediated by adipose-derived adult stem cells. Plast Reconstr Surg. 2007; 119(5):1409–1422.

[4] Spear SL, Wilson HN, Lockwood MD. Fat injection to correct contour deformities in the reconstructed breast. Plast Recon- str Surg. 2005;116:1300–1305.

[5] Serra-Renom, J. M, Muñoz-Olmo, J. L, & Serra-Mestre, J. M. Treatment of tuberous breasts grade III with puckett's technique (modified) and fat grafting to correct the constricting ring. Aesthetic Plast Surg. 2011 Oct; 35(5):773-81.

[6] Serra-Renom, J. M, Muñoz-Olmo, J. L, & Serra-Mestre, J. M. Endoscopic-assisted aesthetic augmentation of tuberous breasts and fat grafting to correct the double bubble. Aesthetic Plast Surg. 2012 (in press).

[7] Ribuffo D, Atzeni M, Serratore F, et al. Cagliari University Hospital (CUH) protocol for immediate alloplastic breast reconstruction and unplanned radiotherapy. A preliminary report. Eur Rev Med Pharmacol Sci. 2011 Jul;15(7):840-4.

[8] Petit JY, Lohsiriwat V, Clough KB, et al. The oncologic outcome and immediate surgical complications of lipofilling in breast cancer patients: a multicenter study--Milan-Paris-Lyon experience of 646 lipofilling procedures. Plast Reconstr Surg. 2011 Aug;128(2):341-6.

[9] Sarfati I, Ihrai T, Kaufman G, et al. Adipose-tissue grafting to the post-mastectomy irradiated chest wall: preparing the ground for implant reconstruction. J Plast Reconstr Aesthet Surg. 2011 Sep;64(9):1161-6.

[10] Salgarello M, Visconti G, Barone-Adesi L. Fat grafting and breast reconstruction with implant: another option for irradiated breast cancer patients. Plast Reconstr Surg. 2012 Feb;129(2):317-29.

[11] Gutowski KA; ASPS Fat Graft Task Force. Current applications and safety of autologous fat grafts: a report of the ASPS fat graft task force. Plast Reconstr Surg. 2009 Jul; 124(1):272-80.

[12] Padoin, A. V, Braga-Silva, J, Martins, P, et al. Sources of processed lipoaspirate cells: influence of donor site on cell concentration. Plast Reconstr Surg. 2008 Aug; 122(2): 614-8.

[13] Fraser JK, Wulur I, Alfonso Z, et al. Differences in stem and progenitor cell yield in different subcutaneous adipose tissue depots. Cytotherapy. 2007, 9:459.

[14] Keck M, Zeyda M, Gollinger K et al. Local Anesthetics Have a Major Impact on Viability of Preadipocytes and Their Differentiation into Adipocytes. Plast. Rec. Surg. 2010, 126:1500.

[15] Erdim M, Tezel E, Numanoglu A, et al. The effects of the size of liposuction cannula on adipocyte survival and the optimum temperature for fat graft storage: an experimental study. J Plast Reconstr Aesthet Surg. 2009, 62:1210.

[16] Coleman S, Mazzola R. Fat Injection From Filling to Regeneration. St Louis, MO: Quality Medical Publishing; 2009.

[17] Ferraro GA, De Francesco F, Tirino V, et al. Effects of a new centrifugation method on adipose cell viability for autologous fat grafting. Aesthetic Plast Surg. 2011 Jun; 35(3):341-8.

[18] Kurita M, Matsumoto D, Shigeura T, et al. Influences of centrifugation on cells and tissues in liposuction aspirates: optimized centrifugation for lipotransfer and cell isolation. Plast Reconstr Surg 2008 Mar;121(3):1033-41; discussion 1042-3

[19] Matsumoto D, Shigeura T, Sato K, et al. Influences of preservation at various temperatures on liposuction aspirates. Plast Reconstr Surg. 2007, 120:1510.

[20] Carvalho PP, Yu G, Wu X et al. Processing and pas- saging of human adipose-derived stromal/stem cells: use of anima free products and extended storage at room temperature. IFATS proceedings, Dallas, 2010.

[21] Serra-Renom, J. M, & Fontdevila, J. New marking designs for vertical scar breast reduction. Aesthet Surg J. 2004; 24(2):171-5.

[22] Georgiade NG. Aesthetic Breast Surgery. Baltimore. Williams 6 Wilkins; 1983.

[23] Graf RM. Reduction mamaplasty and mastopexy using the vertical scar and the thoracic Wall flap technique. Aesth Plast Surg. 2003; 27:06-12.

[24] Serra-Renom, JM , Fontdevila J, Monner J. Mammary reconstruction using tissue expander and partial detachment of the pectoralis major muscle to expand inferior breast quadrants. Ann Plast Surg. 2004;53:317–321.

[25] Serra JM. Retractor with mobile endoscope. Plast Reconstr Surg. 1997;100:529–531.

[26] Serra-Renom, J. M, Guisantes, E, Yoon, T, et al. Endoscopic breast reconstruction with intraoperative complete tissue expansion and partial detachment of the pectoralis muscle. Ann Plast Surg. 2007;58:126–130.

[27] Cordeiro, P. G, & McCarthy, C. M. A single surgeon's 12-year experience with tissue expander/implant breast reconstruction: part I. A prospective analysis of early complications. Plast Reconstr Surg. 2006 Sep 15;118(4):825-31.

[28] Alderman AK, Wilkins EG, Kim HM, et al. Complications in postmastectomy breast reconstruction: Two-year results of the Michigan Breast Reconstruction Outcome Study. Plast Reconstr Surg. 109: 2265, 2002.

Chapter 6

Robotic Harvest of the Latissimus Dorsi Muscle for Breast Reconstruction

Jesse Selber

Additional information is available at the end of the chapter

http://dx.doi.org/10.5772/55040

1. Introduction

Robotic technology has assumed a prominent position in minimally invasive surgery throughout the surgical subspecialties1234. Enhanced precision, tremor elimination, motion scaling, high resolution, 3-D optics and an intuitive interface have permitted wide adoption of robotic surgical techniques across a range of intra-corporeal procedures.

As experience with robotics has grown and permeated main stream surgery, applications in plastic surgery have emerged. Trans-oral robotic reconstruction of oropharyngeal defects has gained momentum, and is now performed in select academic centers in the United States.56789 Robotic microsurgery is a burgeoning field that has great potential for growth as robotic technology and instrumentation improves.101112

Because plastic surgeons are infrequently involved with intracorporeal procedures, there is not a rich history of minimally invasive training in the specialty. Muscle flaps are one of the few reconstructive procedures in which plastic surgeons bypass the skin entirely to gain access to deeper tissue planes. For that reason, there exists the opportunity for a minimally invasive approach to muscle flap harvest.

The latissimus dorsi muscle has been a workhorse of reconstructive surgery since its original description by Iginio Tansini in 1906.13 Its diverse applications range from breast reconstruction with implants, partial breast reconstruction, chest wall and intra-thoracic reconstruction, scalp and extremity coverage, and functional muscle transfer.14,15,16,17,18,19,20 Traditional harvest technique requires a posterior donor-site incision that can be between 15 cm and 45 cm in length, in addition to an axillary incision for pedicle harvest or transfer (Figure 1). The reason for this length is that the incision must accommodate access to the thoracodorsal pedicle in the axilla, as well as the origin of the muscle along the thoracolumbar fascia.

Minimally invasive harvest of the latissimus flap has long been a desirable goal. Endoscopic harvest has been attempted by multiple groups, and is still practiced in certain centers.21,22,23 But because of technical challenges such as line of sight around the curvature of the back, limitations of endoscopic instrumentation, and difficulty maintaining an optical window, all but a few centers have abandoned this technique.24,25

The robotic platform has specific advantages that make it superior to traditional endoscopy. One is the high resolution, three-dimensional optics. The incredible picture clarity and magnification at the point of surgery allow for better identification and control of perforating blood vessels, which has been a problem for the endoscopic approach, evidenced by a high rate of conversion to the open procedure. Another advantage is instrumentation. The robotic instruments have motion in 7 degrees of freedom at the very tips. Not only does this allow for incredible precision in controlling small vessels and maintaining a consistent plane, but it allows negotiation around the curvature of the back. This feature is absent in "straight-stick" endoscopy, which has no real versatility at the tips of the instruments. Finally, surgeon comfort and positioning removes much of the awkwardness of the endoscopic approach to muscle harvest, where the surgeon can find herself struggling in a mechanical disadvantage.

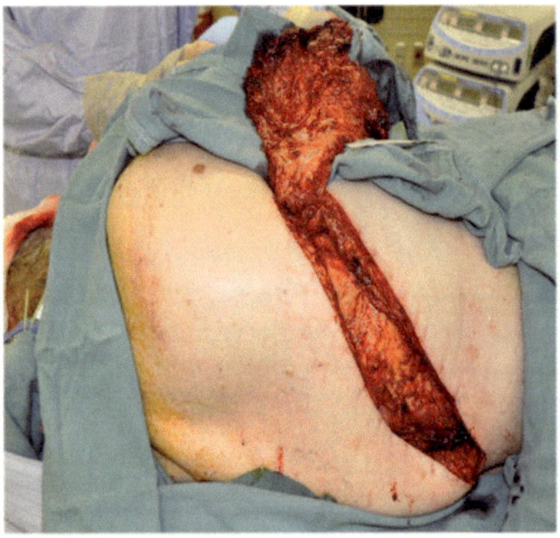

Figure 1. Traditional incision for harvest of the latissimus dorsi muscle can be very long, to access both the pedicle and the muscle origin

2. Operative procedure

2.1. Positioning and defining landmarks

The muscle harvest is performed, like a standard latissimus dorsi harvest, with the patient in the decubitus position with the ipsilateral arm prepped and placed on a sterile Mayo stand. An axillary roll is used to prevent contralateral, brachial plexopathy. The borders of the LD muscle are marked on the patient: the anterior border is palpated preoperatively during active muscle contraction, the superior border is marked from the tendinous insertion, along the tip of the scapula to the posterior border, and the posterior border is marked about 4 cm lateral to the spine.

The bed can be retroflexed in the middle to help open the space between the iliac crest and the lower border of the ribcage. This is important because at the extremes of dissection, as the arms line up with one another, they will frequently bump into the hip or shoulder. Retroflexion obviates some of this problem.

2.2. Incision and port locations

Figure 2 demonstrates the markings for the axillary incision and port placement. When the harvest is performed for breast reconstruction, the sentinel lymph node or axillary node dissection incision is used, without the need for an additional incision. If a new axillary incision is required, then it is designed to facilitate pedicle dissection, dissection of the subcutaneous space anterior to the muscle, and placement of a port at the inferior end of the incision. In such cases, a 5-8 cm incision is oriented along a line between the posterior axilla and the nipple areolar complex. This vector accomplishes two things: 1) it allows the incision to be oblique to the plane of dissection anterior to the muscle, affording a broader initial dissection view 2) it allows a port to be placed in the distal end of the axillary incision, because it is an adequate distance from both the muscle edge and pedicle.

The first port is placed at the end of the axillary incision, which is later closed temporarily with a running stitch to maintain insufflation. The second and third ports are then placed approximately 8 cm apart from each other and from the 1st port, and 8 cm anterior to the anterior border of the muscle. This places the central port at the infra-mammary fold in women, concealing this 12 mm port site. The distal, 8 mm port remains the only visible scar with the arm in repose. The port in the axillary incision can be double cannulated with an 8 mm port inside a 12 mm port. This has two benefits: 1) the inner port can be removed and a laporacopic instrument such as a grasper, a clip applier or a suction irriagator can be placed by the bedside assistant, and 2) and a smoke evacuator can be attached to the insufflations port which helps with visualization. Isufflation can be tolerated at up to 15 mm Hg.

2.3. Initial dissection and port placement

The axillary incision is opened, and the thoracodorsal pedicle is identified, isolated and marked with a vessel loop for identification under endoscopic vision. This is important because when in the console, although detail is very good, orientation can be challenging. Having the pedicle marked helps avoid it at the proximal extent of the dissection and prevents inadvertent pedicle damage. The subcutaneous space anterior to the anterior border of the muscle is then dissected using a long-tip electrocautery and a lighted retractor, in order to place additional ports. The axillary incision, the two additional ports and the anterior border of the muscle must form a hemi-octagon (as shown in Figure 2) that must be completely dissected through the axillary incision to create the confluent subcutaneous space to facilitate placement of instruments and initiation of the dissection.

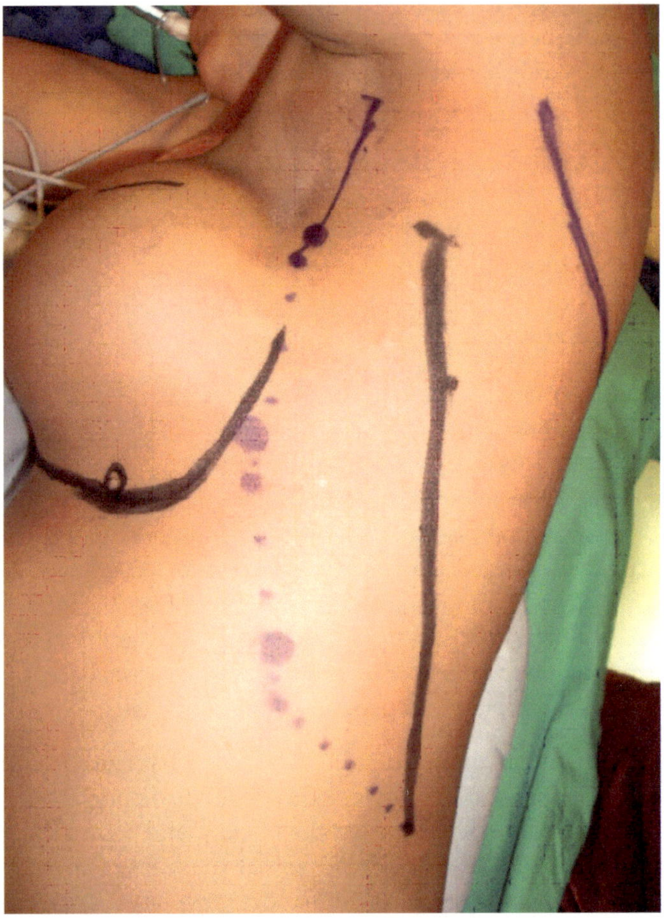

Figure 2. Port placement and axillary incision design for robotic harvest of the LD is shown in relation to the anterior border of the muscle. A hemioctagonal, subcutaneous area is dissected for optimal exposure and ergonomics.

The open dissection through the axillary incision is optimized in the following two ways to ensure a smooth transition to the initial robotic dissection: 1) the deep muscular plane is dissected under direct vision through the axilla as far as technically feasible. This dissection is easily performed under direct vision, and requires less precision, cutting down on unnecessary robotic time. 2) Approximately 4 cm of the superficial plane over the muscle is dissected through the axilla, releasing the anterior border of the muscle so that it is suspended loosely enough that the initial robotic subcutaneous dissection is facilitated, but not released to an extent that obscures the robotic view of the sub-muscular plane of dissection. This is a very helpful technical point. If the muscle is not released at all, then it is very difficult to do robotically, because the machine has to look almost straight up at the muscle. If the edge hangs down, the dissection can be brought into a better orientation for the angle of the arms. If the muscle is released too much, it makes it hard to get in and out of the submuscular space during this part of the dissection.

http://dx.doi.org/10.5772/55040

A 1 cm incision is then made for the second port. A digit is introduced through the axillary incision to palpate the port as it enters the subcutaneous space and a 12 mm camera port is introduced. An small incision is then made over the other port site. A zero-degree endoscope is placed in the 12 mm port and an 8 mm port is placed at the third port site under endoscopic vision. The axillary incision is then temporarily closed using a running suture around 12 mm port to maintain insufflation.

2.4. Robotic docking and dissection

Following port placement, the robotic side cart (Da Vinci, Intuitive Surgical, Sunnyvale, CA) is positioned posterior to the patient with the two robotic arms and the endoscope extending over the patient in proximity to the ports. The distance from the bed is determined by the camera arm being flexed at more or less 90 degrees at the elbow. The other arms can then be brought into position, opening the elbows as much as possible to avoid conflicts during dissection. The robot is then docked to the cannulas, bringing the arms into a position that is nearly parallel to the floor.

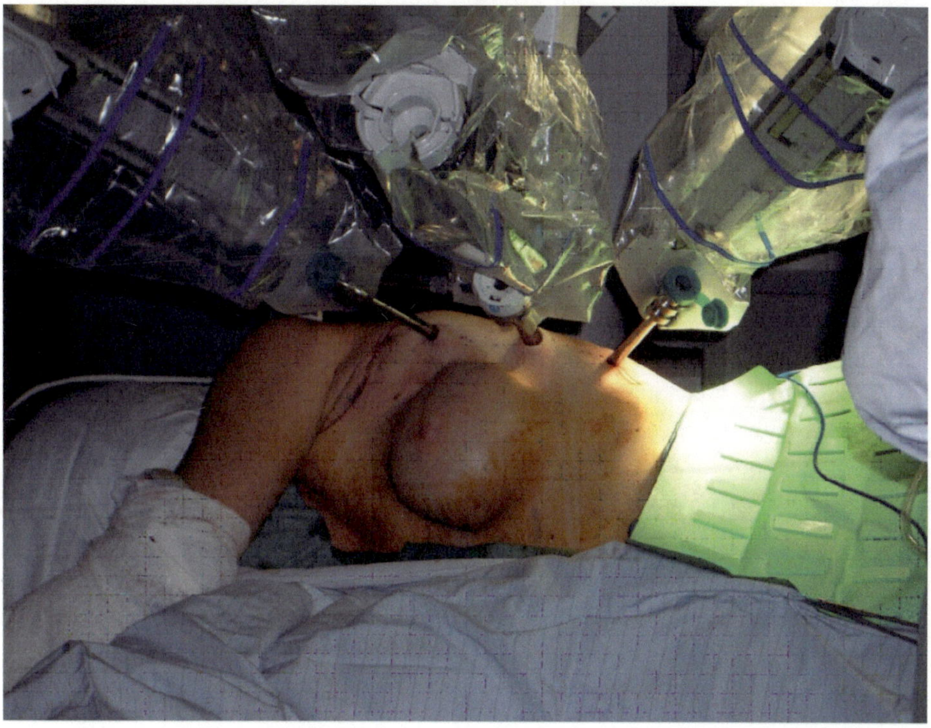

Figure 3. The robot is docked with the Patient-Side Cart behind the patient and the arms nearly parallel with the floor.

Once the patient side cart is docked to the cannulas, insufflation is applied at 10 mm Hg. Dissection begins along the under surface of the muscle.[1] Monopolar scissors and Cadière grasping forceps (Intuitive Surgical, Sunnyvale, California) are used for the dissection. Blood vessels can be clipped using a laparoscopic clip applier through one of the ports, or using a robotic clip applier. When the curvature of the back is encountered, the horizon will get too low for appropriate visualization. At that point, I recommend switching to a 30 degree down scope to better view this portion. Allow your bedside assistant to guide the extent of your dissection by comparing the space created with the preoperative markings. After the undersurface of the muscle is dissected to the borders, the 0 degree scope is replaced and the grasper is used to direct the anterior edge of the muscle towards the chest wall. Dissection then proceeds over the superficial surface of the muscle. The same process of switching to the 30 degree down scope is repeated when the curvature of the back becomes difficult to negotiate. Ideally, the deep and superficial dissection reach the same borders to that at the end, all that is left is the attachment to the thoracolumbar fascia inferiorly and posteriorly.

It is extremely helpful to have an assistant at the bedside familiar with the mechanics of robotic surgery. At the inferior and superior extremes of the dissection, the robotic arms and camera are nearly parallel, and may conflict with one another or the prominences of the patient's hip or shoulder. These undesirable interactions need to be monitored, and subtle modifications of arm positioning over the course of the case will be necessary to prevent them. In addition, as the dissection moves posteriorly, arm position will have to be adjusted to account for the curvature of the back. Specifically, the skin will need to be tented up by lifting the arms straight up. This is called "bumping" the arms. It's important to have the bed all the way to the floor for these adjustments, or the robotic arms will run out of room in the vertical dimension. These adjustments can be made without undocking the robot, but require experience.

Once dissection is complete in both the deep and superficial planes, the monopolar scissors is used to release the muscle at the infero-posterior border. A 30 degree-down scope is useful at this juncture to "look over" the curvature of the back. As the muscle is divided, it is continually "gathered" towards the axilla in order to maintain an optical window and tension at the point of dissection. Once the muscle has been liberated beyond the tip of the scapula, it will be easily accessible through the axillary incision. It is critical to visualize directly the thoracodorsal pedicle and insure that it is not in danger as the dissection approaches the axilla. Identification is made easier by the presence of a vessel loop.

2.5. Undocking and extraction of the muscle

At this stage, the robot can be undocked, and pushed back from the bed. The robotic portion of the procedure is now over. The axillary incision is then re-opened, and the muscle is delivered. An endoscope is reintroduced to confirm adequate hemostasis. Drains are placed though the two lower port sites, positioned in the donor site, and sutured into place.

The tendinous insertion can be released further through the axillary incision under direct visualization. Any remaining attachments are divided postero-superiorly. Usually there is some attachment to the teres major in this area that can be addressed open. If the muscle is being transferred as a pedicled flap for breast reconstruction, the majority of the posterior

---

1 If dissection began along the subcutaneous plane, it would be impossible to maintain the optical window beneath the muscle because insufflation would press the muscle down against the chest wall.

insertion is divided, and the muscle is delivered through the axillary incision, and then into the mastectomy space in preparation for a change to the supine position (Figure 4).

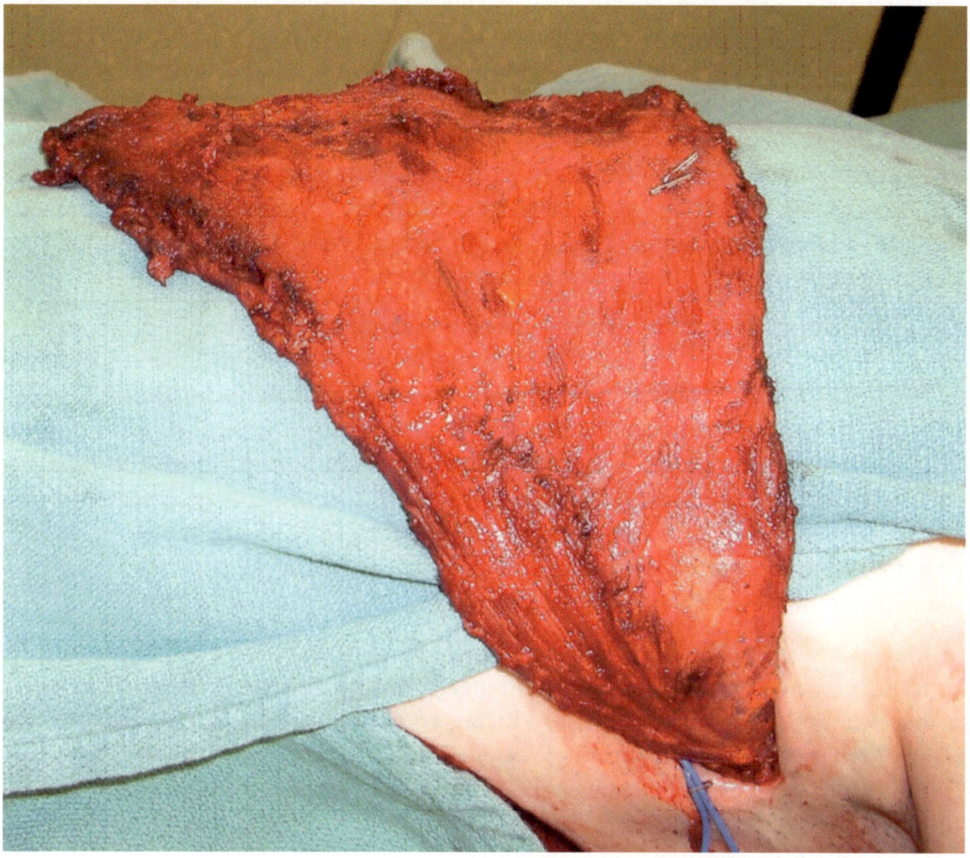

Figure 4. The muscle is delivered following the robotic harvest through the short axillary incision

2.6. Uses of the robotic LD for breast reconstruction

For use as a pedicled flap, the advantages of a muscle only LD with a barely visible donor site are tremendous. Breast reconstruction is more like cosmetic surgery than many other areas of reconstructive surgery in the sense that patients are very sensitive to esthetic outcomes and much more discriminating and informed about how advances in the field apply to their individual treatment plan. Partial breast reconstruction and nipple-areolar-complex (NAC) sparing mastectomy represent two advances in the field that reflect this reality. Robotic assisted LD harvest can enhance and expand the indications of both these procedures.

In the case of lateral lumpectomy defects, if no contralateral procedure is required or desired, then the optimal option for the index breast is volume replacement. If a latissimus muscle can be introduced using the sentinel lymph node biopsy site and two additional ports, this volume replacement can be achieved with minimal donor cost to the patient and without additional breast incisions, incisions on the contralateral breast, or altering the tumor bed. If a patient who is concerned with donor esthetics is presented with the option of a LD flap where a back incision is necessary, her decision might more easily swing away from the LD flap volume replacement procedure and towards local tissue rearrangement based on reduction mammoplasty principles and a contralateral balancing procedure. This potentially compromises her goal of breast volume preservation and commits the patient to a bilateral procedure increasing the potential for complications in the contralateral breast and overall post-radiation asymmetry. Robotic assisted LD harvest has changed the clinical algorithm for partial breast reconstruction in my practice for patients with large, lateral lumpectomy defects.

For NAC sparing mastectomies, implant based results that rival breast augmentations can be achieved; however, the challenge to the reconstructive surgeon is considerable, because the breast mound needs to be centered perfectly under the NAC for a good result. This requires release of the pectoralis major so the expander or implant can descend to the natural position of the breast, which subsequently requires some lower pole support, usually in the form of a serratus flap or bioprosthetic. The serratus is small for this purpose and bioprosthetic is expensive and prone to complication. 26,27 The esthetic benefits related to contour of having muscle under the lower pole instead of allograft or xenograft are substantial (Figure 5 and 6).

In addition, since the NAC complex is present in such cases (in distinction to a skin sparing mastectomy), the need for a skin island is completely mitigated, adding an additional rational for a muscle only LD in this setting. Introducing an LD into the lower pole without a back incision allows for direct to implant single stage reconstruction without the need for bioprosthetic mesh. This technique maximizes the esthetic outcomes in both the breast and back, reduces complications and the cost associated with bioprosthetics and optimizes the outcomes in NAC sparing mastectomy reconstructions (Figure 7).

Another use for the muscle only latissimus is in the second stage of a two-stage implant based breast reconstruction in which the patient received radiation unexpectedly, but had a complete re-expansion with a preservation of the breast skin envelope. In these patients, the risk of exposure and short and long term complications following the exchange is high. A muscle, placed between the permanent implant and the skin at the time of the exchange is protective in these situations. I have a number of colleagues who have requested robotic muscle harvests for their patients in these clinical scenarios.

Regarding tumor staging, it is important to identify patients who will not require adjuvant radiation therapy for the immediate robotic assisted LD flap. In these patients the LD should be preserved for use in a delayed reconstruction setting. If a patient with a T2 tumor is found to have a positive sentinel lymph node on frozen section then a one stage robotic assisted LD with implant reconstruction is deferred pending final pathology. It is critical to preserve the LD as a salvage option for breast reconstruction in these difficult to predict clinical scenarios involving radiation therapy.

http://dx.doi.org/10.5772/55040

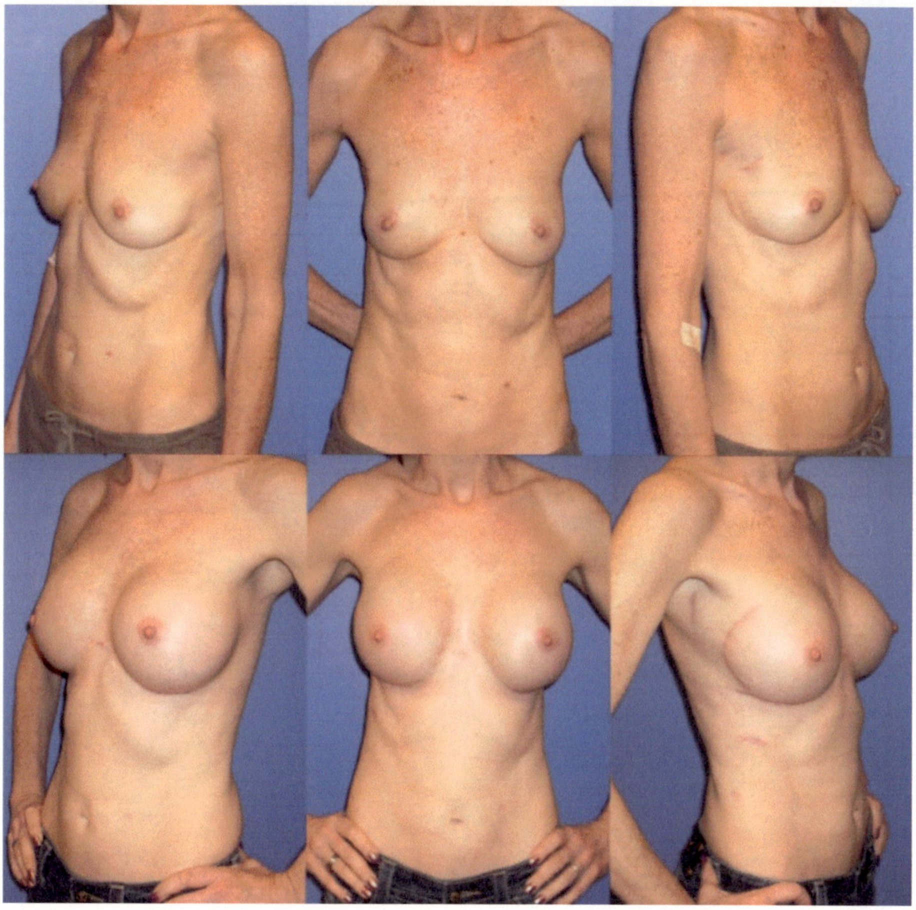

Figure 5. Two stage reconstruction with TE and muscle only LD - For NAC sparing mastectomies, a muscle only LD can be used for lower support with results that rival the contralateral breast augmentation.

3. Results

I have performed 14 robotic latissimus dorsi harvests for breast reconstruction over the past year. The average set up time, which includes the initial axillary incision, port placement, and docking of the robot is about 30 minutes. The actual harvest itself takes a little over an hour. There have been no conversions to the open technique for any of the flaps, and all flaps were harvested and transferred in their entirety. One patient was explanted due to a fungal infection while she was on chemotherapy, months following her procedure. This was considered unrelated to the method of surgery. There have been no other recipient site or donor site complications, including seroma, hematoma or overlying skin injury. One port site was revised to improve esthetics.

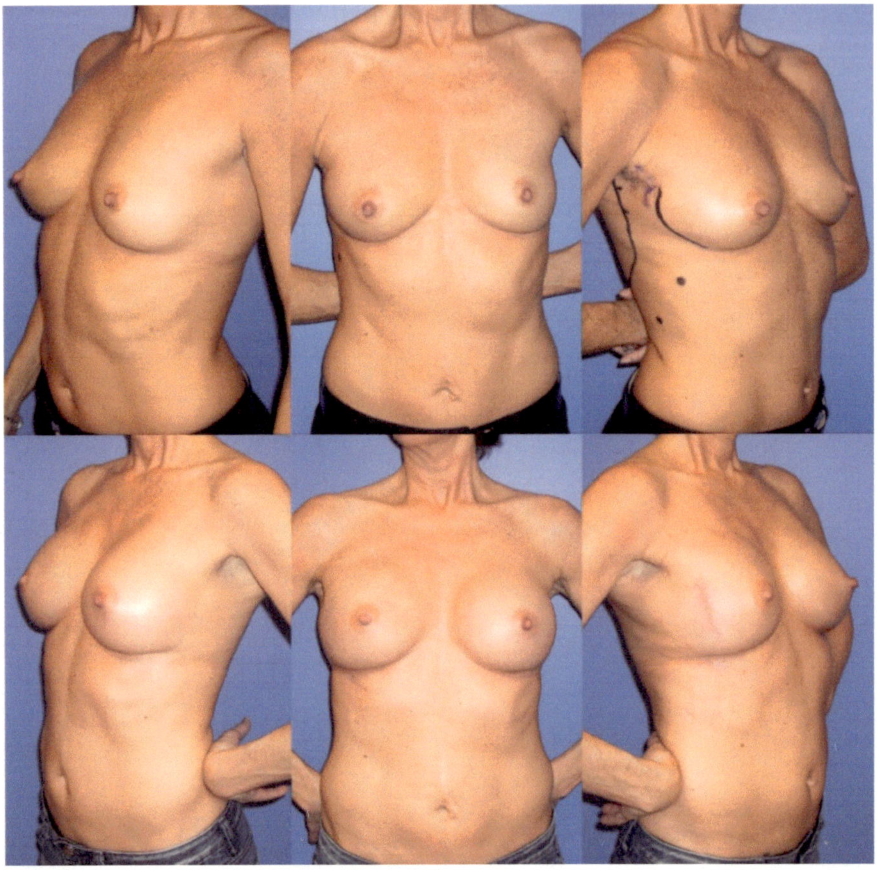

Figure 6. Single stage reconstruction with muscle only LD - For NAC sparing mastectomies, a muscle only LD can be used for lower support with results that rival the contralateral breast augmentation.

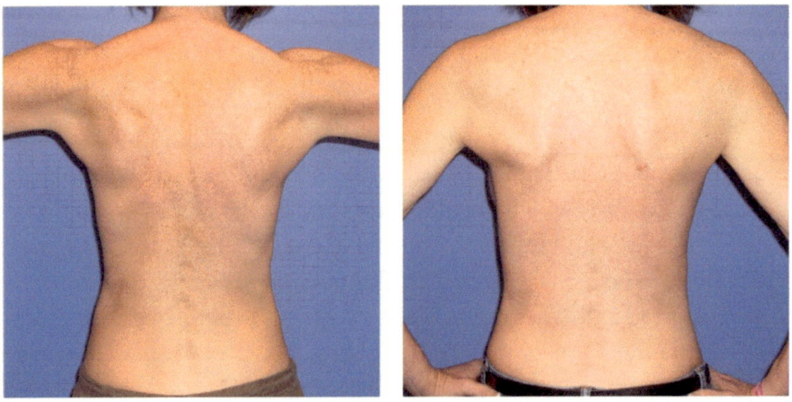

Figure 7. The donor site from a muscle only LD is functionally and esthetically difficult to distinguish from the normal side.

4. Discussion

The goal of minimally invasive surgery is to reduce the esthetic and functional morbidity of open procedures. Robotic technology has many advantages to standard minimally invasive approaches - high resolution, three dimensional optics, intuitive motion and greatly enhanced precision have combined to catapult robotic surgery into minimally invasive surgical mainstream. Plastic surgeons are late adopters of this technology, partly because we frequently operate on the skin itself, and partly because we lack the training and thought process from which to develop minimally invasive robotic concepts and techniques.

The latissimus dorsi muscle flap is one of our most reliable reconstructive options for a variety of indications, and I have demonstrated that this muscle can be reproducibly harvested using a surgical robot. The main advantage of the robotic technique is in sparing the patient a visible incision on the back. Instead, the patient has a short incision hidden in the axilla, with two additional port sites, one of which is obscured in the inframammary fold. Eliminating the "cost" of the donor site incision increases the versatility of an already versatile flap. In my practice, the muscle only LD has, in select cases, replaced bioprosthetic mesh in supporting the lower pole in implant-based breast reconstruction, replaced local tissue rearrangement for partial breast, and lowered the threshold for adding muscle coverage in radiated implant reconstructions.

As we move forward with this and other robotic procedures, our specialty must face the practical considerations of disseminating robotic techniques to a broader population of surgoens. One important concern is cost. A new, dual console, DaVinci SI costs approximately 2.2 million dollars. This is a major capital cost, but it is important to understand that the robotic platform is being purchased by hospitals in order to attract high volumes of patients undergoing established robotic procedures such as prostatectomy. The marginal cost of using the robot for a plastic surgery procedure is only the additional OR time, and the cost of the instruments, which is distributed over 10 uses (the life of the DaVinci instruments). In our setting, a robotic LD harvest costs an additional $800 to $900 compared to an open LD flap harvest. This is about the same cost as a CT scan, which many surgeons routinely get for free flap breast reconstruction. This is not intended as a formal or comprehensive cost-benefit analysis, but only to provide an estimate of the "cost" of eliminating the back incision in an LD harvest.

The other important question impacting dissemination of this technique is its "teachability." There are important barriers to teaching this technique to a wider audience. One is that plastic surgeons need to have a training pathway to learn how to use the surgical robot, separate from any specific technique. Operating the surgical robot has many nuances associated with it, and the surgeon must be comfortable, not only with its basic functionality, but how to manage the machine itself if the procedure is not proceeding optimally. This requires an initial investment of personal time and energy on the part of the learner. The second barrier is that the robotic LD harvest has a multitude of small technical nuances, which if well considered can make for a smooth operative experience, but if poorly accounted for can make it nearly impossible. Moving forward, the success of the operation will rely on standardizing the operative sequence and robotic technique so that it can be taught in an advanced training module and the knowledge can be transferred to other surgeons.

5. Conclusions

Robotic applications now dominate many areas of minimally invasive surgery. The harvest of muscle flaps represents a novel plastic surgery application for this technology. Because of the esthetic sensitivity of breast reconstruction patients in general, eliminating an incision on the back for this very versatile flap has real benefit to patients. The robotic LD mitigates many of the challenges posed by endoscopic harvest by providing a platform with precise instrumentation and high resolution, three-dimensional optics. The technique itself is not simple, but with some experience, is both reliable and reproducible. The most practical applications are for partial breast reconstruction of lateral lumpectomy defects, implant based reconstruction in the context of NAC sparing mastectomies, and in patients with expanders who receive radiation.

Author details

Jesse Selber M.D., M.P.H.

Assistant Professor and Adjunct Director of Clinical Research, Department of Plastic Surgery, The University of Texas, M.D. Anderson Cancer Center, Houston, TexasUSA

References

[1] Yuh, B. E, Hussain, A, Chandrasekhar, R, et al. Comparative Analysis of Global Practice in Urologic Robot-Assisted Surgery. J Endourol. (2010). Sep

[2] Meehan, J. J, Elliott, S & Sandler, A. The Robotic Approach to Complex Hepatobiliary Analies in Children: Preliminary Report. J Pediatr Surg. (2007) Dec;42(12)2110-4.

[3] Jacobsen, G, Berger, R, & Horgan, S. The role of robotic surgery in morbid obesity. J Laparoendosc Adv Surg Tech A (2003), 13:279-83.

[4] Zacharopoulou, C, Sananes, N, Baulon, E, Garbin, O, & Wattiez, A. J Robotic Gynecologic SurgeryL State of the Art.Review of the Literature. Gynecol Obstet Biol Reprod. (2010) Aug 6

[5] Selber JC. Transoral Robotic Reconstruction of Oropharyngeal Defects: A Case Series. Plast Reconstr Surg 126(6):1978-1987, 12/2010). 126(6), 1978-1987.

[6] Genden, E. M, Kotz, T, Tong, C. C, et al. Transoral robotic resection and reconstruction for head and neck cancer. J Laryngoscope (2011). Aug;121(8), 1668-74.

[7] Garfein, E. S. Greaney PJ Jr, Easterlin B, et al. Transoral robotic reconstructive surgery reconstruction of a tongue base defect with a radial forearm flap. Plast Reconstr Surg (2011) Jun;127(6), 2352-4.

[8] Ghanem, T. A. Transoral robotic-assisted microvascular reconstruction of the oropharynx. J Laryngoscope (2011) Mar;121(3), 580-2.

[9] Genden, E. M, Park, R, Smith, C, & Kotz, T. The role of reconstruction for transoral robotic pharyngectomy and concomitant neck dissection. Arch Otolaryngol Head Neck Surg (2011).Feb;137(2), 151-6.

[10] Parekattil, S. J, & Brahmbhatt, J. V. Robotic approaches for male infertility and chronic orchialgia microsurgery. Curr Opin Urol (2011) Nov;21(6), 493-9. Review

[11] Mantovani, G, Liverneaux, P, Garcia, J. C, et al. Endoscopic exploration and repair of brachial plexus with telerobotic manipulation: a cadaver trial. J Neurosurg (2011) Sep;115(3), 659-64. Epub 2011 Apr 8.

[12] Harada, K, Minakawa, Y, Baek, Y, et al. Microsurgical skill assessment: Toward skill-based surgical robotic control. Conf Proc IEEE Eng Med Biol Soc (2011). Aug;2011, 6700-3.

[13] Tansini I Sopra il mio muovo processo di amputazione della mammilla. Gazetta MedicaI Italiana. (1906), 67:141-142.

[14] McCraw, J. B, Dibbell, D. G, & Carraway, J. H. Clinical definition of independent myocutaneous vascular territories. Plast Reconstr Surg (1977) Sep;60(3), 341-52.

[15] Schneider, W. J. Hill HL Jr, Brown RG. Latissimus dorsi myocutaneous flap for breast reconstruction. Br J Plast Surg (1977) Oct ;30(4), 277-81.

[16] Bostwick, J. 3rd, Vasconez LO, Jurkiewicz MJ. Breast reconstruction after a radical mastectomy. Plast Reconstr Surg (1978) May;61(5), 682-93.

[17] Bartlett, S. P. May JW Jr, Yaremchuk MJ. The latissimus dorsi muscle: a fresh cadaver study of the primary neurovascular pedicle. Plast Reconstr Surg (1981) May;67(5), 631-6.

[18] Maxwell, G. P, Mcgibbon, B. M, & Hoopes, J. E. Vascular considerations in the use of a latissimus dorsi myocutaneous flap after a mastectomy with an axillary dissection. Plast Reconstr Surg (1979) Dec;64(6), 771-80.

[19] Germann, G, Waag, K. L, Selle, B, & Jester, A. Extremity salvage with a free musculocutaneous latissimus dorsi flap and free tendon transfer after resection of a large congenital fibro sarcoma in a 15-week-old infant. A case report. Microsurgery (2006), 26(6), 429-31.

[20] Seitz, I. A, Adler, N, Odessey, E, Reid, R. R, & Gottlieb, L. J. Latissimus dorsi/rib intercostal perforator myoosseocutaneous free flap reconstruction in composite defects of the scalp: case series and review of literature. J Reconstr Microsurg. (2009). Nov; 25(9), 559-67.

[21] Pomel, C, Missana, M. C, & Lasser, P. Endoscopic harvesting of the latissimus dorsi flap in breast reconstructive surgery. Feasibility study and review of the literature Ann Chir. (2002) May;127(5), 337-42. French

[22] Lin, C. H, Wei, F. C, Levin, L. S, & Chen, M. C. Donor-site morbidity comparison between endoscopically assisted and traditional harvest of free latissimus dorsi muscle flap Plast Reconstr Surg (1999) Sep; 104(4), 1070-7; quiz 1078. Review. Erratum in: Plast Reconstr Surg (2000) Feb;105(2):823.

[23] Miller, M. J. Robb GL Endoscopic technique for free flap harvesting. Clin Plast Surg (1995) Oct;22(4), 755-73. Review

[24] Fine, N. A, Orgill, D. P, & Pribaz, J. J. Early clinical experience in endoscopic-assisted muscle flap harvest. Ann Plast Surg (1994). Nov;469-72, 33(5), 465-9. Discussion

[25] Ramakrishnan, V. V, Southern, S, & Villafane, O. Endoscopic harvest of the latissimus dorsi muscle using the balloon dissection technique. Plast Reconstr Surg (1997) Mar;99(3), 899-903; discussion 904-5.

[26] Liu, A. S, Kao, H. K, Reish, R. G, et al. Postoperative complications in prosthesis based breast reconstruction using acellular dermal matrix. Plast Reconstr Surg (2011) May;127(5), 1755-62.

[27] Lanier, S. T, Wang, E. D, Chen, J. J, et al. The effect of acellular dermal matrix use on complication rates in tissue expander/implant breast reconstruction. Ann Plast Surg (2010) May;64(5), 674-8.

Section 3

Microsurgical Reconstruction

Chapter 7

Mastering the Deep Inferior Epigastric Artery Perforator Flap (DIEP): Refining Techniques and Improving Efficiency

Joshua L. Levine, Julie V. Vasile, Hakan Usal,
Heather A. Erhard and John J. Ho

Additional information is available at the end of the chapter

http://dx.doi.org/10.5772/56074

1. Introduction

1.1. Patient selection

Most women seeking breast reconstruction are candidates for Deep Inferior Epigastric Perforator (DIEP) flaps. The only absolute contraindication is prior abdominoplasty [1]. Other types of abdominal surgery including liposuction are relative contraindications [2], and need to be evaluated with respect to the extent of the abdominal surgery and the result of the magnetic resonance angiogram (MRA.) If a patient is too thin and simply does not have enough abdominal tissue for the breast reconstruction (one or two breasts), she can either have a low-volume reconstruction with the intent to augment the reconstruction later, or use another donor site, like the thighs or buttocks. We tend not to operate on patients with BMI over 36, and require that they lose weight prior to elective DIEP surgery. We also require that patients quit smoking for three months prior to surgery, but exceptions may be made in select patients.

2. Preoperative imaging

Our technique for MRA of the abdomen has been published [3-5]. We obtain MRA on all patients undergoing perforator flap procedures. This includes patients who have expanders or implants in place at the time of MRA. In our experience, there have not been adverse effects from performing MRA on patients with expanders or implants. The appropriate vessels are selected preoperatively and the patient is marked either the day before surgery or the in the holding area the day of surgery. It is important to evaluate the MRA and to mark the patient preoperatively in order to think about and understand the anatomy. This allows for excellent planning and the ability to predict possible pitfalls and back-up plans. An example of a MRA showing a DIEP is Figure 1. We have found preoperative imaging to be vitally important for planning and execution of perforator flap surgery. The MRA enables the surgeon to evaluate perforators with respect to their location in the abdominal flap, intramuscular course and size. The key perforators are selected preoperatively and marked on the patient's abdomen according to measurements from the umbilicus. A handheld Doppler ultrasound is used to confirm the locations of the perforating vessels at the time of marking.

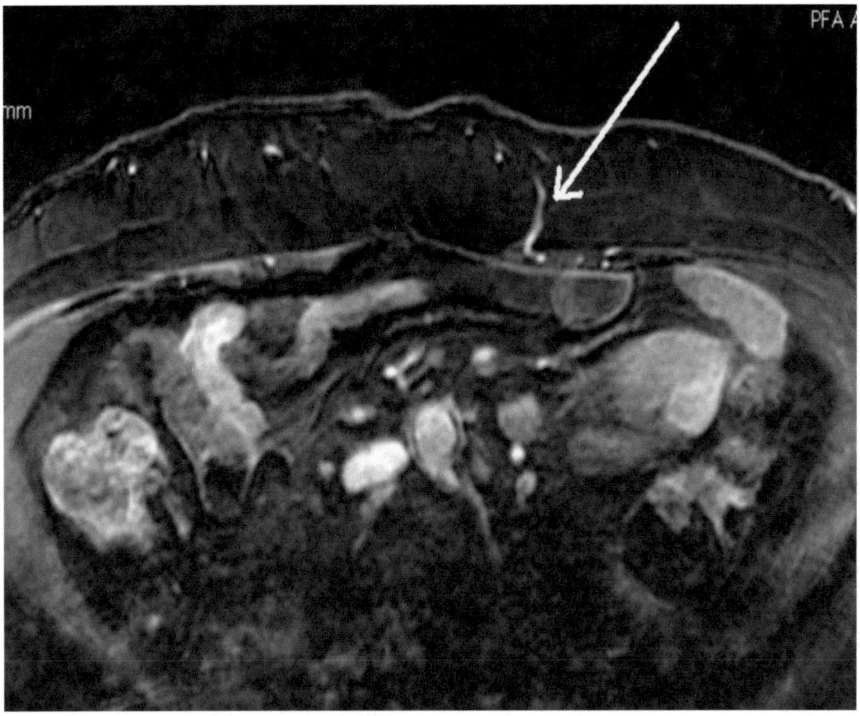

Figure 1. MRA of the abdomen with arrow pointing to a DIEP.

3. Flap harvesting and tips for success

The patient is placed on the table supine with arms prepped and wrapped with gauze roll or stockinette (Figure 2). The arms are placed on arm boards and covered with sterile arm drapes in order to bring the arms in later during the procedure when the microscope is brought in for vessel anastomosis (Figure 3).

http://dx.doi.org/10.5772/56074

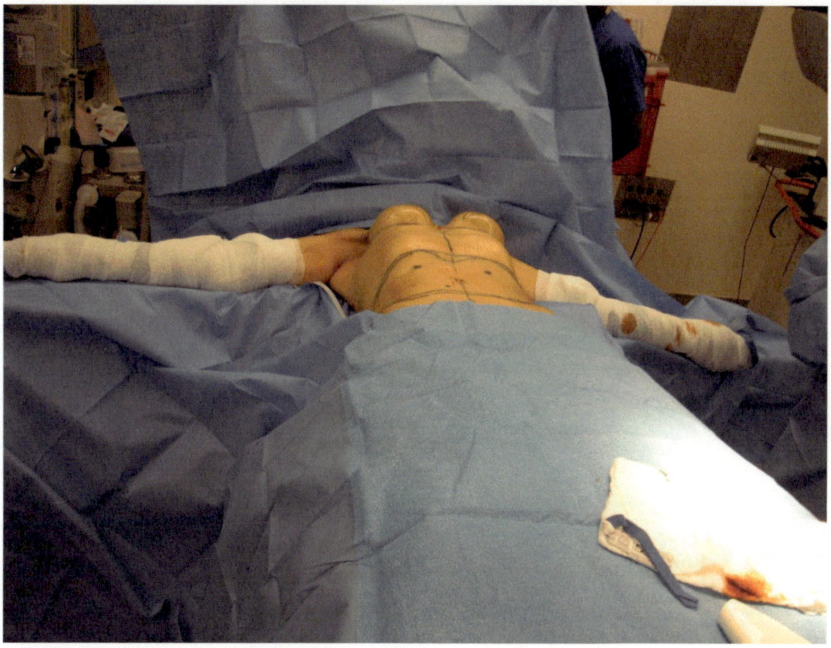

Figure 2. Sterile drape of the arms

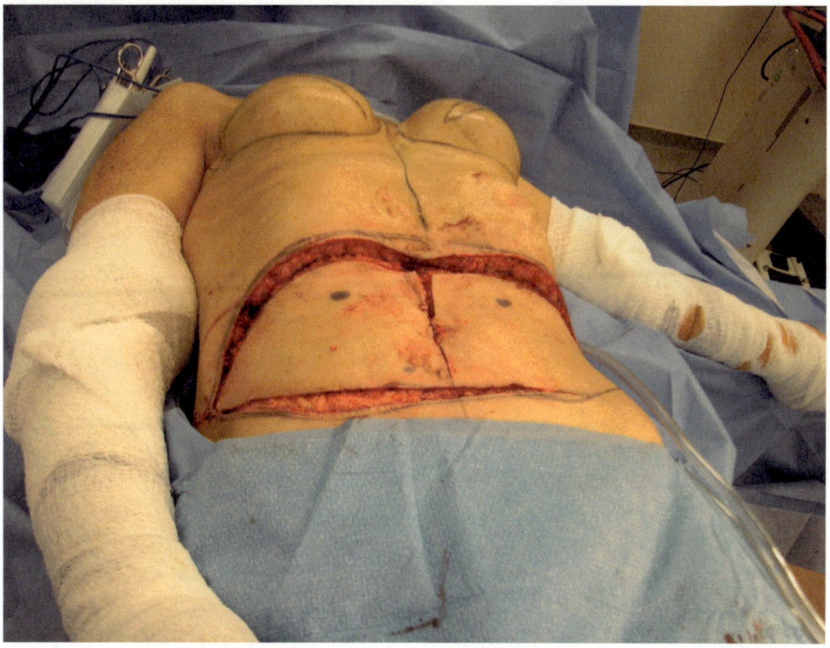

Figure 3. Sterile drape of the arm in adducted position.

In delayed breast reconstruction, three surgeons can start at the same time (where availability of personnel permits). One surgeon will start harvesting the internal mammary vessels while the other two surgeons harvest the abdominal flaps simultaneously.

4. Abdominal flap dissection

Abdominal incisions are made according to the preoperative markings. If a large flap is desired, beveling is used to capture as much fat as possible in the upper abdomen [6]. The upper abdominal flap is turned over superiorly so that the skin edges can be stapled pulling the upper abdominal skin/fat in static cephalad retraction (Figure 4). The lower, suprapubic incision is initially made very superficially in order to evaluate and possibly preserve superficial vessels (Figure 5).

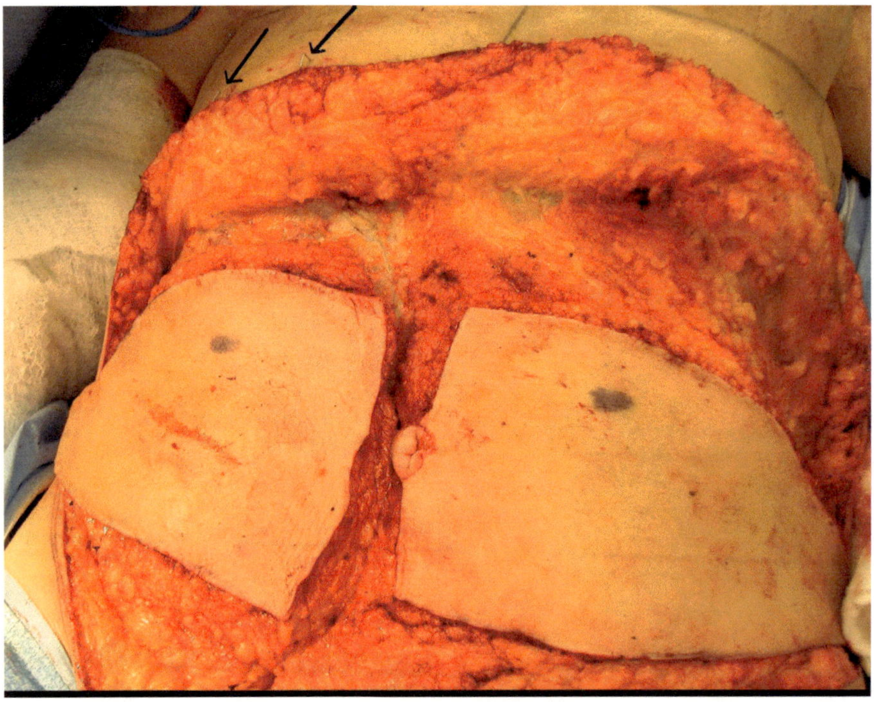

Figure 4. The stapled cephalad skin edge provides a static cephalad retraction.

The surgeon has knowledge about the caliber of superficial vessels from the MRA, but it is always a good idea to reevaluate them in-situ. Once the superficial vessels are identified, a decision can be made as to whether they should be used, and if so, how much length should be harvested. Generally, a large Superficial Inferior Epigastric Vein (SIEV) (>2mm) and Superficial Inferior Epigastric Artery (SIEA) (>1mm) should be preserved as a back-up drainage for the flap. A few extra centimeters are adequate for the vein, but remember that the

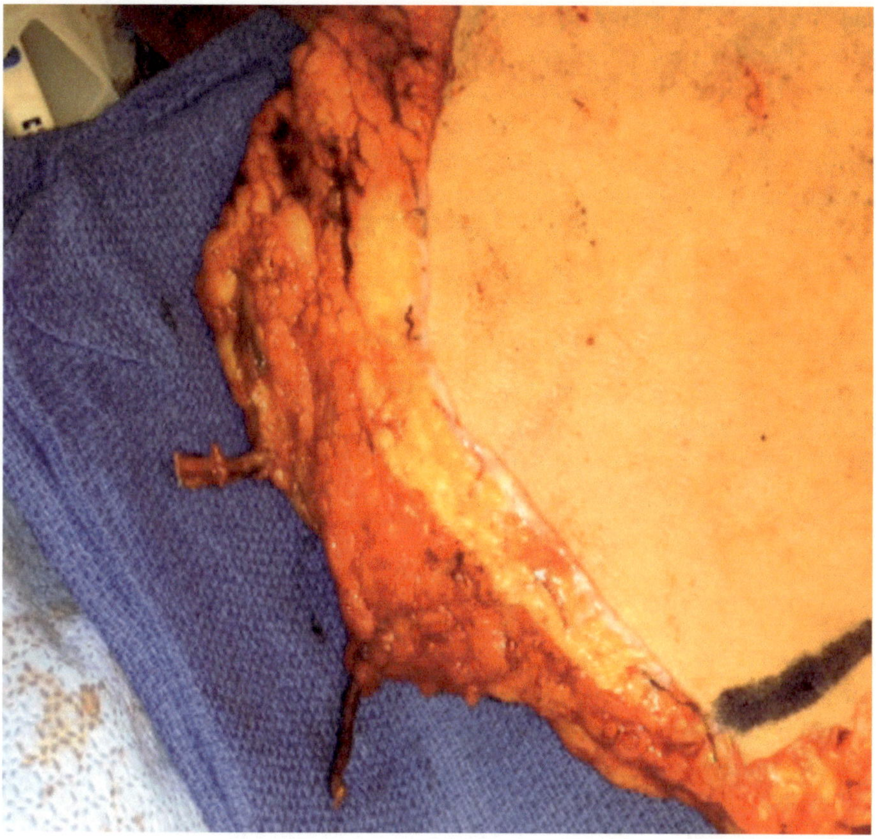

Figure 5. Preservation of SIEA and SIEV

more you get, the easier it will be to use the vessel if needed. If the flap becomes congested after anastomosis to the DIEP perforator pedicle, the superficial vein will become engorged and easy to find. If the length is inadequate, further dissection into the flap can be easily done on the enlarged vein. If the SIEA is to be considered as a pedicle or a back-up inflow system, its dissection should be postponed until after the perforator has been selected. This is because the SIEA dissection is very tedious and time consuming, and an adequate perforator pedicle is almost always preferable to an SIEA pedicle [7]. Of course, choosing a perforator pedicle obviates the need for the SIEA dissection. Keep in mind, leaving the suprapubic flap too thin will create the risk of prolonged seroma formation and a defect of the abdominal wall contour. Therefore, after finding the superficial epigastric artery and vein, adequate fat thickness should be left within the distal (suprapubic) skin flap. This is done by coning the dissection as you proceed toward the harvested end of the vessels, leaving more and more fat behind.

To enable two surgeons to harvest in tandem, the best technique is to start from the midline and harvest simultaneously. After the midline incision is made, the umbilicus is incised circumferentially down to the abdominal wall. The two abdominal flaps can then be elevated at the level of the fascia under loupe magnification with bipolar electrocautery from medial to lateral. It may be necessary to elevate from any of the other three edges of the flap in order to proceed to the perforators of choice. Constant repositioning and resetting of retraction devices may be necessary. Even a lateral-row perforator can be dissected by raising the abdominal flap from medial to lateral, but it may require burning medial row perforator options. This should only be done after the lateral row perforator of choice had been evaluated under direct vision and selected as the perforator of choice. A large perforator on the MRA usually correlates with a large perforator in-situ, but not always. Thus, it may be necessary to look at more than one option if there is no clearly dominant perforator on MRA. Constant communication with the other surgeon is imperative so that one does not get in the other's way.

Once the appropriate perforator has been selected, a small incision is made superiorly and inferiorly around the perforator in the anterior rectus fascia. This will begin the intramuscular muscular dissection, and also allow the surgeon to further evaluate the quality of the perforator. The perforator is then dissected free from the anterior abdominal wall fascia circumferentially. A small cuff of fascia may be left around the perforator as trying to dissect the vessels from the fascia may cause damage to these fragile vessels. The fascia incision is carried out generously both superiorly and inferiorly to allow adequate exposure.

Muscle fibers are delicately separated with bipolar diathermy in a longitudinal direction within the natural septum through which the perforator emerges. The muscle fibers are gently teased away until reaching the deep inferior epigastric vessels. There will be branches off of the perforator requiring cauterization or ligation and division. Intraoperative reference to the MRA will be extremely helpful in predicting the intramuscular course of the perforator. A short intramuscular course may be associated with a fast and safe dissection. However if the perforator emerges through an inscription, it may be quite challenging.

Retraction and exposure are extremely important, and thus should be constantly evaluated and improved as the dissection progresses. During muscle dissection, muscle fibers are initially retracted with "fish hook" retractors secured to a clamp on skin staples or drapes. As the dissection continues larger Gelpi retractors replace the "fish hooks." Examples of static retraction is shown in Figures 6-8.

During dissection, the large bulky abdominal wall flaps should be handled with great care. Skin edges can be folded over and secured with skin staples. An assistant holding the bulky and often slippery flap may inadvertently pull the flap and may cause intimal damage to perforator vessels or even rupture them. Therefore, static, mechanical retraction is preferred as described above.

With imaging we have been able to reliably select the best perforator for each flap, increasing the likelihood of selecting only one dominant perforator per flap. When a perforator is of medium or small size, more perforators can be harvested if they are in line with the others. The superior continuation of the deep inferior epigastric vessels are ligated and divided and the dissection continues inferiorly until there is adequate pedicle length and diameter of the vessels.

http://dx.doi.org/10.5772/56074

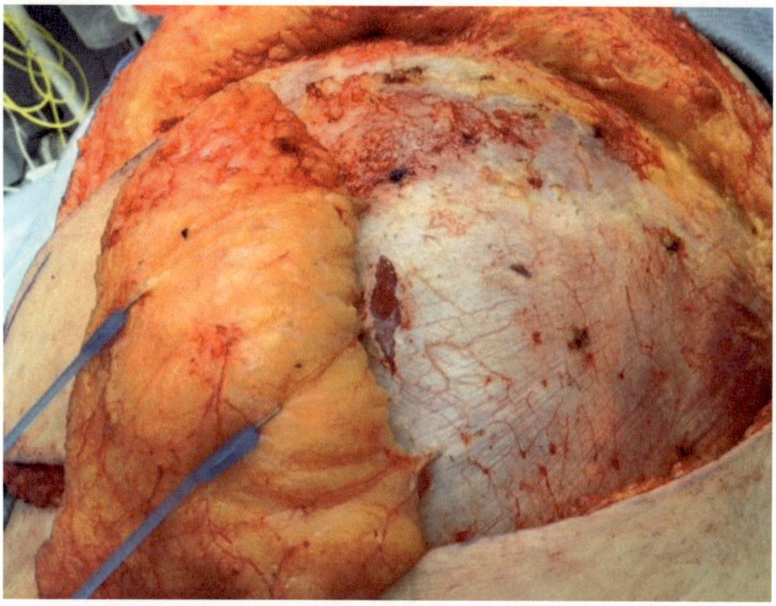

Figure 6. Fish hook providing adjustable static retraction.

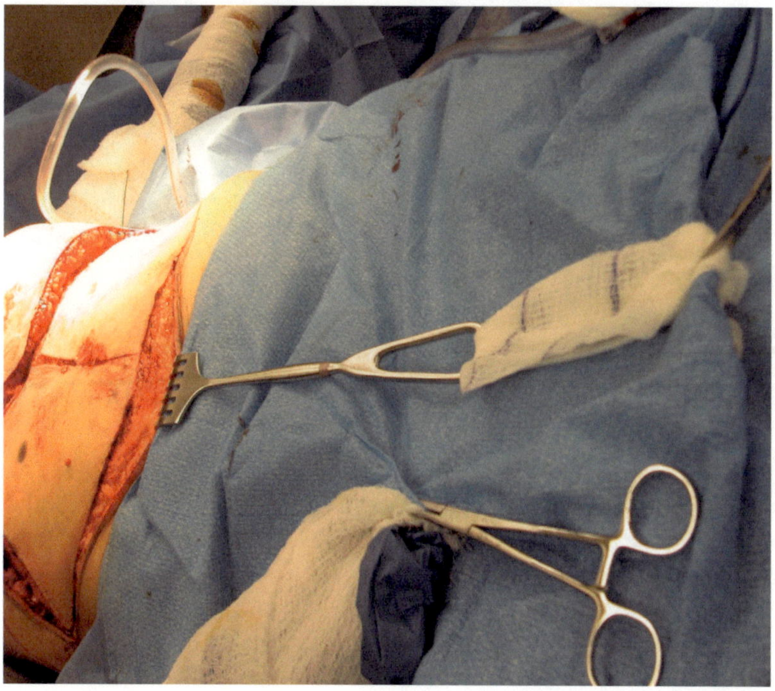

Figure 7. Rake retractor providing static tissue retraction.

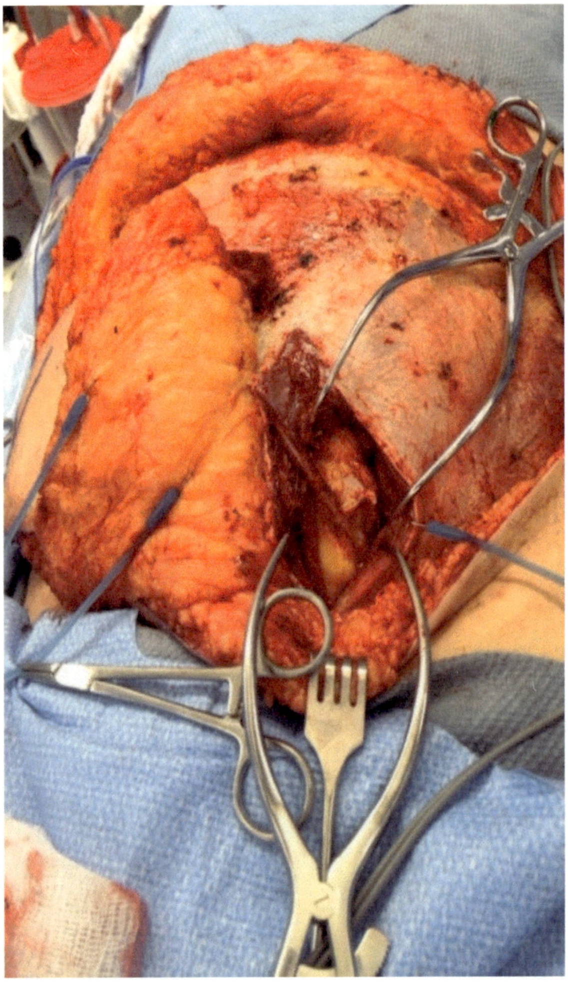

Figure 8. Use of both "fish hook" and Gelpi retractors.

5. Third surgeon: Internal mammary vasculature dissection

The third surgeon prepares the chest wall for anastomosis. For a delayed procedure with explantation of implants, the skin over the implants is elevated off the pectoralis muscle and internal capsule, creating a large space for the flap. The space between the skin and muscle is created up to the clavicle superiorly, and should be about 1.5X the predicted size of the flap. The implant is then removed, and the pectoralis muscle is tacked back down on the chest all (where it belongs). We prefer the second or third intercostal space since the vessels are 1.5-2.5 mm in diameter and a good size match with DIEP vessels.

At the second or third intercostal space, a transverse incision is made parallel to the fibers of the pectoralis muscle exposing two consecutive rib cartilages. An incision is made in the perichondrium longitudinally in each rib. The perichondrium is stripped off with a Freer

http://dx.doi.org/10.5772/56074

elevator and the intervening intercostal muscle is removed. At the costochondral junction, rib is sometimes removed to provide enough space for anastomosis. The internal mammary vessels can be found in a thin layer of fat under the intercostal muscle and are dissected. A branching point of the internal mammary vein is identified and can allow for greater diameter for improved size match with a DIEP vein. Care is taken to leave enough distal artery and vein stump of internal mammary vessels in case an anastomotic revision becomes necessary. These vessels can be successfully used for retrograde anastomosis in case of an anastomotic failue or damage to proximal vessels.

Previous implants with or without radiation therapy can result in a significantly thick posterior capsule making the initiation of the internal mammary dissection more difficult; once through this capsule and into the proper plane below the intercostal muscle, dissection proceeds more easily. An internal mammary lymph node can frequently be encountered. Although it may demonstrate inflammatory changes only, the identified node should be sent for permanent pathology in patients with a cancer history, as this can change stage and treatment. Of note, the internal mammary vessels are typically smaller in caliber on the left than the right side[8].

6. Flap harvest

Before division of the DIEP vessel we mark the anterior surface of the vessels with ink for later anatomic orientation and to avoid kinking of the vessels during insetting. It is also helpful to reconfirm the position of the Doppler signal on the skin prior to harvest.

After the dissection is finished, the abdominal flap is harvested and weighed. The abdominal flap weight can be compared with the mastectomy specimen weight. The flap is held up above the chest wall and the vessels are dangled free over the chest to find the natural orientation of this long pedicle. The ink mark on the anterior wall of DIEP vessels may help with orientation. The flap is secured to the chest wall with sutures. At this point, the arms, which had been prepped into the field are brought into adduction and clamped to the sheets. The arm boards are removed. This allows for two microsurgeons to approach the table and work together under the microscope. The table is slid caudally so that there is room for the surgeons' knees when sitting for the microsurgery. The microscope pedal is used so that the scope can be adjusted while operating with two hands.

7. Under the microscope

The vein is coupled with the coupler (Synovis, Microcompanies Alliance, Inc. Birmingham, AL) and the artery is hand sewn. Arterial coupling can also be done. Once the anastomosis is complete, skin signals are marked on the flap and flap is carefully placed under chest wall skin flaps. Careful positioning of the flap is done under direct vision of the pedicle. Many failures can be attributed to pedicle kink at the anastomosis due to long pedicle length.

8. Insetting

The excess skin on the flap is de-epithelized and adequate bleeding is evaluated. The flap is tacked into position to avoid movement, and to cover the depression created medially at the anastomosis. In cases of nipple sparing mastectomy, a skin paddle is left in the mastectomy incision for monitoring. This skin paddle can be excised 4 days later and closed before the patient leaves the hospital.

Author details

Joshua L. Levine[1*], Julie V. Vasile[2], Hakan Usal[2], Heather A. Erhard[3] and John J. Ho[4]

*Address all correspondence to: jlevine@diepflap.com; jvasilemd@gmail.com; heathererhard@optonline.net

1 Department of Plastic Surgery The Center for the Advancement of Breast Reconstruction at New York Eye & Ear Infirmary New York, NY, USA

2 The Center for the Advancement of Breast Reconstruction at New York Eye & Ear Infirmary New York, NY, USA

3 Division of Plastic and Reconstructive Surgery, Montefiore Medical Center, Albert Einstein College of Medicine, Bronx Plastic Surgery, NY, USA

4 Northern Westchester Hospital, Mount Kisco, NY, USA

References

[1] Massey, M. F, Spiegel, A. J, Levine, J. L, Craigie, J. E, Kline, R. M, Khoobehi, K, Erhard, H, & Greenspun, D. T. Allen Jr. RJ, Allen Sr. RJ. Perforator flaps: recent experience, current trends, and future directions based on 3974 microsurgical breast reconstructions. Plastic and Reconstructive Surgery (2009). , 124(3), 737-751.

[2] Granzow, J. W, Levine, J. L, & Chiu, E. S. LoTempio MM, Allen RJ. Breast reconstruction with perforator flaps. Plastic and Reconstructive Surgery (2007). , 120(1), 1-12.

[3] Zou, Z, Lee, H. K, Cerilles, M, Levine, J. L, Greenspun, D. T, Allen, R. J, Vasile, J, Rohde, C, Chen, C. M, & Prince, M. R. Gadofosveset trisodium enhanced abdominal perforator MRA. Journal of Magnetic Resonance Imaging (2012). Mar;Epub 2011 Oct 26, 35(3), 711-16.

[4] Newman, T. M, Vasile, J, Levine, J. L, Greenspun, D. T, Allen, R. J, Chao, M. T, Winchester, P, & Prince, M. R. Perforator flap magnetic resonance angiography: a review

of 25 deep inferior epigastric and gluteal perforator artery flap patients. Journal of Magnetic Resonance Imaging (2010). May;, 31(5), 1176-84.

[5] Vasile, J. V, Newman, T. M, Prince, M. R, Rusch, D. G, Greenspun, D. T, Allen, R, & Levine, J. L. Contrast-enhanced magnetic resonance angiography. Clinics in Plastic Surgery (2011). , 38(2), 263-275.

[6] Gill, P. S, Hunt, J. P, Guerra, A. B, Dellacroce, F. J, Sullivan, S. K, Boraski, J, Metzinger, S. E, Dupin, C. E, & Allen, R. J. A. year retrospective review of 758 DIEP flaps for breast reconstruction. Plastic and Reconstructive Surgery (2004). , 113(4), 1153-1160.

[7] Granzow, J. W, Chiu, E. S, Levine, J. L, Gautam, A, Hellman, A, Rolston, W, Kuo, B, Saullo, T, Heitland, A. S, & Allen, R. J. Autologous breast reconstruction using the superficial inferior epigastric flap revisited. Plastic Surgery (2005). Abstract Supplement; 116(3) 133

[8] Dupin, C. L, Allen, R. J, Glass, C. A, & Bunch, R. The internal mammary artery and vein as a recipient site for free-flap breast reconstruction: a report of 110 consecutive cases. Plastic and Reconstructive Surgery (1996).

Chapter 8

Double Venous System Drainage in Deep Inferior Epigastric Artery Perforator Flap Breast Reconstruction

Scott Reis, Jules Walters, Jason Hall and
Sean Boutros

Additional information is available at the end of the chapter

http://dx.doi.org/10.5772/55296

1. Introduction

The field of breast reconstruction has evolved rapidly since the advent of the first silicone gel-filled prosthesis by Cronin and Gerowin in 1963. [1] Over the past decades, we have seen remarkable advances in the field with microsurgical techniques becoming the gold standard for breast reconstruction. The deep inferior epigastric artery perforator (DIEP) flap has many advantages when compared to other methods of autologous breast reconstruction, namely reliability, malleability of soft tissue, and limited donor site morbidity. It is primarily for these reasons that the DIEP flap has become the preferred autologous option of many microsurgeons.

The main disadvantage of the DIEP flap is the technical difficulty, especially during the early experience of the microsurgeon. Even in experienced hands, there is a small yet significant incidence of flap compromise and loss. Gill et al. reported a partial flap loss rate of 2.5% and total flap loss rate of < 1% in their 10-year review of 758 DIEP flaps. They also reported a 5.8% flap re-exploration rate. [2] Other large series have reported similar results with respect to major complications. [2-7,13,16]

With regards to vascular problems, venous congestion tends to be the primary concern for microsurgeons who perform DIEP flap breast reconstruction. Complications due to the venous drainage or venous anastomosis have been shown to be eight times more common than issues arising from arterial insufficiency or arterial anastomotic complications. [2] These problems can lead not only to the rare total flap failure but more commonly to the need to return to the operating room in the immediate postoperative period to correct venous insufficiency and even partial flap failure and fat necrosis in the long-term. [3-7] Anatomic studies have shown that the deep inferior epigastric vein (DIEV) connects with the superficial inferior epigastric vein (SIEV) through a system of choke vessels within the flap. [8] In numerous studies, the superficial venous system has been used to adequately decongest the flap in cases where venous congestion was clinically observed [9-13]. We have found that routinely anastomosing both the superficial and deep venous systems has resulted in significantly fewer operative take-backs and decreased venous complications with use of the DIEP flap.

2. Surgical technique

We begin the harvest of the DIEP flap with the inferior incision in a central to lateral direction. Our focus is first to identify a usable superficial vein. All reasonable superficial veins are preserved and compared to one another. The largest superficial vein is chosen, with preference given to veins more central in the flap. There is a consistent superficial vein which is present in unoperated abdominal wall flaps that is located approximately 5-10cm from the midline and a few millimeters deep to the dermis. In patients with prior low transverse incisions, this vein usually lies just lateral to the incision and most likely represents a smaller vein that has dilated over time. At the inferior portion of the flap, these veins are typically 1 to 2 mm in diameter. Dissection continues caudally for approximately 5 to 8 cm, or until a large side branch joins this more central vein. A venae comitans of the superficial inferior epigastric artery (SIEA) is typically not our vein of choice as it usually has more branches, thus requiring a longer time of dissection. In unilateral cases, the superficial veins are dissected bilaterally, and their location is typically consistent from one side to the other.

We typically do not obtain preoperative imaging to localize the DIEA perforators, unless the patient has had prior abdominal or pelvic surgery that would affect the patency of the perforating vessels. Upon dissection of the flaps, we choose the largest perforator on which to harvest the flap, and typically take any other reasonable perforators that require minimal extra rectus dissection. Typically 1-3 perforators are taken. In bilateral cases, we give slight preference to the lateral row perforators, as they are more central in the flaps. In unilateral cases, we give stronger preference to the medial row perforators.

In immediate reconstruction cases, the breast surgeon is advised to use hemoclips to control any medial bleeding rather than electrocautery. This bleeding is typically from internal mammary venous perforators (IMVPs). Once the mastectomy is competed, we identify any sizable transected IMVPs. If no usable transected vein is identified in the mastectomy dissection field, the mastectomy skin flap is further dissected superiorly and medially to search for an IMVP. These IMVPs are dissected through the pectoralis muscle down to the intercostal level. In our experience, after communication with the oncologic surgeon, adequate caliber venous perforators are routinely identified and spared during the initial mastectomy procedure. These veins tend to be very large and thin walled, thus making them ideal for venous coupling.

In cases of delayed reconstruction, we elevate the mastectomy skin flaps and search for IMVPs. If a large IMVP is found in the second or third interspace, it is dissected a short distance through the pectoralis muscle to the intercostal level. If no usable IMVP is identified, the lowest interspace which is wide enough to allow dissection without removing a portion of rib is chosen. This technique allows a greater chance of finding two internal mammary venae comitantes since there is more often both a medial and lateral venae comitantes in the lower interspaces. Selecting the lowest interspace also decreases the likelihood of causing an upper inner quadrant soft tissue depression due to division of the pectoralis muscle. The intercostal muscles are elevated from the rib directly over the internal mammary artery (IMA) and vein (IMV). Each vessel is dissected well below the inferior rib margin to gain as much pedicle length as possible. It is also advantageous to include any side branches, as even small side branches afford the option of opening the vein through the branch to make the vein larger and thus allow a larger coupler to be used.

Once the flap is harvested, it is taken to the back table. The artery is cannulated with a 24 gauge angiocatheter, and the flap then irrigated with heparinized saline. Typically 60-80cc is flushed through the flap divided between three syringes. With the first flush, the pedicle is inspected for any obvious leaks and controlled accordingly. With the second and third, the veins are closely observed. With both veins left free to drain, the amount draining will typically be similar through both systems. However, occasionally we will note a deep or superficial dominance where the drainage is predominantly through one of the systems.

In the vast majority of DIEP reconstructions, a good caliber IMVP is present. In these cases, the IMA to DIEPA and IMV to DIEPV anastomoses are performed first. The superficial vein is then allowed to dilate after being controlled with a microvascular clamp. With the vein dilated, the second venous anastomosis is then performed. If the second venae comitant of the IMA is to be used for superficial system drainage, the DIEPV is anastomosed to the more lateral IMV, and the superficial vein is anastomosed to the more medial IMV. If there is no IMVP, only one IMV, and the flap is superficially dominant, we will anastomosethe secondary vein to one of the DIEPVs. Before performing this superficial to deep vein anastomosis,we irrigate through one of the DIEPVs inretrograde fashion to verify anterograde flow in other, in order to ensure that there are no problematic venous valves. All venous anastomosesare performed with the Synovis microvascular anastomotic coupler.

Finally, the DIEP flap is inset. It is sutured to the chest wall at the inframammary fold and lateral breast margin with incorporation of pectoralis fascia in the lateral chest wall stitch. Medially, we tack the flap to both the undersurface of the mastectomy skin flap and superiorly to the highest point within the pocket. We do not use any implantable monitoring devices for the DIEP flaps. Monitoring of the flap is by means of a small skin paddle and bedside doppler exam. In patients who do not require a skin paddle, we make a cruciate incision in the mastectomy skin flap over an audible Doppler signal and then suture the four edges down to a deepithialized portion of the DIEP flap creating a small patch of exposed dermis to monitor for signs of venous congestion. Our patients are placed on bed rest for four days and are usually discharged on postoperative day four. While in the hospital, patients are given low molecular weight heparin and sequential compression devices for DVT prophylaxis. Intraoperatively, 1500 units of heparin is given intravenously one hour into surgery, also for DVT prophylaxis.

A recent study published in Plastic and Reconstructive surgery (accepted for publication) reviewed 352 consecutive DIEP flaps performed by the senior author (SGB). In this study, 311 flaps underwent double venous anastomosis while 41 underwent one venous system anastomosis. There were no flap losses in either group. There was one operative exploration for venous congestion in the double system group (0.32%) and 2 in the single system group (4.9%). This difference was statically significant. The single system group take back rate was almost identical to prior published results.

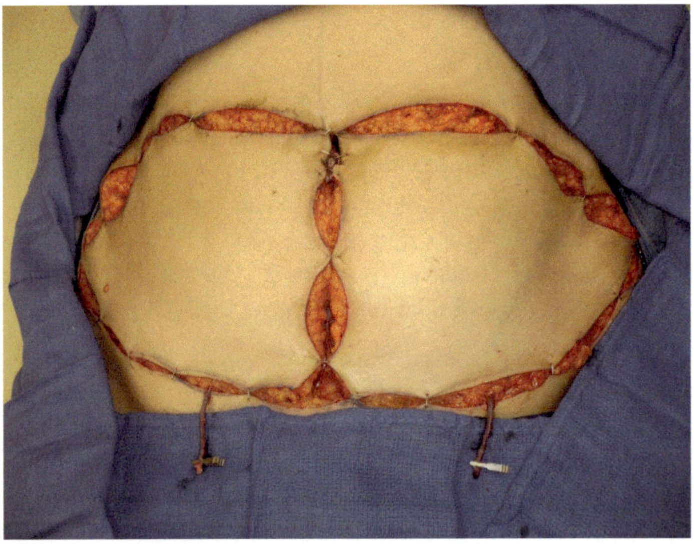

Figure 1. Location of typical superficial vein for secondary venous system drainage

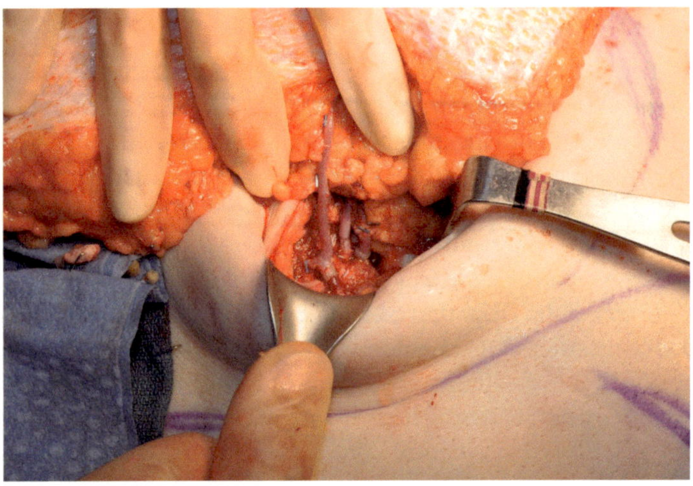

Figure 2. Superficial vein to the IMVP flap orientation

http://dx.doi.org/10.5772/55296

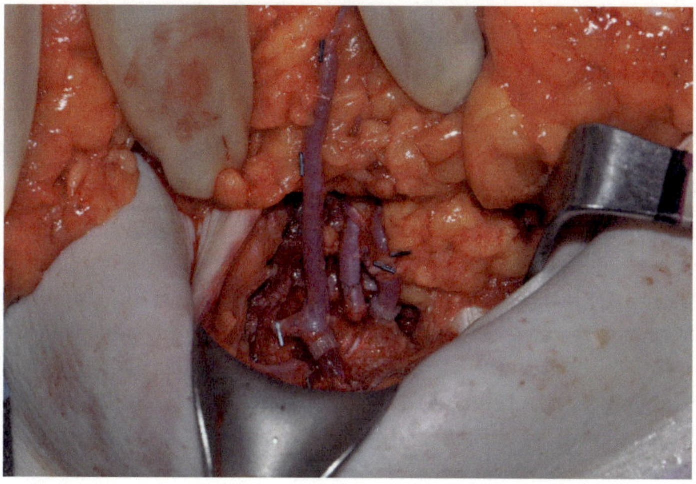

Figure 3. Closer view of the vascular layout for typical dual venous system drainage

3. Discussion

DIEP flaps are commonly performed in large academic hospitals or certain specialized microsurgical centers. The rapid availability of "in house" physicians and residents and the large volume of procedures performed in these settings contribute to excellent outcomes at many facilities [2-7,13,16].With some exceptions, community-based hospitals tend not to be equipped for rapid return to the operating room should vascular complications arise. In these instances, referring physicians may then be more encouraged to refer to plastic surgeons who perform procedures with fewer short-term complications even if their long-term reconstructive outcomes are less optimal. Thus, the typical community reconstructive plastic surgeon may perform microsurgical breast reconstruction less often than those in academic settings.

One of the most common complications of DIEP flaps is venous insufficiency, which is likely multifactorial in nature. The superficial inferior epigastric vein (SIEV) is often the dominant venous drainage of the lower abdominal skin and subcutaneous tissue. It is typically located halfway between the anterior superior iliac spine and pubic symphysis and lies below the dermal vascular plexus but above Scarpa's fascia. A system of choke vessels exists between the superficial inferior epigastric vein and the deep inferior epigastric system; however, certain variations in anatomy may exist. [8] Venous branches crossing the midline have been found to be absent in 36% of cases [4, 14]. This paucity of crossing branches explains why survival of Zone IVof the flap can be quite unpredictable.

During the standard harvest of an elliptical transverse fasciocutaneous island, the SIEV is transected. Venous drainage is thus rerouted to the perforating veins through choke vessels [8]. However, there are cases where the DIEP flap is more dependent on superficial drainage. Consequently, venous drainage through the DIEP system may be insufficient to adequately drain the entire flap. Anatomic studies have shown that in certain patients, the drainage of the abdominal flap can be preferentially through the superficial system with little communication to the deep system [15]. Patients who have had preoperative imaging showing the absence of communication between the two systems were more likely to have venous problems intraoperatively. This anatomic variant may be a significant cause of venous insufficiency when surgeons rely on the DIEP system alone.

Despite the many advantages the DIEP flap has to offer, there may be a higher incidence of fat necrosis and venous congestion [16]. Several authors have reported various techniques to treat the congested breast DIEP flap. The DIEV and SIEV have been anastomosed to the internal mammary and thoracodorsal vessels by Cohn and Walton [17]. Niranjan et al describe using a vein graft to connect the DIEV to the cephalic vein [18]. Another option described by Tutor et al involved connecting a venae comitantes of the DIEP pedicle to an intercostal branch of the IMV [19]. Additionally, with routine harvest of a superficial vein, the superficial venous system may be used for venous augmentation of the congested DIEP flap. This may be accomplished by anastomosing the superficial vein to an internal mammary vein perforator (IMVP),a secondary IMV, to the distal end of the IMV in a retrograde fashion, to the deep system directly, or even to the basilic vein [20-22]. The SIEV is present in 95% of patients, and preservation of this vein can be very beneficial with minimal additional operative time and morbidity [23].

A possible negative aspect of the double venous system technique is the additional operative time required. However, many surgeons routinely dissect the superficial vein as a lifeboat in the event of venous congestion, thus mitigating a portion of the additional operative time required. With experience, the added time is less than 15 minutes per flap. We believe that this time added in a routine basis is insignificant in comparison to the time required for an operative take back.

4. Conclusion

The dual venous system technique adds minimal additional time to the operation and adds an additional layer of security by augmenting the venous drainage of the flap. In our experience, the use of the dual-venous technique has successfully minimized returns to the operating room for venous complications in the early postoperative period. Microsurgeons who routinely perform DIEP breast reconstructions should be familiar with this technique, as it has proved valuable in our own practice.

Author details

Scott Reis, Jules Walters, Jason Hall and Sean Boutros*

*Address all correspondence to: drseanboutros@drseanboutros.com

Houston Plastic & Craniofacial Surgery, Houston, TX, USA

References

[1] Cronin TD, Gerow FJ. Augmentation mammaplasty: A new "natural feel" prosthesis. Transactions of the Third International Congress of Plastic and Reconstructive Surgery 1963: 41-49.

[2] Gill P, Hunt J, Guerra A, et al. A 10-year retrospective review of 758 DIEP flaps for breast reconstruction. Plast Reconstr Surg 2004:113(4) 1153-60..

[3] Scheer AS, Novak CB, Neligan PC, Lipa JE. Complications Associated With Breast Reconstruction Using a Perforator Flap Compared With a Free TRAM Flap. Ann Plast Surg 2006:56(4) 355-8.

[4] Blondeel PN, Arnstein M, Verstraete K, Depuydt K, Van Landuyt KH, Monstrey SJ, Kroll SS. Venous congestion and blood flow in free transverse rectus abdominis myocutaneous and deep inferior epigastric perforator flaps. Plast Reconstr Surg 2000:106(6)1295-9.

[5] Nahabedian MY, Momen B, Galdino G, Manson PN. Breast reconstruction with the free TRAM or DIEP flap: patient selection, choice of flap, and outcome. Plast Reconstr Surg 2002:10(2) 466-75.

[6] Chen CM, Halvorson EG, Disa JJ, McCarthy C, Hu QY, Pusic AL, Cordeiro PG, Mehrara BJ. Immediate postoperative complications in DIEP versus free/muscle-sparing TRAM flaps. Plast Reconstr Surg 2007:120(6) 1477-82.

[7] Tran NV, Buchel EW, Convery PA. Microvascular complications of DIEP flaps. Plast Reconstr Surg 2007:119(5) 1397-405.

[8] Schaverien M, Saint-Cyr M, Arbique G, Brown SA. Arterial and venous anatomies of the deep inferior epigastric perforator and superficial inferior epigastric artery flaps. Plast Reconstr Surg 2008:121(6) 1909-19.

[9] Xin Q, Luan J, Mu H, Mu L.J. Augmentation of venous drainage in deep inferior epigastric perforator flap breast reconstruction: efficacy and advancement. ReconstrMicrosurg 2012:28(5) 313-8.

[10] Sbitany H, Mirzabeigi MN, Kovach SJ, Wu LC, SerlettiJM. Strategies for recognizing and managing intraoperative venous congestion in abdominally based autologous breast reconstruction. Plast Reconstr Surg 2012:129(4) 809-15.

[11] Momeni A, Lee GK. A case of intraoperative venous congestion of the entire DIEP-flap--a novel salvage technique and review of the literature. Microsurgery 2010:30(6) 443-6.

[12] Ali R, Bernier C, Lin YT, Ching WC, Rodriguez EP, Cardenas-Mejia A, Henry SL, Evans GR, Cheng MH. Surgical strategies to salvage the venous compromised deep inferior epigastric perforator flap. AnnPlast Surg 2010:65(4) 398-406.

[13] Enajat M, Rozen W , Whitaker I, Smit J, Acosta R. A single center comparison of one versus two venous anastomoses in 564 consecutive DIEP flaps: Investigating the effect on venous congestion and flap survival. Microsurgery 2010:30(3) 185-91.

[14] Carramenha e Costa MA, Carriquiry C, Vasconez LO. An anatomic study of the venous drainage of the transverse rectus abdominis musculocutaneous flap. Plast Reconstr Surg 1987:79(2) 208-217.

[15] Schaverien MV, Ludman CN, Neil-Dwyer J, Perks AG, Raurell A, Rasheed T, McCulley SJ. Relationship between venous congestion and intraflap venous anatomy in DIEP flaps using contrast-enhanced magnetic resonance angiography. PlastReconstr Surg 2010:126(2) 385-9.

[16] Kroll SS. Fat necrosis in free transverse rectus abdominis myocutaneous and deep inferior epigastric perforator flaps. Plast Reconstr Surg 2000:106(3) 576-583.

[17] Cohn AB, Walton RL. Immediate autologous breast reconstruction using muscle-sparing TRAM flaps with superficial epigastric system turbocharging: a salvage option. J Reconstr Microsurg 2006:22(3) 153–156.

[18] Niranjan NS, Khandwala AR, Mackenzie DM. Venous augmentation of the free TRAM flap. Br J Plast Surg 2001:54(4) 335–337.

[19] Tutor EG, Auba C, Benito A, et al. Easy venous superdrainage in DIEP flap breast reconstruction through the intercostals branch. J Reconstr Microsurg. 2002:18(7) 595–598.

[20] Kerr-Valentic MA, Gottlieb LJ, Agarwal JP. The retrograde limb of the internal mammary vein: an additional outflow option in DIEP flap breast reconstruction. Plast Reconstr Surg 2009:124(3) 717-21.

[21] Wechselberger G, Schoeller T, Bauer T, Ninkovic M, Otto A, Ninkovic M. Venous superdrainage in deep inferior epigastric perforator flap breast reconstruction. Plast Reconstr Surg 2001:108(1) 162-6.

[22] Guzzetti T, Thione A. The basilic vein: an alternative drainage of DIEP flap in severe venous congestion. Microsurgery 2008:28(7) 555-8.

[23] Reardon CM, Ceallaigh SO, O'Sullivan ST. An anatomical study of the superficial inferior epigastric vessels in humans. Br J Plast Surg 2004:57(6) 515–519.

[24] Hanasono MM, Kocak E, Ogunleye O, Hartley CJ, Miller MJ. One versus Two Venous Anastomoses in Microvascular Free Flap Surgery. Plast Reconstr Surg 2010:126(5) 1548-57.

Chapter 9

Septocutaneous Gluteal Artery Perforator (Sc-GAP) Flap for Breast Reconstruction: How We Do It

Stefania Tuinder, Rene Van Der Hulst, Marc Lobbes,
Bas Versluis and Arno Lataster

Additional information is available at the end of the chapter

http://dx.doi.org/10.5772/56224

1. Introduction

In 1976 the first free flap for breast reconstruction was reported bij Fujino: he used the gluteus maximus myocutaneous flap. A skin-fat-muscle flap, including the superior gluteal artery and veins, was dissected and anastomosed to the thoracoacromial artery and vein [1]. In 1983 Shaw published a series of 10 patients undergoing the superior gluteal myocutanous free flap [2]: technical refinements were added to the work of Fujino. Only in 1993 Allen introduced the superior gluteal artery perforator (S-GAP) flap for breast reconstruction [3]. The pedicle of the flap was longer than that of the gluteus maximus myocutaneous flap because of the intra-muscular dissection: as a consequence a vein graft was not necessary to perform the micro-anastomosis: moreover no muscle was sacrified giving less donor site morbidity. In 2010 LoTempio and Allen published a review of the latest 17 years with gluteal flaps [4]: over the years the donor site is just improved, positioning the scar in the upper buttock superior from medial to lateral and beveling superior to reduce the contour deformity. Their experience showed a complication rate of 2 % of flap loss. The improvement in technique and results is also due to the introduction of new technologies such as MRA (magnetic resonance angiog-raphy) en CTA (computed tomography angiography) supporting the identification of the best perforator.

Within the first years of development of perforator flaps confusion arose about the nomen-clature: for example the flap based on paraumbilical perforators, originating from the deep inferior epigastric artery, was called PUP (paraumbilical perforator flap) by Koshima [5] and DIEP (deep inferior epigastric perforator) flap by Allen and Treece [6]. Attempts were made to unify the perforator flap nomenclature:

1. In 2001, during the fifth international course on perforator flaps in Gent, Belgium [7]
2. The Canadian proposal, summarized in an article by Geddes et al. [8].
3. The Asian microsurgical community proposal, with a tendency to use a more complex terminology [9].

Discussion however is still open regarding the nomenclature of perforator flaps and the last proposal is published in 2010 by Sinna et al. [10]. In 2012 Taylor commented that with the advent of modern imaging techniques, the true subcutaneous course of a perforator has to be considered in the classification and in the flap design [11].

Clinically it is really important to distinguish perforators running through the muscle (in this chapter indicated as musculocutaneous) and perforators running between two muscles (septocutaneous) because they have different clinical implications, particularly with respect to the S-GAP flap. The evolution from the S-GAP (superior gluteal artery perforator) flap to the Sc-GAP (septocutaneous gluteal artery perforator) flap reflects the above mentioned concept. We published a preliminary anatomical study [12] and later on a clinical study [13] on this concept showing that the use of septocutaneous perforators can make the dissection of the flap easier with an improvement in the aesthetic results of the donor site.

1.1. Topographical and functional anatomy of the gluteal region

This paragraph is partly based on Gray's Anatomy [14], Moore Clinically Oriented Anatomy [15] and Stone and Stone's Atlas of Skeletal Muscles[16].

The gluteal region or buttock is bounded cranially by the iliac crest and caudally by the oblique border of the gluteus maximus muscle. The horizontal skin fold of the buttock, indicated as gluteal fold (sulcus glutealis, ruga glutealis horizontalis), is often mistaken for this caudal border. It is important clinically to define the exact borders of the gluteal region in order to achieve skin projections of underlying bony landmarks, muscles, nerves and blood vessels as accurately as possible. The crena analis or crena ani is the vertical cleft, leading to the anus, between the left and right buttock. It is also called (crena) clunium, gluteal furrow, intergluteal or natal cleft, rima ani or rima clunium. Besides the iliac crest, the anterior superior iliac spine (ASIS) and the posterior superior iliac spine (PSIS), at the beginning and end of the iliac crest, are important bony landmarks. The PSIS is marked by a skin dimple. Caudomedially the ischial tuberosity can be palpated, deep to the gluteus maximus muscle. Laterally the greater trochanter is an important, palpable landmark. The prominence of the buttock is not only formed by the gluteus maximus muscle, but in the craniolateral part also by the gluteus medius.

In the gluteal region two muscle layers can be distinguished: (1) a superficial layer containing the gluteus maximus, and (2a-e) a deep layer containing the gluteus medius, gluteus minimus, piriformis, triceps coxae and quadratus femoris muscles (fig 1). The gluteus muscles are mainly extensors and abductors in the hip joint, the piriformis, triceps coxae and quadratus femoris are mainly lateral rotators.

http://dx.doi.org/10.5772/56224

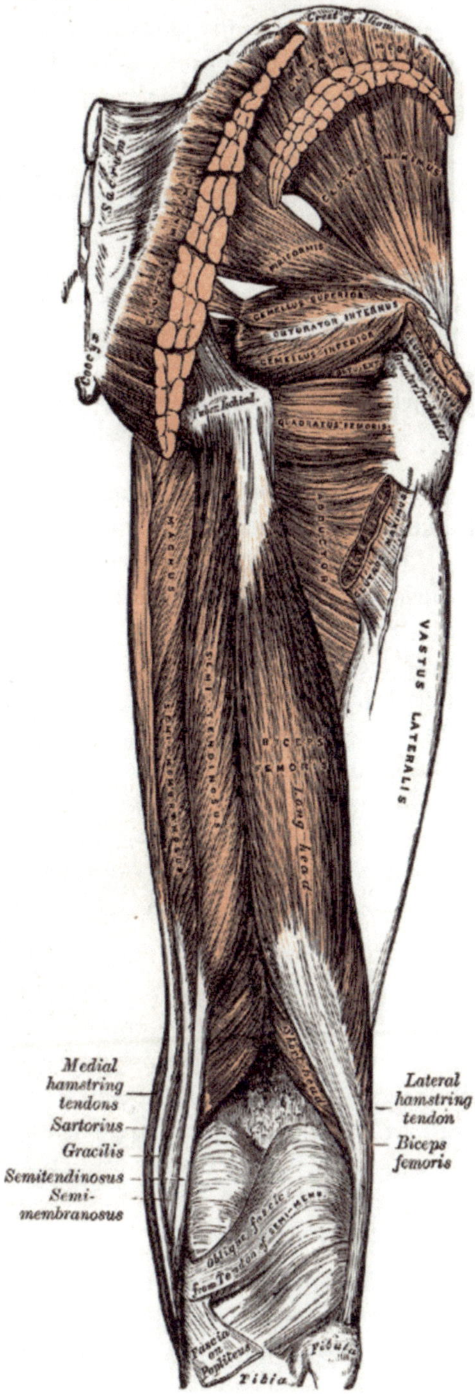

Figure 1. Muscles of the gluteal region and the posterior thigh.

(1) The gluteus maximus muscle is the largest, thickest and most superficial muscle in the buttock. It originates from the outer surface of the ilium, dorsally from the posterior gluteal line, from the adjacent dorsal surface of the lower sacrum and from the lateral coccyx. Connective tissue muscle origins are the sacrotuberal ligament, the erector spinae aponeurosis and the gluteus medius fascia. Muscle fibers descent obliquely and laterally, where the thicker and larger cranial part of the muscle merges with the superficial fibers of the caudal part to continue over the greater trochanter as the iliotibial tract, a reinforcement of the deep fascia lata of the thigh. The tensor fasciae latae muscle, originating from the outer edge of the iliac crest, between the ASIS and the iliac tubercle, also continues in the iliotibial tract, steadying the femur on the tibia during walking, in conjunction with the gluteus maximus muscle. When taking the fixed point at the pelvis, the cranial part of the gluteus maximus is active in abduction and lateral rotation of the thigh and the caudal part extends and also laterally rotates the thigh. When taking the fixed point distally, it stabilizes the trunk during bipedal gait and, together with the hamstrings, raises it.

(2a) The gluteus medius muscle is a broad, thick, fan-shaped muscle. It originates from the outer surface of the ilium caudal to the iliac crest and inserts at the lateral surface of the greater trochanter. Optionally a deep slip of muscle may be attached to the cranial end of it. The caudal part of the gluteus medius muscle is covered by the gluteus maximus, divided from it by a thin connective tissue septum, and bordered (and sometimes partly covered) by the piriformis muscle. The cranial part of the gluteus medius is covered by a strong deep gluteal fascia, on which the gluteus maximus muscle fibers attach caudally and the gluteus medius muscle fibers attach from the inner side. The craniomedial origin of the gluteus maximus doesn't reach the midline and is quite thin. More to the lateral side the muscle becomes thicker. Therefore it easier to find an intermuscular septum between the gluteus maximus and medius muscles at a distance of about 7 cm from the midline. The gluteus medius is a strong abductor at the hip joint and important in stabilizing the pelvis: it is largely responsible for pelvic tilt during walking. The caudal part of the muscle, inserting more to the anterior of the greater trochanter, also medially rotates the thigh.

(2b) The gluteus minimus muscle is the smallest and thinnest of the gluteus muscles. Like the gluteus medius it is a fan-shaped, triangular muscle. It originates from the outer surface of the ilium, between the middle (anterior) and lower (inferior) gluteal lines and, behind, from the margin of the greater sciatic notch. The muscle fibers converge to an aponeurosis that is continuous with the cranial part of the triangular iliofemoral ligament. This aponeurosis finally, as a capsular expansion, inserts to the anterior surface of the greater trochanter. During locomotion the gluteus minimus exerts the same action as the gluteus medius. The anterior fibers medially rotate the thigh more strongly than the gluteus medius muscle.

The muscles described below (2c-e) are all located caudally and deeper than the region of surgical dissection of the Sc-GAP (see also 'Arterial topography') and are described to complete the muscular anatomy of the gluteal region.

(2c). Yet, the piriformis muscle is an important key-structure in the gluteal region to understanding innervation and vascularization (see below). This pear-shaped muscle arises from the internal (anterior) surface of the sacrum, leaving the lesser pelvis through the greater sciatic foramen. It also originates from the region near the posterior inferior iliac spine (PIIS), the adjacent sacroiliac joint capsule and sometimes the inner (pelvic) part of the sacrotuberous ligament. Its insertion, often blended with that of the triceps coxae muscles, which are attaching more posteriorly and caudally, is on the cranial border of the greater trochanter. Sometimes the piriformis muscle belly is also blended with that of the gluteus medius. It laterally rotates the thigh at the hip joint and abducts the thigh.

(2d) The triceps coxae muscle is composed of the gemellus superior, obturator internus and gemellus inferior muscle.

(2e) The quadratus femoris muscle is a flat, rectangular muscle, located between the gemellus inferior and the cranial border of the adductor magnus.

1.2. Arterial topography of the gluteal region

The gluteal region is supplied by the superior and inferior gluteal arteries (SGA and IGA), both directly branching from the internal iliac artery. The accompanying venous tree shows a similar ramification pattern and finally drains into the internal iliac vein (fig 2).

1.3. The superior gluteal artery

The short and large superior gluteal artery (SGA) is a continuation of the posterior trunk of the internal iliac artery and runs posteriorly between the lumbosacral trunk and the first sacral ventral ramus. Within the lesser pelvis it supplies the piriformis and obturator internus muscles and is a nutritient artery for the hip bone. It leaves the greater sciatic foramen cranial to the piriformis muscle and immediately ramifies into (1) superficial and (2) deep branches (fig 3). The superficial branch of the SGA enters the septal plane between the gluteus medius and gluteus maximus muscles. From that plane there are three clinical important ramifications:

(1a) Muscular branches that only supply the gluteus maximus itself.

(1b) Septocutaneous perforators which reach the subcutis and skin, running through the interseptal plane between the gluteus maximus and medius muscles (fig 4).

(1c) Musculocutaneous perforators which finally reach the subcutis and skin, running through the gluteus maximus muscle.

The superficial branch of the SGA anastomizes with branches of the inferior gluteal artery (IGA), the medial circumflex femoral artery and the lateral sacral artery. Comark and Lamberty [17] also described a superficial branch using the septal connective tissue plane between the gluteus maximus and the gluteus medius to devide into a posterior, intermediate and anterior branch. Anterior end branches pierce the deep fascia in the superolateral edge of the gluteus maximus muscle to supply the (sub)cutis there (septocutaneous perforators, as mentioned above).

(2) The deep branch of the SGA runs between the gluteus medius muscle and the posterior pelvic surface (gluteus minimus and piriformis muscles). It divides into a (2a) superior and an (2b) inferior division.

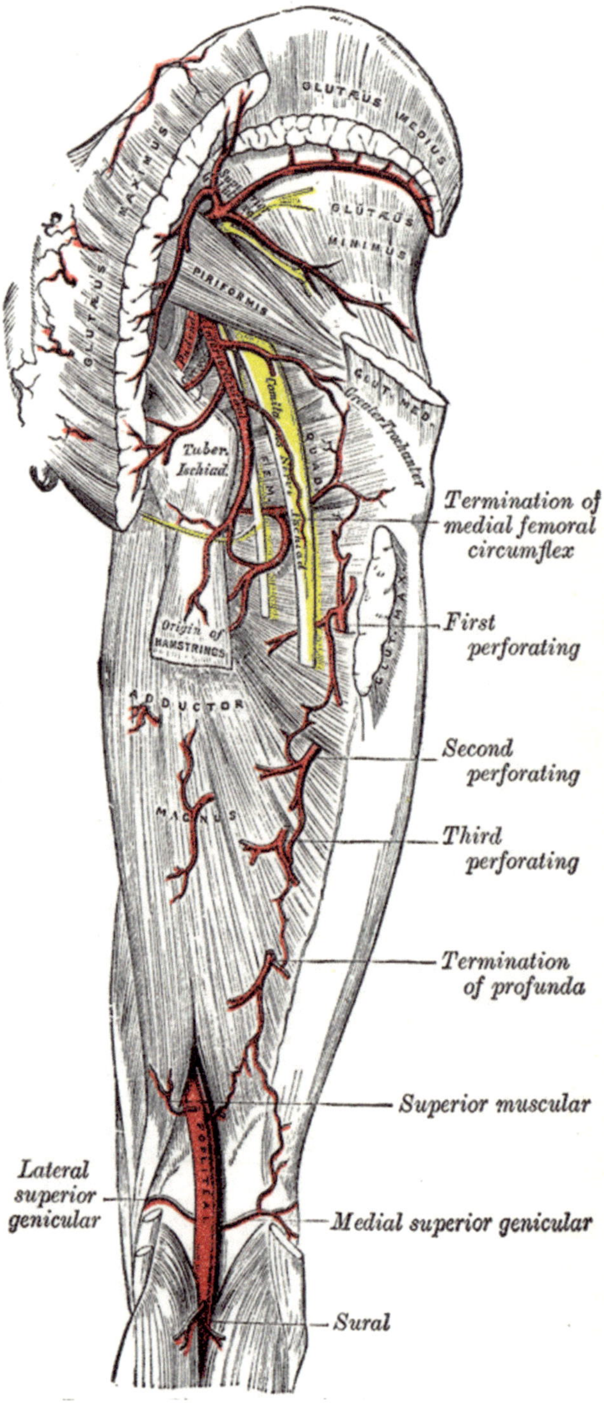

Figure 2. Arteries and nerves of the gluteal region and the posterior thigh.

http://dx.doi.org/10.5772/56224

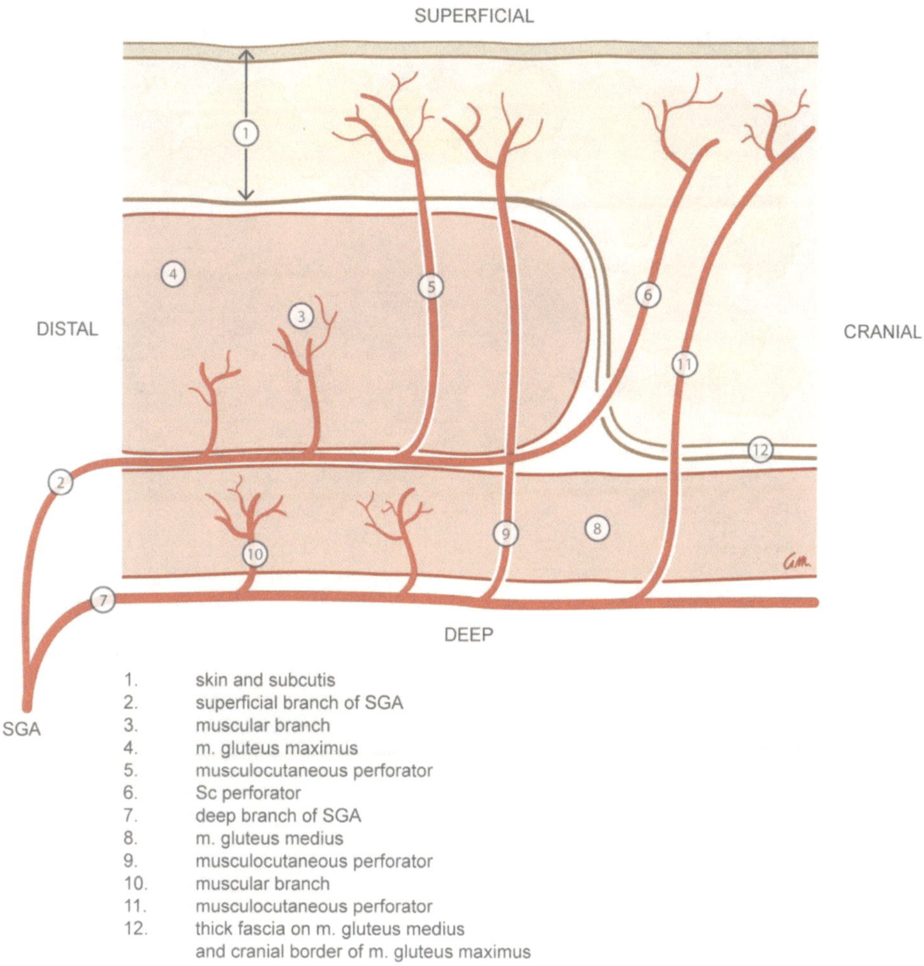

Figure 3. Schematic illustration of the course of perforators and muscular branches originating from the superficial and the deep branch of the superior gluteal artery. Illustration of Greet Mommen, www.greetmommen.be.

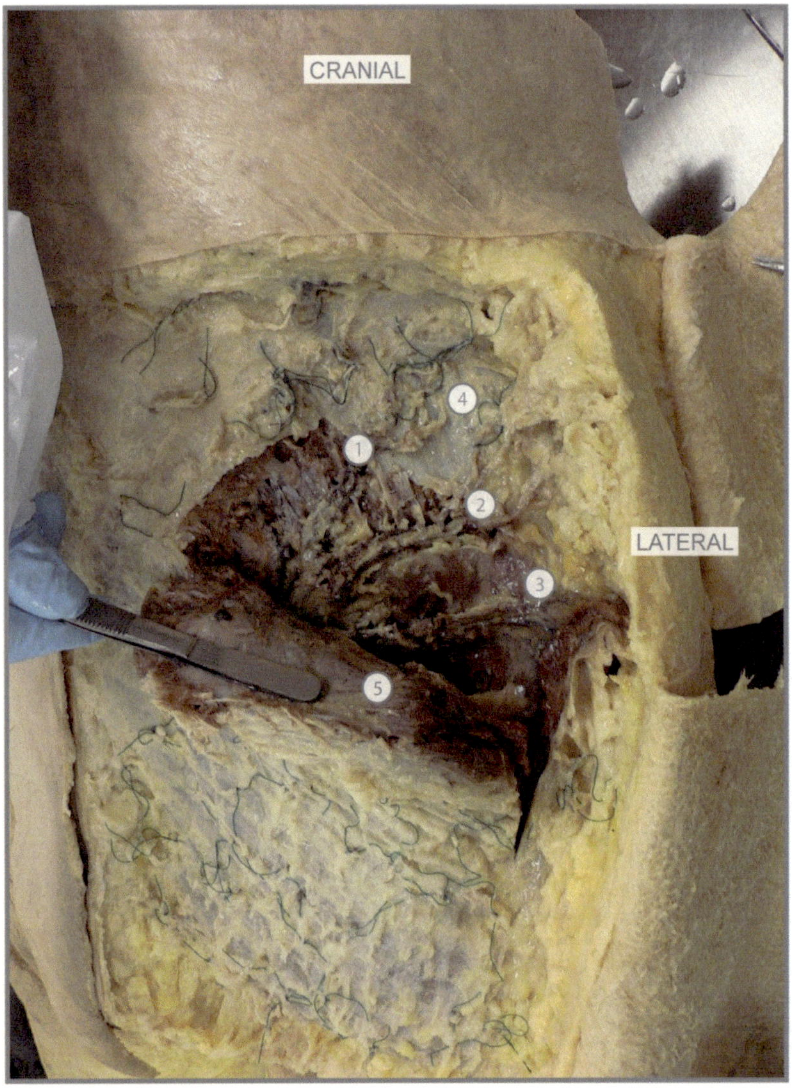

1. Sc perforator
2. Sc perforator
3. Sc perforator
4. fascia on m. gluteus medius
5. m. gluteus maximus

green ligations: gluteal perforators

Figure 4. Cadaveric dissection: musculus gluteus maximus partly detached from its origin to show the septocutaneous perforators underneath.

(2a) The superior division supplies the gluteus medius muscle, continues obliquely along the upper border of the gluteus minimus and supplies also the latter. Finally it runs along the ASIS and anatomizes with the deep circumflex iliac artery and the ascending branch of the lateral circumflex femoral artery.

(2b) The inferior division also runs obliquely between the gluteus medius and minimus muscles, supplies them both and, like the superior division, anatomizes with the lateral circumflex femoral artery. One branch of the inferior division, in the trochanteric fossa, joins the inferior gluteal artery (IGA) and the ascending branch of the medial circumflex artery. Other branches pierce the gluteus minimus muscle into the deep, to supply the hip joint. The deep branch also gives of musculocutaneous perforator, reaching the skin through gluteus medius and maximus muscles. Those branches have to be excluded as pedicle for the S-GAP, because of the difficult dissection through the two muscles.

At the point where the superficial and the deep branch of the SGA meet, near the opening cranial to the piriformis muscle, a venous network of large, fragile bloodvessels is present forming a caput medusae. Clinically the dissection always should stop before reaching this caput medusae.

1.4. The inferior gluteal artery

The inferior gluteal artery (IGA) is the larger terminal branch of the anterior trunk of the internal iliac artery. It descends anterior from the sacral plexus and the piriformis muscle, behind the internal pudendal artery. Inside the pelvis it supplies piriformis, pelvic floor, perianal fat and branches to the fundus of the bladder and to the seminal vesicles and the prostate. It leaves the greater sciatic foramen below the piriformis muscle, supplying gluteus maximus, obturator internus, gemelli, quadratus femoris and upper hamstrings. The extra-pelvic part of the IGA anastomoses with the SGA and with the internal pudendal, obturatory and medial circumflex femoral arteries.

1.4.1. Nerves in the gluteal region

The gluteal region is innervated by many nerves that can be divided into a superficial and a deep group. The deep nerves are the most important clinically.

1.4.2. The superficial gluteal nerves

The skin of the buttock receives cutaneous nerves from several lumbar and sacral segments, called cluneal nerves. They are divided into a (1) superior, (2) middle and an (3) inferior cluneal group.

1.4.3. The deep gluteal nerves

The seven deep gluteal nerves are branches of the sacral plexus. They leave the lesser pelvis through the greater sciatic foramen caudal to the piriformis muscle, except for the superior gluteal nerve, emerging cranial to this muscle.

1.4.4. The superior gluteal nerve

The superior gluteal nerve arises from the dorsal branches of the ventral rami of L4-L5 and S1 and leaves the pelvis cranial to the piriformis muscle together with the SGA. It accompanies the deep branch of the SGA (see above) between the gluteus medius and minimus and divides into a superior branch that supplies the gluteus medius and an inferior branch that supplies the gluteus medius and minimus and the tensor fasciae latae muscles.

1.4.5. The inferior gluteal nerve

This nerve arises from the dorsal branches of the ventral rami of L5 and S1-S2 and leaves the pelvis caudal to the piriformis muscle, superficially from the sciatic nerve and laterally from the pudendal nerve and internal pudendal artery, that, together with the IGA, all issue through the same space.

1.4.6. The sciatic nerve

This largest nerve in the body, the main branch of the sacral plexus, is formed by the ventral rami of L4-L5 and S1-S3. It usually does not supply structures in the pelvis, but is a well palpable landmark in the gluteal region. It usually passes out of the pelvis to enter the gluteal region caudal to the piriformis muscle and consists of a medial tibial and a lateral common peroneal nerve.

1.4.7. The posterior femoral cutaneous nerve

This nerve, supplying a very large skin area, also gives rise to the inferior cluneal nerves. It arises from the dorsal branches of the ventral rami of S1-S2, supplying the skin of the inferior buttock, and the ventral branches of the ventral rami of S2-S3, supplying the skin of the perineum.

1.4.8. The nerve to the quadratus femoris muscle

This nerve arises from the anterior devisions of the ventral rami of L4-L5 and S1 and leaves the pelvis caudal to the piriformis muscle.

1.4.9. The nerve to the obturator internus muscle

This nerve, arising from the anterior devisions of the ventral rami of L5 and S1-S2, leaves the pelvis caudal to the piriformis muscle and medial to the sciatic nerve.

1.4.10. The pudendal nerve

The pudendal nerve, arising from the anterior devisions of the ventral rami of S2-S4, leaves the pelvis caudal to the piriformis muscle as the most medial nerve

http://dx.doi.org/10.5772/56224

2. Preoperative radiological imaging

Numerous radiological imaging modalities are available to identify perforator branches in advance, facilitating surgical planning and shortening operative time [18,23]. At this moment, the most widely applied modalities in the preoperative evaluation and planning of perforator flap procedures are Doppler ultrasound (DUS) and CT angiography (CTA) [18]. Both these imaging techniques are widely available and relatively inexpensive. CT allows for beautiful 3D reconstructions, showing location, size and course of the perforators with high accuracy. Both modalities come with some disadvantages though. Doppler is associated with long imaging times, low accuracy and high interobserver variability [18,24]. CTA, on the other hand, suffers from exposure to ionizing radiation, which is an important drawback in the often (relatively) young patients, especially as the ovaries are within the field of view [25,27].

Magnetic resonance angiography (MRA) might overcome these disadvantages. Several authors have recently demonstrated that MR angiography is suitable as preoperative imaging modality to evaluate the perforator branches of the DIEA en SGA [18-20-22-28,29]. Excellent soft-tissue contrast and the absence of ionizing radiation are important advantages of MRI. Disadvantages of MRI, however, include limited availability and relatively long acquisition times. For now, experience with contrast-enhanced MR angiography (CE-MRA) in the preoperative workup of patients undergoing DIEP or S-GAP flap procedures is still scarce. Although studies comparing MRA and CTA/DUS generally report excellent results for MRA, the diversity in applied MRA techniques is large. Spatial resolution, applied contrast media (conventional extracellular contrast agents versus blood pool contrast agents), field strength (1,5 Tesla versus 3 Tesla magnets) and the application and method of fat-suppression techniques differ between studies. These differences, combined with the fact that most studies included only limited numbers of patients, make it difficult to determine the most optimal MRA protocol. In general, a higher spatial resolution will improve the sensitivity for detecting perforator branches at the cost of longer acquisition times and lower image quality (increased noise-levels). Blood pool contrast agents can be used for steady-state imaging to acquire high-resolution images with excellent signal-to-noise ratios. However, these agents suffer from limited availability and are relatively expensive compared to conventional extracellular contrast agents. Acquisition times are longer compared to first-pass imaging sequences using conventional contrast agents.

Higher field strength generally provides better signal-to-noise ratios and improved image quality. MRI scanners with field strengths of 3 Tesla or above are less widely available than 1.5 Tesla scanners. In addition, homogenous fat suppression is much more difficult to obtain at higher field strengths, which could result in unwanted image artifacts or decrease in vessel-to-background contrast ratios, as the perforator branches are located within the subcutaneous abdominal fat. To optimize contrast between the perforator branches and surrounding fat tissue, fat suppression can be very useful. Fat suppression requires a homogenous magnetic field, and is negatively influenced by patient movement (breathing and bowel movements), resulting in longer acquisition times. Given these variables, the most suitable MRA sequence to evaluate the perforator branches for each institution will depend on the local availability of MRI hardware, contrast agents and the allowed acquisition time.

As an example, the imaging in our institution is in general performed using 15 mL gadobutrol 1.0 mmol/mL (Gadovist®, Bayer Healthcare Pharmaceuticals), administered through the antecubital vein. An automatic injector is used, ensuring a constant flow rate of 1.5 mL/sec, followed by a saline flush. The field strength of our scanner is 1.5 Tesla and a four-channel SENSE body coil is used for imaging.

After the necessary survery and reference scans, we perform several sequences which are listed below. The sequence parameters of the sequences used in our hospital are also provided. Although these might differ between vendors and field strengths, we think they can serve as a basis for introducing this kind of MR imaging in the reader's own department.

Firstly, the transverse, balanced, T1-weighted FFE is performed, which has a field-of-view of 400x400 mm, and a slice thickness of 6 mm. Voxel size is 1.32 x 1.32 mm. Remaining scan parameters for this sequence are: TE 1.80 ms, TR 3.6 ms, flip angle 65 degrees (fig 5).

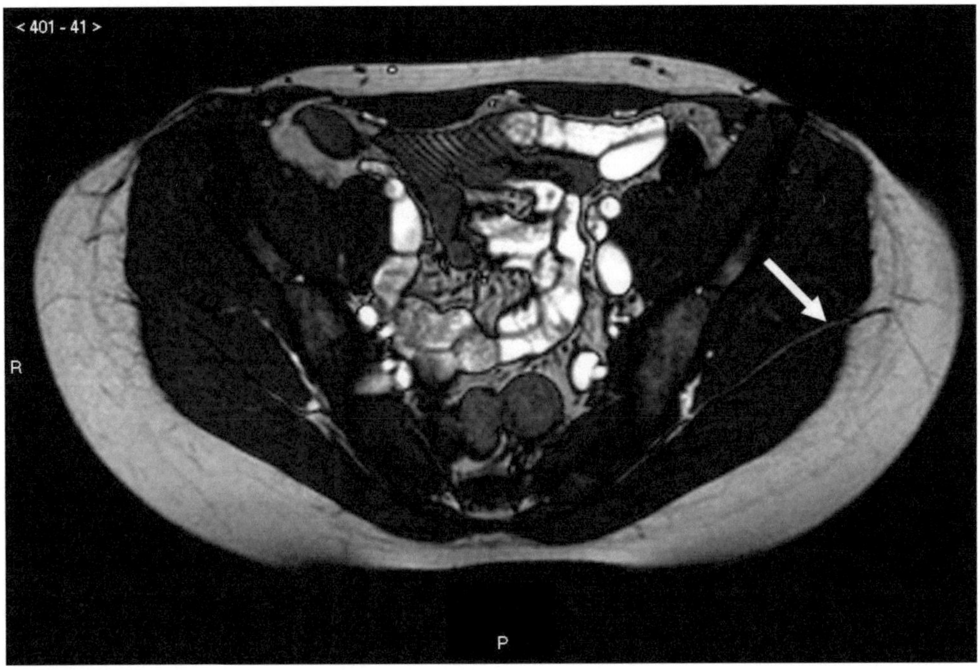

Figure 5. Transverse, balanced, T1-weighted FFE sequence on MRA. The arrow shows the perforator vein(s) running between gluteus maximus and medius muscle.

http://dx.doi.org/10.5772/56224

This is followed by a sagittal, balanced, T1-weighted fast field echo (FFE) is performed with a field-of-view 430x430 mm, and a slice thickness of 10 mm. Voxel size is 1.68 x 1.68 mm. The remaining scan parameters are: TE 1.56 ms, TR 3.1 ms, flip angle 65 degrees.

Next, a bolus tracker sequence is performed to assess the optimal time period of enhancement of the vessels of interest. This is followed by a coronal, three-dimensional T1-weighted FFE sequence, which has a field-of-view of 400x360 mm and a slice thickness of 2 mm. Voxel size is 1.0x1.36 mm. The remaining scan parameters are: TE 1.53 ms, TR 5.0 ms, flip angle 40 degrees.

Finally, a transverse, three-dimensional T1-weighted FFE sequence ('THRIVE') is acquired, which has a field-of-view of 380x304 mm and a slice thickness of 3 mm. Voxel size is 0.95x0.95 mm. The remaining scan parameters are: TE 3.9 ms, TR 7.8 ms, flip angle 10 degrees (fig 6).

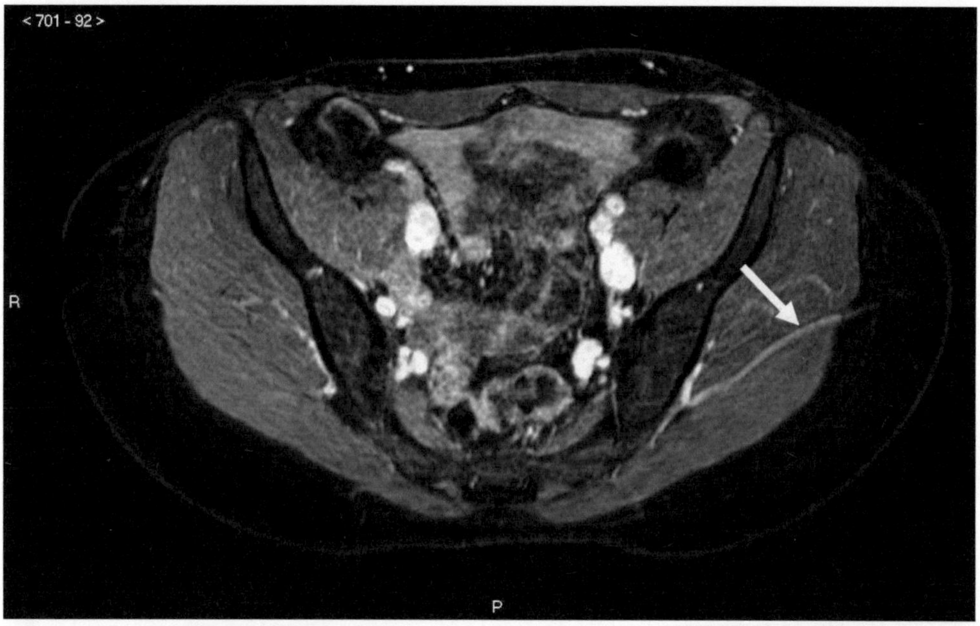

Figure 6. Transverse, three-dimensional T1-weighted FFE sequence ('THRIVE') on MRA. The arrow shows the comitant perforator artery running between gluteus maximus and medius muscle.

3. Preoperative landmarks

Step 1: Every patient undergoes preoperative imaging before surgery. Only patients with a suitable septocutaneous perforator are scheduled for breast reconstruction with Sc-GAP (75%). In MRA a septocutaneous perforator is considered suitable for surgery if the pedicle length is 6 cm or more.

Step 2: On the MRA the projection of the septocutaneous perforator on the surface of the patient is identified: because the gluteal region is not flat (as for example is the abdominal region) the distance of the perforator from the midline is calculated on the curvature of the gluteal region (x axis) (fig 7).

The projection of the umbilicus on the patient's dorsal midline is identified as a landmark to determine the craniocaudal position of the perforator itself (y axis) (fig 8, A,B,C).

Step 3: To determine the position of the perforator as accurately as possible, a number of lines is drawn on the patient's skin. The patient's position should be the same as in surgery (see pitfalls). The midline is indicated with line A and the cranial end of the crena analis with a horizontal line B With a color doppler (Esaote MyLab 25 Color Doppler with a LA523, 4-13 MHz probe) the cranial margin of the gluteus maximus muscle, where it originates from the thick gluteus medius fascia, is also identified, positioning the probe approximately parallel to this margin (fig 9A). It is marked on the skin as line C. Finally the iliac crest is identified and marked on the skin as a curved line D. The probe then is rotated 90° (fig 9B) and every perforator is identified and drawn on the skin: it is possible to identify perforators emerging from the septal plane between the gluteus maximus and medius muscles, though it is not possible to follow them to their origin from the SGA (fig 10).

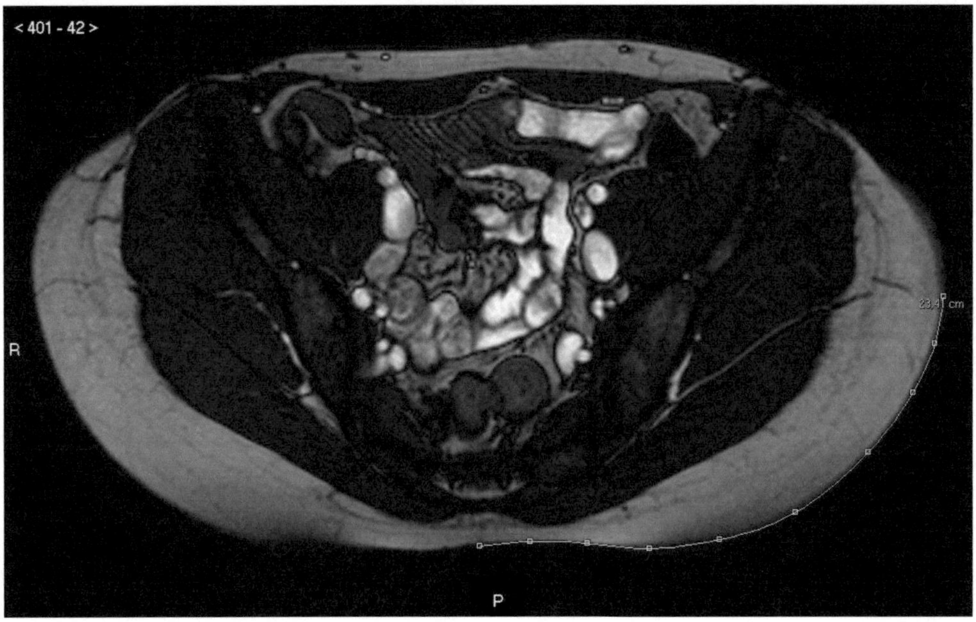

Figure 7. MRA imaging showing the measurement of the distance from the midline to the skin projection of the perforator chosen as pedicle for the Sc-GAP.

http://dx.doi.org/10.5772/56224

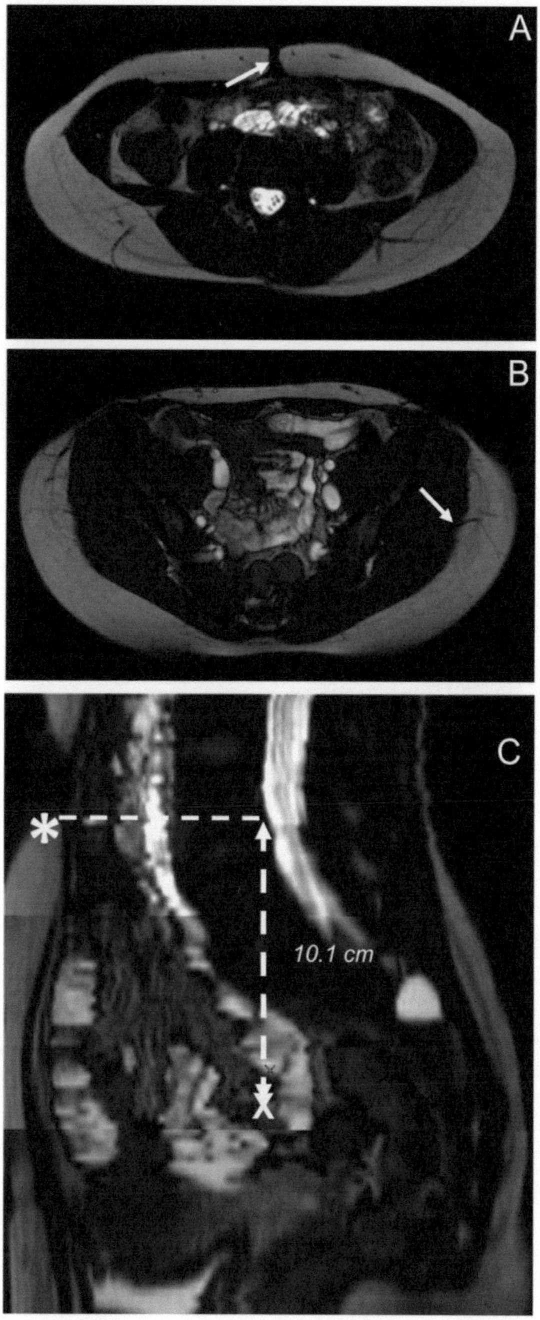

Figure 8. An example of how to assess the anteroposterior length. Firstly, the location of umbilicus is determined (A, arrow). Secondly, the location of the exit of the perforator between the gluteal muscles into the subcutaneous fat is determined (B, arrow). Finally, the position of the umbilicus, determined on the sagittal reconstructed images (C, asterisk), and the site of the perforator exit of B are marked by the crosshair (C, arrow). In this way, the craniocaudal length from the umbilicus to the site of the perforator exit can be determined. It was 10.1 cm in this example.

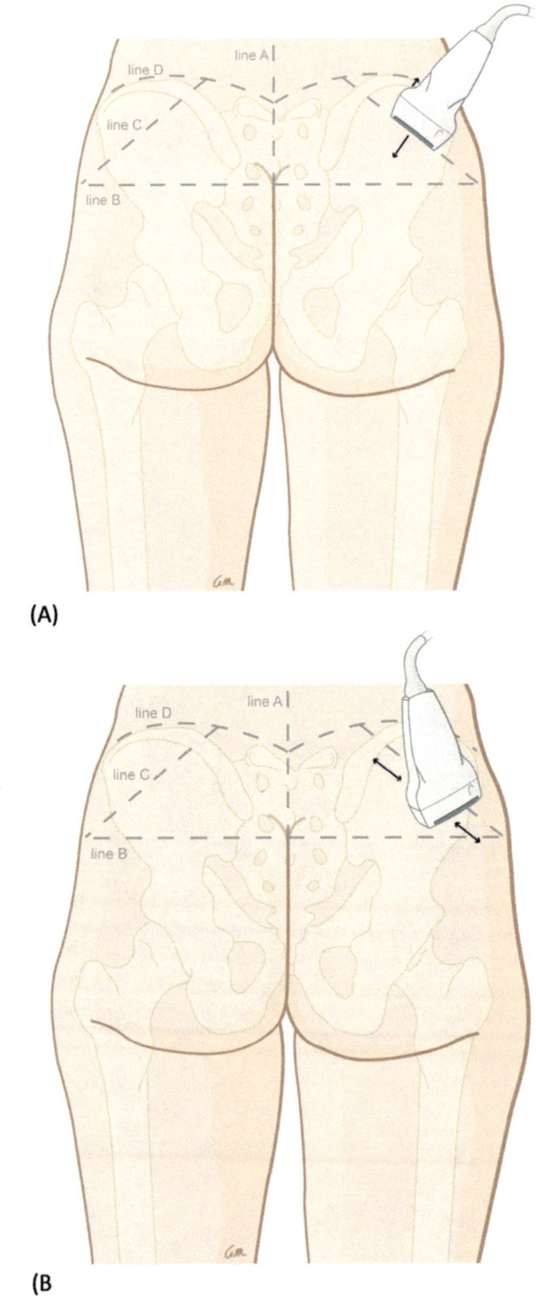

Figure 9. Schematic illustration of the identification of the cranial margin of the gluteus maximus muscle. line A: midline, line B: cranial end of the crena analis, line C: cranial border of m. gluteus maximus, line D: iliac crest. (A): probe positioned parallel to the margin of the gluteus maximus. (B): probe rotated 90 degrees and positioned perpendicularly to the margin of the gluteus maximus to identify the perforators. Illustration of Greet Mommen, www.greetmommen.be.

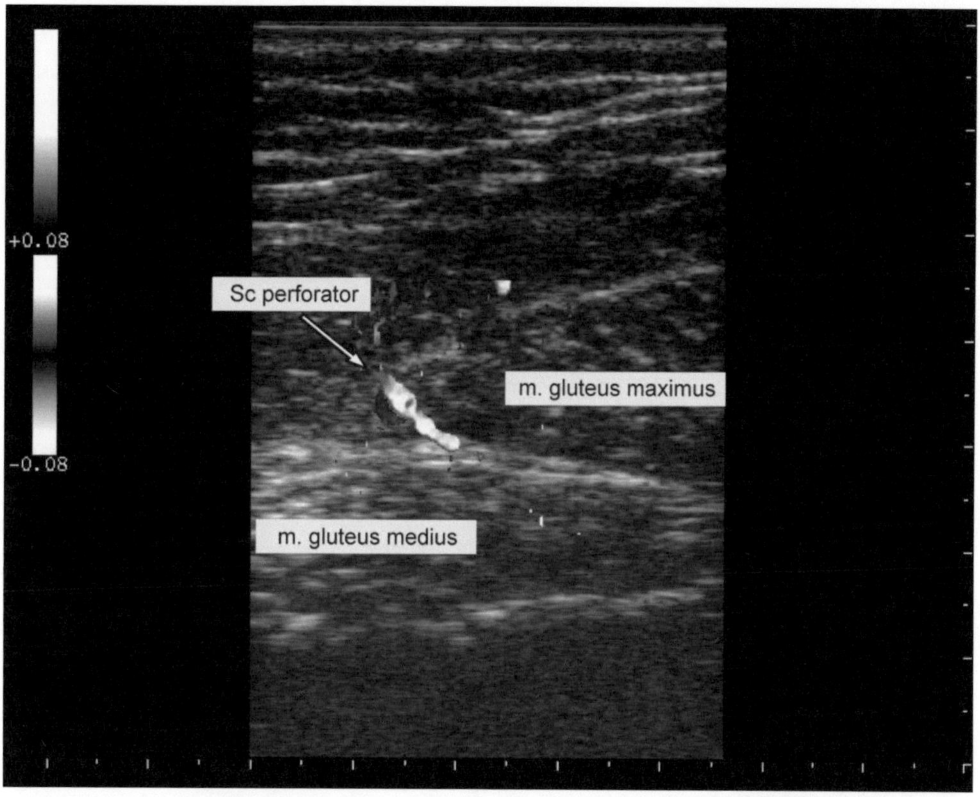

Figure 10. Visualization with Color Doppler of a perforator emerging between gluteus maximus and medius muscles.

Step 4: Adding all this information enables a precise identification of the perforator with the preferred location and length. In our first cases the flap contour, centered on this perforator, was always drawn elliptically completely on the superficial projection of the intermuscular septum between gluteus maximus and medius muscle. This ensures that, when marking proves not to be exact enough or the perforator chosen at first instance is damaged, alternative septocutaneous perforators, if present, can be used as pedicle for the flap. Out of experience the elliptical skin island now is changed in an S-shape to avoid undesirable dog ears medially and laterally (fig 11A, B).

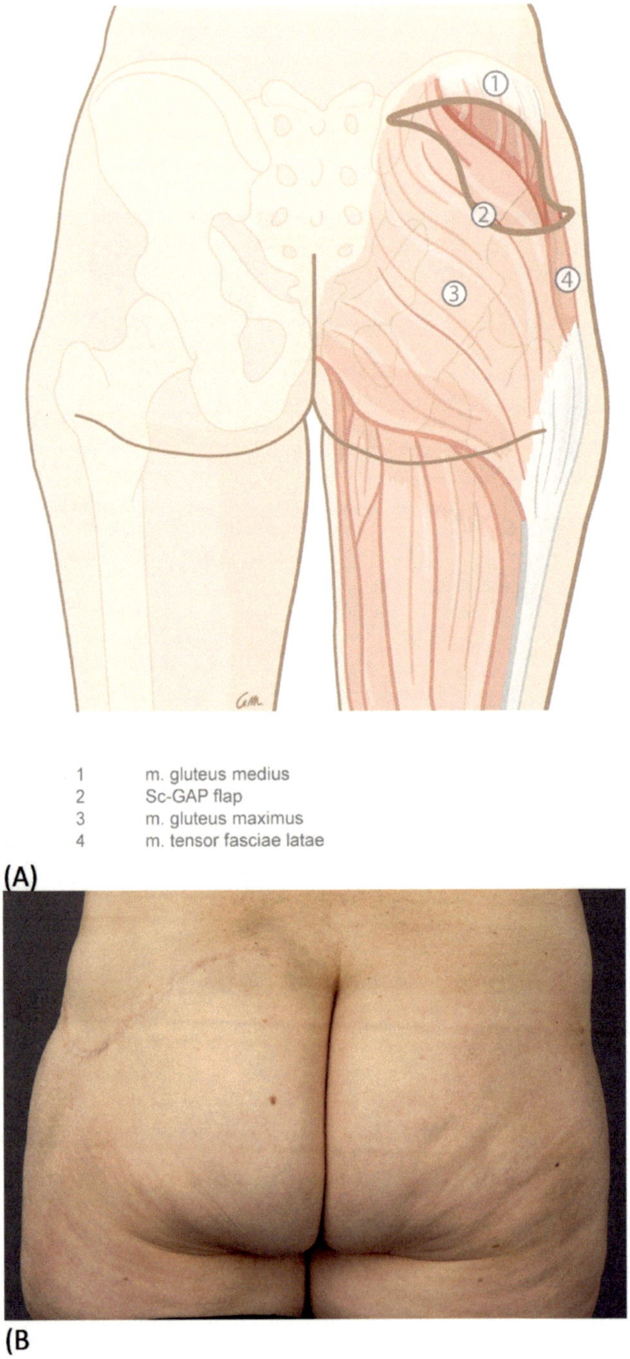

Figure 11. S-shaped design of the flap: (A) schematic visualization. (B) example on a patient. Illustration of Greet Mommen, www.greetmommen.be.

The pinch test is used to identify the maximal width of the flap. The flap is just orientated a bit more cranial than the standard drawing of an S-GAP flap (fig 12).

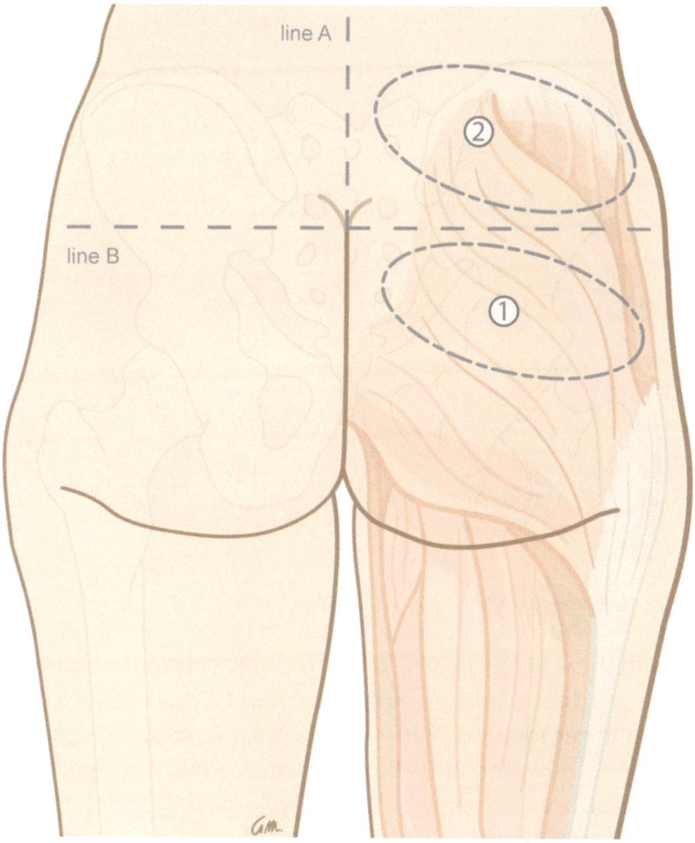

Figure 12. Schematic illustration of (1) region where a standard S-GAP is usually drawn and (2) region where the Sc-GAP is drawn. Illustration of Greet Mommen, www.greetmommen.be.

4. Surgical technique

The patient is initially supine. The internal mammary (thoracic) vessels are identified first, to reduce the ischemic time of the flap later on, especially in bilateral reconstructions.

The patient then is turned in prone position. The dissection starts at the craniomedial (fig 13), thin origin of the gluteus maximus muscle. Medially is the best starting point because perforators 6-8 cm from the midline, being too short, are not suitable as pedicle for the flap. The craniomedial edge of the gluteus maximus is identified and the fascia is opened.

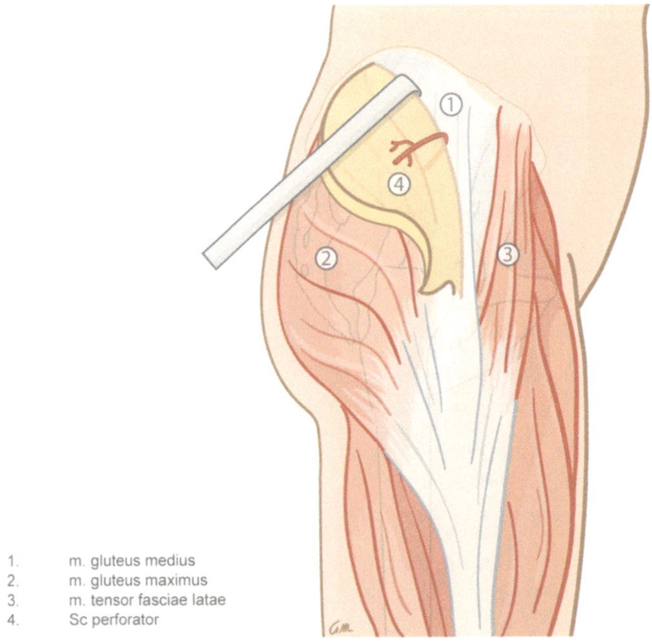

Figure 13. Craniomedial dissection of the Sc-GAP flap. Illustration of Greet Mommen, www.greetmommen.be.

Actually, underneath the thin medial origin of the gluteus maximus muscle, it is very easy to develop in a blunt way a dissectional plane between the gluteus maximus and medius muscles and, introducing the finger into this plane, sometimes the pulsation of the perforator can be felt: this offers the opportunity to identify the exact location where the perforator emerges from the tight cranial fascial border between the gluteus maximus and medius muscles. The dissection continues in a retrograde way from medial to lateral, paying attention not to damage perforators emerging from the septum between the gluteus maximus and medius. The fascia of the gluteal muscles is very tight in this region and the approach of the septal plane between the gluteus maximus and medius is sometimes not easy: therefore this approach is a key point in the dissection. When the perforator(s) are identified the complete flap is incised and isolated.

The dissection continues, lifting the gluteus maximus muscle (fig 14 A, B) with the aid of a light hook. When the muscle is very tight it is difficult to lift it enough. In that case the gluteus maximus can partially be dissected at its origin on the sacrum and later on be sutured back. The perforator is followed between the gluteus maximus and medius paying attention to ligate every muscular or musculocutaneous branch. In the intermuscular septal plane the perforators join the superficial branch of the SGA (see anatomy). Near the sacrum the perforator continues retrogradely, running deep from the gluteus medius to reach its origin at the SGA. There the caput medusae of veins is present. These veins have usually a caliber above the 3 mm and are very fragile, having a very thin wall. To avoid problems the dissection is finished just before the caput medusae.

http://dx.doi.org/10.5772/56224

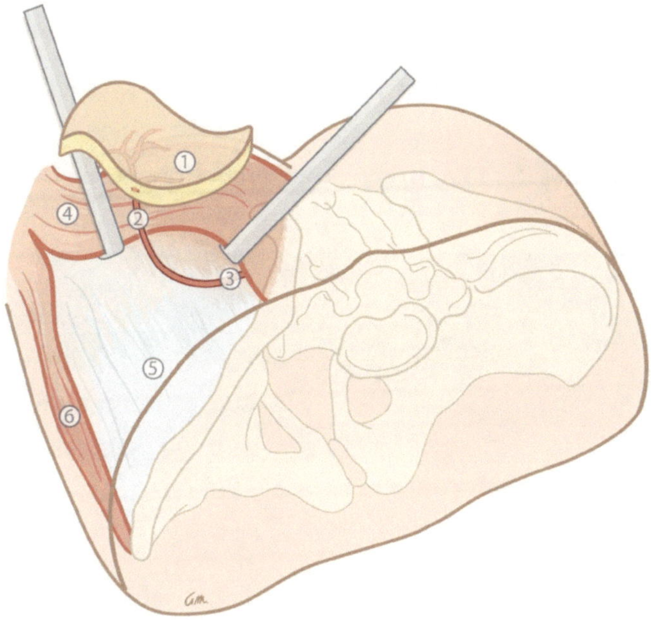

1. Sc-GAP flap
2. Sc perforator
3. SGA: superficial branch
4. m. gluteus maximus
5. m. gluteus medius
6. m. tensor fascia latae

(A)

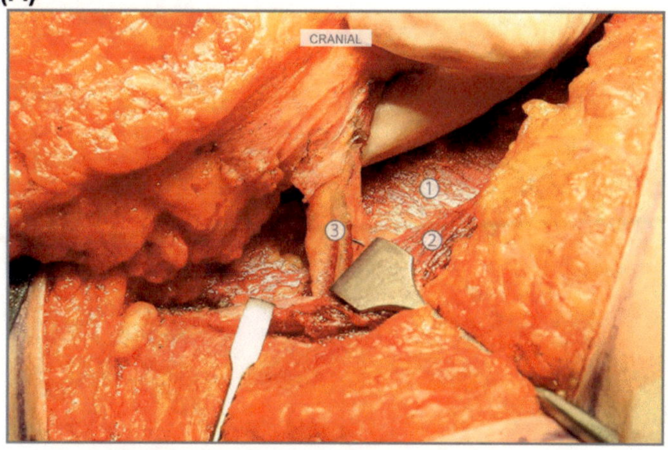

1. m. gluteus medius
2. cranial border m. gluteus maximus
3. Sc perforator

(B

Figure 14. Musculus gluteus maximus lifted up, showing interseptal course of septocutaneous perforator, (A) schematic illustration and (B) intraoperative finding. Illustration of Greet Mommen, www.greetmommen.be.

The flap is then removed from the gluteal region and the ischemia time starts. The donor site is closed, 2 drains are positioned and the patient is turned in supine position.

The anastomosis to the internal mammary (thoracic) vessels proceeds in the same way as for a DIEP flap.

Some preoperative pictures (fig 15 A, B) and postoperative results (fig 16 A, B) are shown.

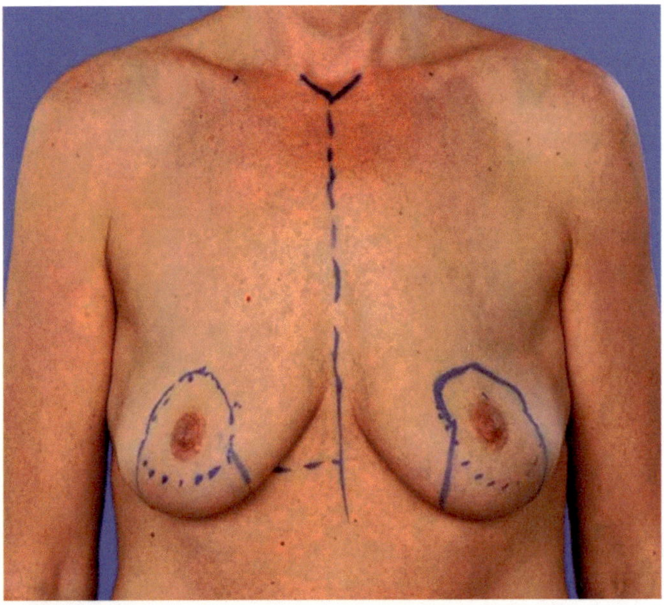

(A)

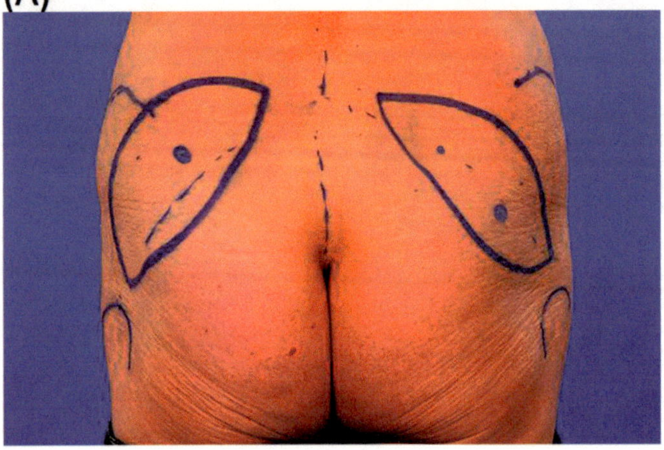

(B

Figure 15. Preoperative pictures of (A) breasts and (B) gluteal region: bony landmarks and drawing of the flaps with perforators at the cranial border of the gluteus maximus muscle are visible.

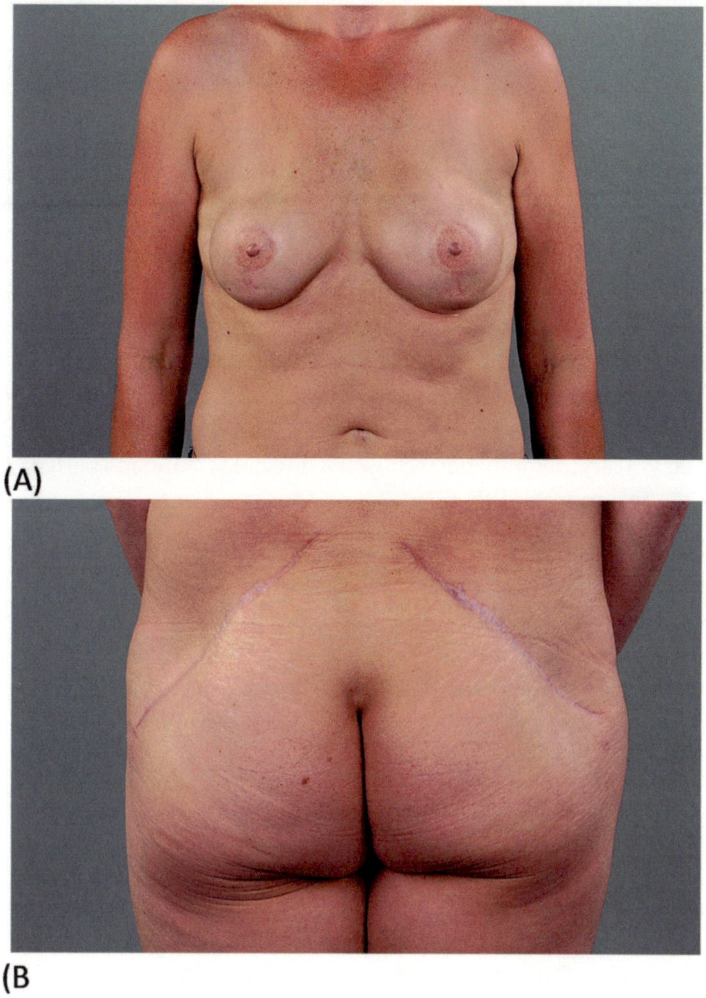

Figure 16. Postoperative pictures of (A) breasts and (B) gluteal region.

5. Pitfalls

1. Do not consider suitable for surgery a perforator with a pedicle length measured on MRA less than 6 cm: the anastomosis with the mammary vessels will be very difficult.

2. Draw your patient in the exact same position as she will have during the operation (in our practice patients will have a pillow underneath the abdomen in the operative theatre): the skin of the gluteal region can move very easily with respect to the muscles because of the presence of a lot of subcutaneous tissue. A different position during drawing and operation can lead to a shift in the position of the septal plane and the perforator.

3. The identification of the septal plane between the gluteus maximus and medius muscles is essential: actually it is the key point of the dissection.

4. Lift the gluteus maximus muscle carefully because you can damage muscular or musculocutaneous branches of the superficial branch of the SGA.

5. If a clear visualization of the perforator is not possible, the gluteus maximus can partially detached from his origin from the sacral bone and at the end be reattached.

6. To be sure to include the perforator, chosen with the MRA, the flap is oriented just cranial to the edge of the gluteus maximus muscle: getting more experienced in the exact identification of the perforator offers the opportunity to change the flap orientation to improve aesthetic results. Because of the large number of perforators in this area it is not difficult to identify one of them with a standard Doppler, but you still don't know if it is a septocutaneous or a musculocutaneous one. The dissection especially will be very difficult when you accidentally have chosen a musculocutaneous perforator running into the gluteus medius muscles (see fig 3).

7. Septocutaneous perforators, compared to musculocutaneous ones, are surrounded by a greater amount of fat and connective tissue. Therefore they are more compact than musculocutaneous ones and, as a consequence, less flexible: the plastic surgeon has to pay more attention to maintain the original orientation of the pedicle to avoid torsion or kinking during positioning of the flap on the breast. The orientation can be maintained visually by marking the upper surface of the pedicle with ink.

Acknowledgements

We would like to give special thanks to Greet Mommen, medical scientific illustrator at Maastricht University, Department of Anatomy and Embryology, for the realization of the illustrations in this chapter. Her ideas and active contribution were essential to make clear the concepts, described above.

Author details

Stefania Tuinder[1*], Rene Van Der Hulst[1], Marc Lobbes[2], Bas Versluis[2] and Arno Lataster[3]

*Address all correspondence to: nervofaciale@yahoo.it

1 Department of Plastic and Reconstructive Surgery, MUMC+, Maastricht, The Netherlands

2 Department of Radiology, MUMC++, Maastricht, The Netherlands

3 Department of Anatomy & Embryology, Maastricht University, Maastricht, The Netherlands

References

[1] Fujino, T, Harashina, T, & Enomoto, K. Primary breast reconstruction after a standard radical mastectomy by a free flap transfer (case report). Plast Reconstr Surg. (1976). , 58(3), 371-4.

[2] Shaw, W. W. Breast reconstruction by superior gluteal microvascular free flaps without silicone implants. Plast Reconstr Surg. (1983). , 72(4), 490-501.

[3] Allen, R. Tucker C Jr. Superior gluteal artery perforator free flap for breast reconstruction. Plast Reconstr Surg. (1995). , 95(7), 1207-12.

[4] LoTempio MMAllen RJ. Breast reconstruction with SGAP and IGAP flaps. Plast Reconstr Surg. (2010). Review., 126(2), 393-401.

[5] Koshima, I, Moriguchi, T, Fukuda, H, Yoshikawa, Y, & Soeda, S. Free, thinned, paraumbilical perforator-based flaps. J Reconstr Microsurg. (1991). , 7(4), 313-6.

[6] Allen, R. J, & Treece, P. Deep inferior epigastric perforator flap for breast reconstruction. Ann Plast Surg. (1994). , 32(1), 32-8.

[7] Blondeel, P. N, Van Landuyt, K. H, Monstrey, S. J, Hamdi, M, Matton, G. E, Allen, R. J, Dupin, C, Feller, A. M, Koshima, I, Kostakoglu, N, & Wei, F. C. The "Gent" consensus on perforator flap terminology: preliminary definitions. Plast Reconstr Surg. (2003). quiz 1383, 1516; discussion 1384-7., 112(5), 1378-83.

[8] Geddes, C. R, Morris, S. F, & Neligan, P. C. Perforator flaps: evolution, classification and application. Ann Plast Surg (2003). Review., 50(1), 90-9.

[9] Blondeel, P. N, Morris, S. F, Hallock, G. G, & Neligan, P. C. eds. Perforator flaps: Anatomy, Technique and Clinical Application. St. Louis: Quality Medical; (2006).

[10] Sinna, R, Boloorchi, A, Mahajan, A. L, Qassemyar, Q, & Robbe, M. What should define a "perforator flap"? Plast Reconstr Surg. (2010). Review., 126(6), 2258-63.

[11] Taylor, G. I, Rozen, W. M, & Whitaker, I. S. Establishing a perforator flap nomenclature based on anatomical principles. Plast Reconstr Surg. (2012). e-9e.

[12] Tuinder, S, Van Der Hulst, R, Lataster, A, & Boeckx, W. Superior gluteal artery perforator flap based on septal perforators: preliminary study. Plast Reconstr Surg. (2008). e-8e.

[13] Tuinder, S, Chen, C. M, & Massey, M. F. Allen RJ Sr, Van der Hulst R. Introducing the septocutaneous gluteal artery perforator flap: a simplified approach to microsurgical breast reconstruction. Plast Reconstr Surg. (2011). , 127(2), 489-95.

[14] Warwick, R, & Williams, P. L. (1973). Gray's Anatomy, 35th Edition, Edinburgh: Longman Group Ltd.

[15] Moore, K. L. (1992). Clinically Oriented Anatomy, 3rd Edition, Baltimore: Williams & Wilkins.

[16] Stone, R. J, & Stone, J. A. (2000). Atlas of Skeletal Muscles, 3rd Edition, Boston: McGraw- Hill Companies Inc.

[17] Cormack, G. C, & Lamberty, B. G. H. (1994). The Arterial Anatomy of Skin Flaps, 2nd Ed. New York: Churchill Livingstone:, 218-22.

[18] Mathes, D. W, & Neligan, P. C. Current techniques in preoperative imaging for abdomen-based perforator flap microsurgical breast reconstruction. J Reconstr Microsurg. (2010). , 26(1), 3-10.

[19] Chernyak, V, Rozenblit, A. M, Greenspun, D. T, et al. Breast reconstruction with deep inferior epigastric artery perforator flap: 3.0-T gadolinium-enhanced MR imaging for preoperative localization of abdominal wall perforators. Radiology. (2009). , 250(2), 417-24.

[20] Rozen, W. M, Phillips, T. J, Ashton, M. W, et al. Preoperative imaging for DIEA perforator flaps: a comparative study of computed tomographic angiography and Doppler ultrasound. Plast Reconstr Surg. (2008). , 121(1), 9-16.

[21] Alonso-burgos, A, Garcia-tutor, E, Bastarrika, G, et al. Preoperative planning of deep inferior epigastric artery perforator flap reconstruction with multislice-CT angiography: imaging findings and initial experience. J Plast Reconstr Aesthet Surg. (2006). , 59(6), 585-93.

[22] Masia, J, Clavero, J. A, Larranaga, J. R, et al. Multidetector-row computed tomography in the planning of abdominal perforator flaps. J Plast Reconstr Aesthet Surg. (2006). , 59(6), 594-9.

[23] Acosta, R, Smit, J. M, Audolfsson, T, et al. A Clinical Review of 9 Years of Free Perforator Flap Breast Reconstructions: An Analysis of 675 Flaps and the Influence of New Techniques on Clinical Practice. J Reconstr Microsurg. (2011). Feb;, 27(2), 91-8.

[24] Giunta, R. E, Geisweid, A, & Feller, A. M. The value of preoperative Doppler sonography for planning free perforator flaps. Plast Reconstr Surg. (2000). , 105(7), 2381-6.

[25] Brenner, D. J, Doll, R, Goodhead, D. T, et al. Cancer risks attributable to low doses of ionizing radiation: assessing what we really know. Proc Natl Acad Sci U S A. (2003). , 100(24), 13761-6.

[26] Hall, E. J, & Brenner, D. J. Cancer risks from diagnostic radiology. Br J Radiol. (2008). , 81(965), 362-78.

[27] Einstein, A. J. Medical imaging: the radiation issue. Nat Rev Cardiol. (2009). , 6(6), 436-8.

[28] Rozen, W. M, Stella, D. L, Phillips, T. J, et al. Magnetic resonance angiography in the preoperative planning of DIEA perforator flaps. Plast Reconstr Surg. (2008). e-3e.

[29] Fukaya, E, Grossman, R. F, Saloner, D, et al. Magnetic resonance angiography for free fibula flap transfer. J Reconstr Microsurg. (2007). , 23(4), 205-11.

Chapter 10

Profunda Artery Perforator (PAP) Flap for Breast Reconstruction

Constance M. Chen, Maria LoTempio and
Robert J. Allen

Additional information is available at the end of the chapter

http://dx.doi.org/10.5772/56332

1. Introduction

Perforator flap breast reconstruction has strong appeal for many women undergoing mastectomies, but the procedure requires adequate donor site tissue. The most common donor site for perforator flap breast reconstruction is the abdomen, such as the deep inferior epigastric perforator (DIEP) or superficial inferior epigastric artery (SIEA) flap, as most women have adequate donor site tissue, the procedure may be performed in the supine position, and the perforating vessels have a dependable caliber and length. In the past, the second line option was usually the buttock, but the buttock as a donor site had multiple disadvantages – most notably a short vascular pedicle, a deforming donor site defect, and a long operative time due to the need to reposition the patient for harvest and inset. Recently, the posterior thigh has emerged as an excellent donor site for perforator flap breast reconstruction. Indeed, the profunda artery perforator (PAP) flap, which uses the skin and fat of the posterior thigh, has surpassed the gluteal artery perforator (GAP) flap in our practice as the second line donor site for microsurgical breast reconstruction.

The PAP flap for breast reconstruction was originated in 2010 by Dr. Robert J. Allen at the 13th International Course on Perforator Flaps in Mexico City. The first patient was a 52-year-old woman who had undergone previous attempts at breast reconstruction with a failed transverse rectus abdominis muscle (TRAM) flap and a failed implant. She wanted autologous tissue reconstruction, and other options considered for her included the superior gluteal artery perforator (SGAP) flap, inferior gluteal artery perforator (IGAP) flap, and the transverse upper gracilis (TUG) flap. Of note, however, the patient had excess posterior thigh tissue, and she did not want to sacrifice her muscle for breast reconstruction. While posterior thigh perforator flaps based on the inferior gluteal artery or profunda femoris artery had previously been described in the literature,[1-3] they had not been performed for breast reconstruction. Cadaver studies had demonstrated that the dominant blood supply to the posterior thigh was the posterior perforators emerging from the profunda femoris artery (Figure 1). Given the patient's history, body habitus, and background work by other surgeons and anatomists, Dr. Allen decided to proceed with the first posterior thigh profunda artery perforator (PAP) flap for microsurgical breast reconstruction.

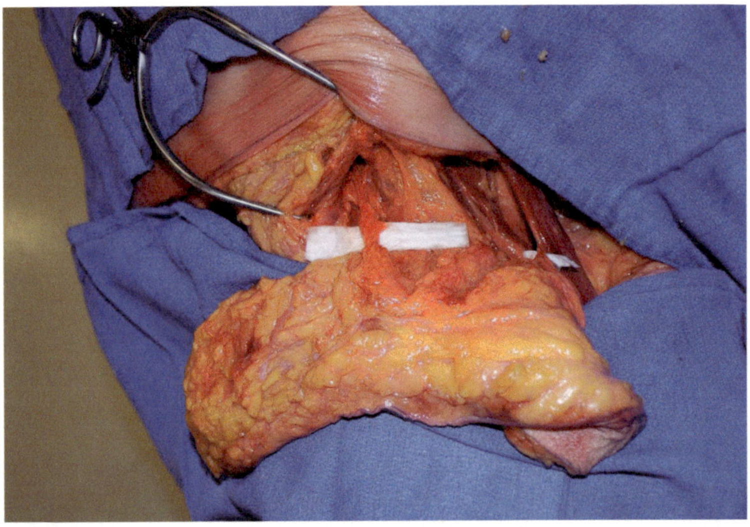

Figure 1. Cadaver studies had demonstrated that the dominant blood supply to the posterior thigh was the posterior perforators emerging from the profunda femoris artery.

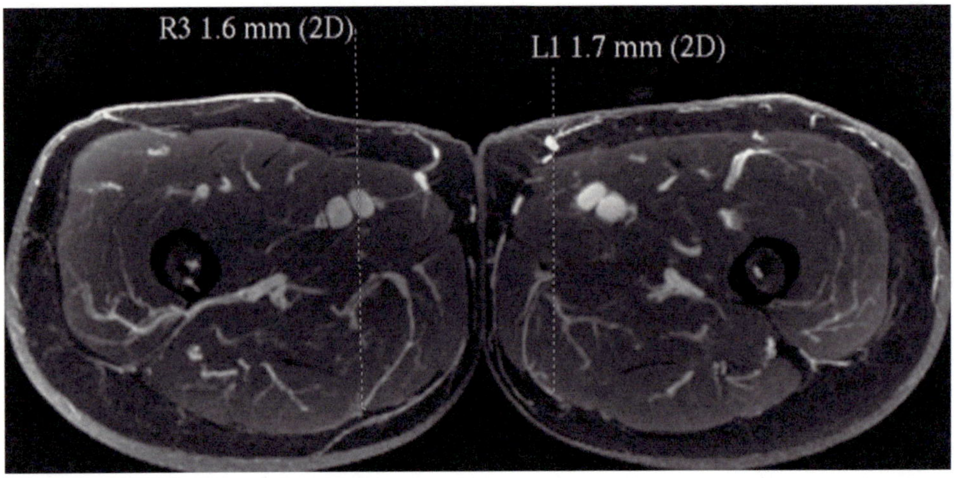

Figure 2. With the midline and inferior gluteal crease as reference points, the largest, most well-placed perforators with the longest vascular pedicle can be identified. In this image, the best perforators have been identified as R3 and L1.

2. Indications

The PAP flap is appropriate for women with insufficient abdominal tissue, previous abdominal liposuction or surgery, a failed TRAM/DIEP/SIEA, pear-shaped body habitus, or who simply have a preference for a non-abdominal donor site. The donor site is the area on the posterior thigh found inferior to the gluteal crease. Excess posterior thigh fat is difficult to address by diet and exercise, and is accentuated in women who are pear-shaped. Even in women who are very thin, there is almost always a "banana roll" of excess skin and fatty tissue located on the back of the thigh below the buttock crease. Removal of the transverse posterior thigh tissue provides contouring and lifting to the thigh area, creates a rounder and more shapely buttock, and does not result in sciatic nerve exposure. The scar is usually concealed within a bathing suit, and the tissue is very soft and pliable.

In breast reconstruction, the PAP flap is coned to create a natural aesthetic breast shape with ample volume for most patients. Even in patients with a BMI < 18, the PAP flap can be successfully used for a very attractive breast reconstruction. The PAP flap skin paddle usually measures 4-7 cm in width and 26 cm in length. Volumes range from 150-900 grams, but in the average patient the volume is between 300-400 grams. Since no muscle is removed, postoperative pain and functional problems are minimized.

3. Preoperative planning

Once the decision has been made to proceed with a PAP flap, each of our patients undergoes a magnetic resonance (MR) or computed tomography (CT) angiogram pre-operatively to determine perforator size and intra-operative course. MR or CT angiography of the pelvis and thigh with contrast is performed in the supine position. Preoperative imaging with MRA or CTA makes it possible to define the intramuscular course of perforators prior to the flap elevation.[4-8] This makes it possible to quickly and accurately identify the size, location, and route of target perforators before the operative procedure. With the midline and inferior gluteal crease as reference points, the largest, most well-placed perforators with the longest vascular pedicle can be identified (Figure 2). Ideally, we choose the medial perforator closest to the inferior gluteal crease and just posterior to the gracilis muscle for ease of dissection in the supine/frog leg position. Three-dimensional MRA reconstruction allows the surgeon to visualize the placement of the perforators prior to marking (Figure 3).

Once the perforators have been selected, the patient is marked one day before surgery. Based on the preoperative imaging, a handheld Doppler probe is used to identify and mark the skin perforators (Figure 4). Typically, there are both medial and lateral perforators, but we usually favor the medial perforators because they are easier to harvest in the supine position. The medial perforator usually enters posterior to the gracilis muscle. There have been some situations in which a more posterior and lateral perforator was dominant and therefore used. The superior marking is at the gluteal fold. The inferior marking is less than 6 cm below the superior marking. The flap is designed in a crescent shape so the scar does not extend onto the visible lateral or medial thigh outside of the gluteal fold. Once the marks are drawn, we listen with a hand held doppler to identify the arterial signal.

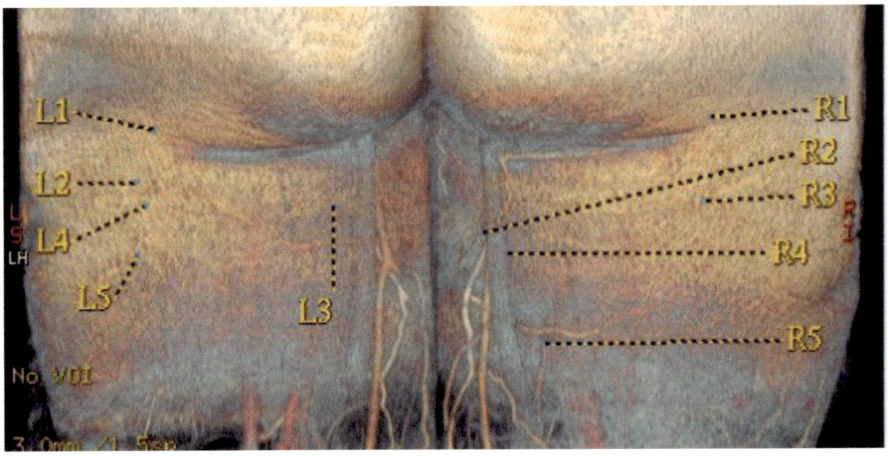

Figure 3. Three-dimensional magnetic resonance angiography (MRA) reconstruction allows the surgeon to visualize perforator placement prior to marking. The best perforator will be chosen on the basis of location and caliber.

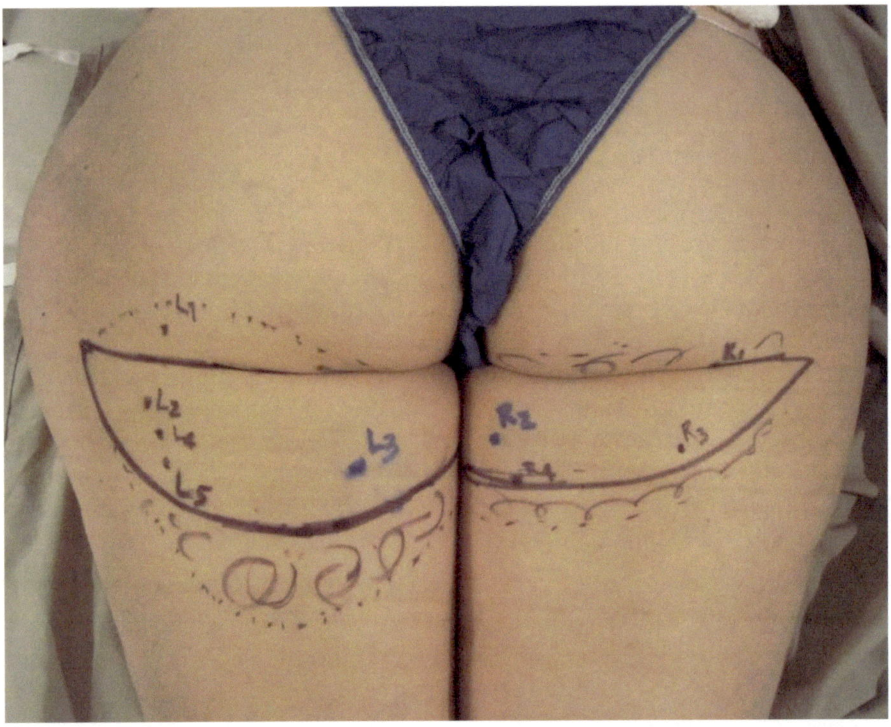

Figure 4. Once the perforators have been selected, we see the patient the day before surgery to apply the marks. Based on the preoperative imaging, the previously identified perforators are transposed onto the patient's body. A handheld Doppler probe is used to confirm and mark the skin perforators one day prior to surgery. The squiggly marks indicate additional fat that will be captured with beveling.

4. Anatomy

The posterior thigh tissue is bordered by the iliotibial tract and adductor muscles horizontally, and the gluteal fold and popliteal fossa vertically. The profunda femoris artery enters the posterior compartment of the thigh and typically gives off three main perforators. The first perforator supplies the adductor magnus and gracilis, and the second and third perforators supply the semimembranosus, biceps femoris, and vastus lateralis.

5. Surgical technique

On the day of surgery each of our patients receive 5000 units of subcutaneous heparin and perioperative intravenous antibiotics. The operation is performed under general anesthesia. Once general anesthesia is administered, the patient is prepped to include the upper thighs into the field. Sequential compression stockings are placed and wrapped with sterile towels and drapes. Flap harvest may be performed in the supine or prone position. The supine frog-leg position offers the advantage of decreased operative time because of rapid dissection from a medial approach and the lack of a need for repositioning. The prone position uses a lateral approach and maintains the possibility of conversion to a transverse upper gracilis flap if no adequate perforators are identified. When the supine approach is used, there is no specific bailout flap, and therefore preoperative imaging is essential.

When in the preferred supine position, the patient's legs are placed in a frog leg position. Using a 10-blade scalpel, the incision is made on the crescent-shaped skin island designed on the thigh down to the subcutaneous fat, and the skin and fat raised above the muscles of the inner thigh. When the most lateral markings need to be incised, the leg is placed medial to access the lateral/posterior thigh region. The leg is placed back into frog leg position and beveling inferior is performed to capture as much fat as possible. In the supine position, the fascia is entered over the gracilis muscle and the vascular pedicle is identified approximately 3 cm posterior to the gracilis muscle. Careful dissection is performed to identify the perforating branch from the profunda femoris artery which supplies the flap with blood. Staying above the fascia until the posterior border of the gracilis is identified, the fascia is incised and the perforator is found in relation to the gracilis muscle. Once the key perforator is identified, standard perforator dissection proceeds to harvest the desired pedicle length and vessel diameter (Figure 5). Creating adequate exposure to ligate the tiny branches that enter the muscle, the pedicle elongates until its caliber is consistent consistent with the internal mammary artery. It is helpful to obtain wide exposure with fish hooks and Gelpi retractors, advancing the Gelpi retractors as the dissection proceeds. The vessel is then followed back toward the main profunda artery to its parent vessel (Figure 6).

After recipient-site preparation, the anastomosis is performed. The internal mammary artery and vein are prepared in the chest and the flap is then harvested, weighed and transferred to the breast. Once on the chest, the PAP flap vessels are anastomosed to the internal mammary vessels using microsurgery. The profunda perforator vein is anastomosed to the internal

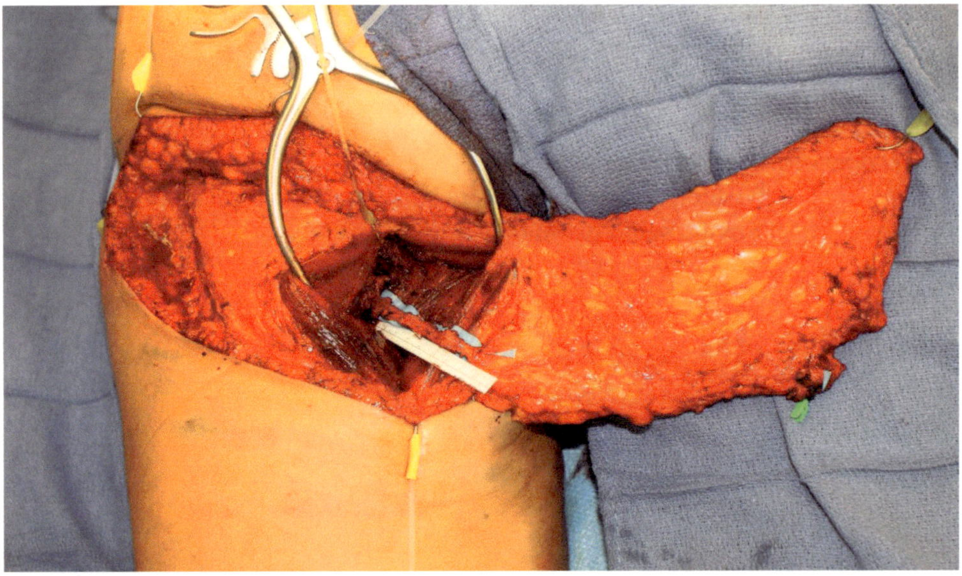

Figure 5. Careful dissection is performed to identify the perforating branch from the profunda femoris artery which supplies the flap with blood. Staying above the fascia until the posterior border of the gracilis is identified, the fascia is incised and the perforator is found in relation to the gracilis muscle. Once the key perforator is identified, standard perforator dissection proceeds to harvest the desired pedicle length and vessel diameter.

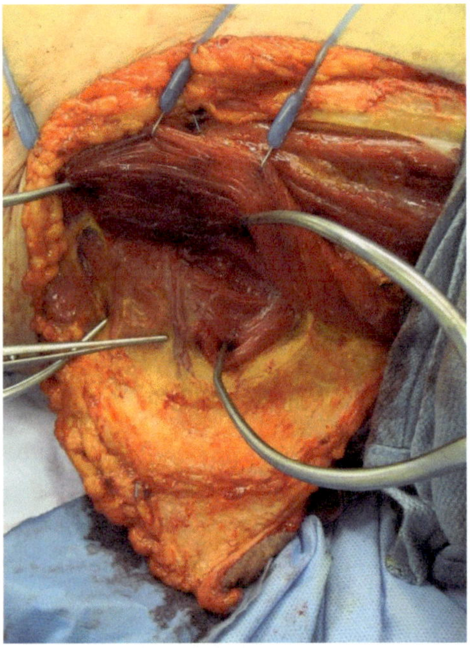

Figure 6. It is helpful to obtain adequate exposure with fish hook retractors and Gelpi retractors, advancing the Gelpi retractors as the dissection proceeds. The vessel is then followed back toward the main profunda artery to its parent vessel.

mammary vein using a venous coupler with sizes ranging from 2.0 to 3.0 mm. The artery is addressed next. Using a 9-0 nylon, the profunda artery is anastomosed to the internal mammary artery with either a continuous suture or interrupted sutures. If the flap is buried, an internal Doppler monitoring device is used. If a skin island is used, an internal Doppler device is usually unnecessary. Either way, the flap is deepithelialized and inset. After blood flow is reestablished, the flap is coned and shaped in a manner similar to the TUG flap for breast reconstruction (Figure 7).

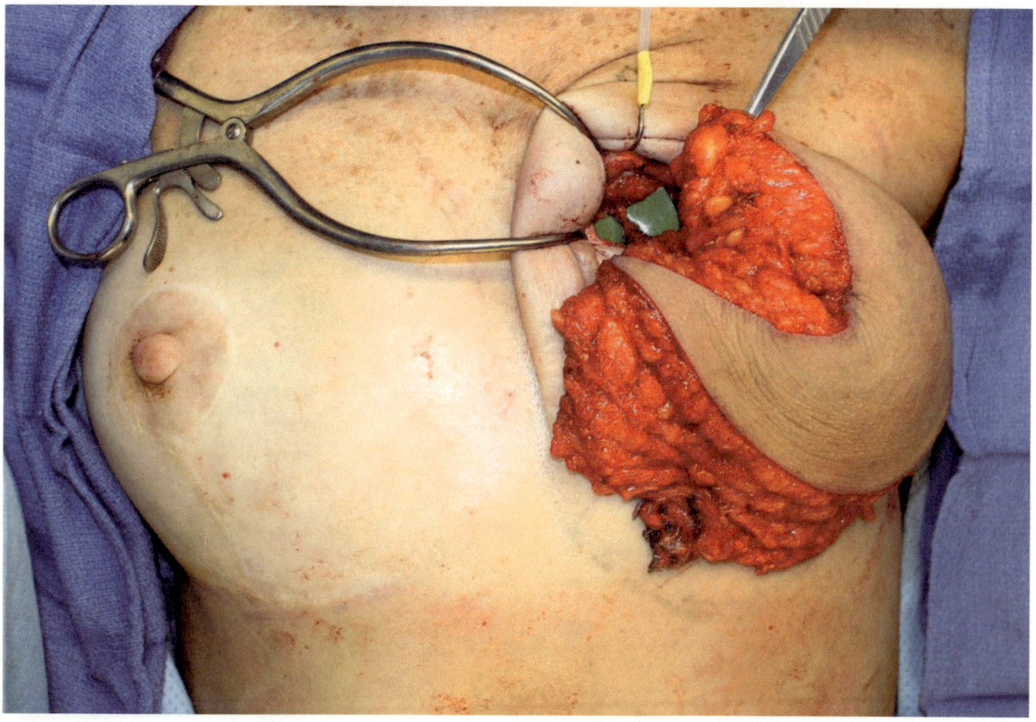

Figure 7. After blood flow is reestablished, the flap is coned and shaped in a manner similar to the TUG flap for breast reconstruction.

The donor site is closed in a multilayer fashion over a drain. Meticulous closure of the posterior thigh donor site must be performed in order to achieve primary wound healing and avoid subsequent wound dehiscence. The superior aspect of the donor site incision needs to be tacked down with 2-0 vicryl to preserve the gluteal crease and to prevent inferior migration of the scar onto the thigh. The postoperative appearance of a PAP flap breast reconstruction creates an uplifted and conical aesthetically pleasing breast shape (Figure 8). The donor site is also usually well-concealed (Figure 9).

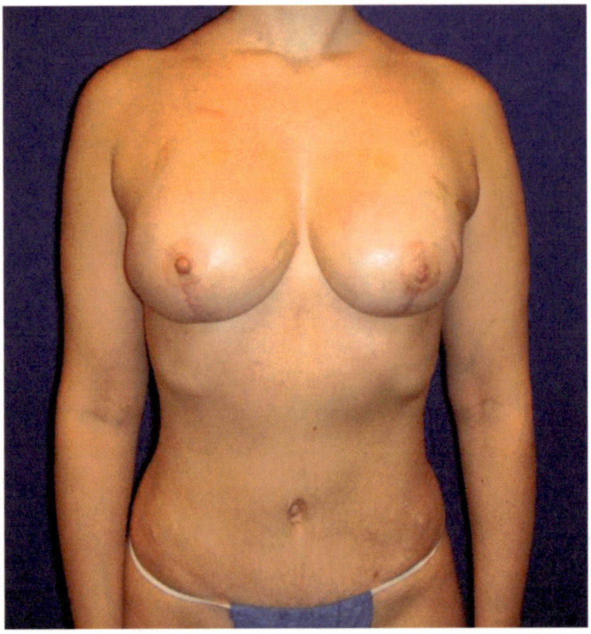

Figure 8. The postoperative appearance of a PAP flap breast reconstruction creates an uplifted and conical aesthetically pleasing breast shape.

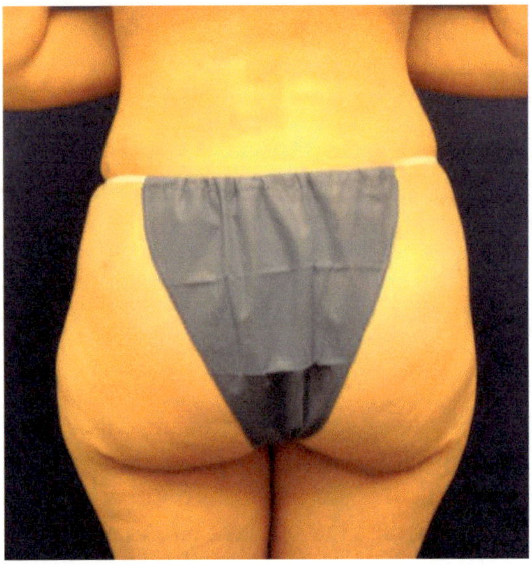

Figure 9. The donor site is also usually well-concealed.

http://dx.doi.org/10.5772/56332

6. Postoperative management

The postoperative care is similar to other perforator flaps such as the DIEP or GAP flaps. On postoperative day one, the Foley catheter, blood pressure cuff, oxygen, and intravenous fluids are discontinued. Patients may start a regular diet. Pain is usually well-controlled by oral medications. Although the patient may ambulate or sit with minimal discomfort, strenuous exercise should be avoided for 6-8 weeks. Patients usually stay in the hospital 3-4 days to monitor the blood flow into the free flap. When discharged, the patient may walk without difficulty, but some have reported temporary tightness in the posterior thigh. Other potential complications include posterior thigh numbness, donor site dehiscence, seroma, hematoma, takeback, flap loss and other potential complications of microvascular surgery.

7. Discussion

Most microsurgeons who perform autologous tissue breast reconstruction select the abdomen as their first choice in donor site. We agree with this choice; we also prefer the abdomen as our primary donor site for autologous tissue breast reconstruction. Our second choice donor site for microsurgical breast reconstruction, however, is the posterior thigh. Like the abdomen, the posterior thigh donor site does not require positioning changes during the operative procedure. The patient can remain supine for both flap harvest and inset, which minimizes the anesthesia time for the patient. Finally, patients report minimal pain at the donor site. Anecdotally, they seem to ambulate and mobilize earlier than patients who undergo abdominal flap harvest.

The advantage to the PAP flap is a natural shape with ample volume in most cases. The scar is usually well-concealed when wearing a bathing suit. The pedicle length usually ranges from 8-10 cm, and is a good size match to the internal mammary vessels. Disadvantages include possible inferior location of the perforator causing the scar to be placed lower on the thigh in a more conspicuous position. This may be revised in a secondary procedure to raise the scar so that it is camouflaged in the gluteal fold. In very large-breasted women, the posterior thigh donor site may not be adequate. In such cases, additional procedures used to obtain volume such as fat grafting or rotational flaps may also be performed at a second stage.

Developments in radiographic imaging have supported preoperative flap design and planning. The ability to identify perforators preoperatively has decreased the level of difficulty for perforator flaps. Intraoperative flap elevation is now more predictable and straightforward, which makes dissection faster and easier. Hypothetically, easier perforator flap dissection should also lead to a lower complication rate. We feel that the PAP flap is a viable technique for autologous tissue breast reconstruction that may be easier to master than the traditional GAP procedures. In conclusion, we recommend the PAP flap as a simple and reliable approach to perforator flaps for microsurgical breast reconstruction.

Author details

Constance M. Chen MD, MPH, FACS[1,2,3], Maria LoTempio MD[1,2,3] and
Robert J. Allen MD, FACS[1,3,4]

1 Plastic & Reconstructive Surgery, New York Eye & Ear Infirmary, New York, NY, USA

2 Plastic & Reconstructive Surgery, Lenox Hill Hospital, New York, NY, USA

3 Plastic & Reconstructive Surgery, New York Downtown Hospital, New York, NY, USA

4 Institute of Reconstructive Plastic Surgery, NYU Medical Center, New York, NY, USA

Authors declare no financial interest or commercial association with information submitted in manuscript. No products, devices, or drugs were used or identified in the manuscript.

References

[1] Hurwitz, D. J. Closure of a large defect of the pelvic cavity by an extended compound myocutaneous flap based on the inferior gluteal artery. *Br J Plast Surg* (1980)., 33, 256-261.

[2] Angrigiani, C, Grilli, D, & Thorne, C. H. The adductor flap: a new method for transferring posterior and medial thigh skin. *Plast Reconstr Surg* (2001)., 107, 1725-1731.

[3] Song, Y. G, Chen, G. Z, & Song, Y. L. The free thigh flap: a new free flap concept based on the septocutaneous artery. *Br J Plast Surg* (1984)., 37, 149-159.

[4] Saint-Cyr, M, Schaverien, M, Arbique, G, et al. Three- and four-dimensional computed tomographic angiography and venography for the investigation of the vascular anatomy and perfusion of perforator flaps. *Plast Reconstr Surg* (2008)., 121, 772-780.

[5] Alonso-Burgos, A, Garcia-Tutor, E, Bastarrika, G, et al. Preoperative planning of deep inferior epigastric artery perforator flap reconstruction with multislice-CT angiography: imaging findings and initial experience. *J Plast Reconstr Aesthet Surg* (2006)., 59, 585-593.

[6] Rosson, G. D, Williams, C. G, Fishman, E. K, et al. D CT angiography of abdominal wall vascular perforators to plan DIEAP flaps. *Microsurgery* (2007)., 27, 641-646.

[7] Neil-Dwyer, J. G, Ludman, C. N, Schaverien, M, et al. Magnetic resonance angiography in preoperative planning of deep inferior epigastric artery perforator flaps. *J Plast Reconstr Aesthet Surg*(2008).

[8] Chernyak, V, Rozenblit, A. M, Greenspun, D. T, et al. Breast Reconstruction with Deep Inferior Epigastric Artery Perforator Flap: 3.T Gadolinium-enhanced MR Imaging for Preoperative Localization of Abdominal Wall Perforators. *Radiology*(2008). , 0.

[9] Tuinder, S, Van Der Hulst, R, Lataster, A, et al. Superior gluteal artery perforator flap based on septal perforators: preliminary study. *Plast Reconstr Surg* 122: 146e-148e, (2008).

Chapter 11

The Use of Proximal and Distal Ends of Internal Mammary Arteries and Veins as the Recipient Vessels for Combined Breast and Chest Wall Reconstruction with Free Bipedicled TRAM or DIEP Flap

Lan Mu and Senkai Li

Additional information is available at the end of the chapter

http://dx.doi.org/10.5772/56612

1. Introduction

Breast reconstruction, after the traditional radical mastectomy, is particularly challenging for a plastic surgeon. For these patients, not only the breast but subclavian and anterior axillary fold deformities need to be reconstructed. The TRAM flap including zone IV is usually required to be used for this complex reconstruction. The design of a TRAM FLAP with bipedicled deep inferior epigastric vessels would insure the perfusion of whole flap. However, it is difficult to find two sets healthy recipient vessels since the thorocodorsal vessels are usually damaged during axillary dissection or radiation therapy.

Fujino first reported the use of the internal mammary artery (IMA) as the recipient artery in breast reconstruction with superior gluteal microvascular free flap in 1975 [1]. The technique of use of the IMA as a recipient artery was modified and popularized by Shaw (1983) [3]. In 1994 [5], Blondeel and colleagus reported a refinement of breast reconstruction by the use of a bilateral deep inferior epigastric perforator flap in one woman with a vertical infraumbilical scar, in which the two arterial pedicles were anastomosed to the proximal IMA by end-end and end-side patterns. However, the procedure is complicated and technically demanding.

Conventionally, the proximal ends of internal mammary artery and vein (IMA, IMV) are usually used as the recipient vessels in breast reconstruction with free flaps. Since 1980s, we have used both the proximal and distal ends of internal mammary vessels as recipient vessels for end-end anastomoses to the vessels of the bipedicled flap and proved that the distal IMA with retrograde flow could be used as one of the supplying arteries for a second anastomoses in the breast reconstruction. [6 - 11]

This chapter will describe the anatomy, arterial pressures of antegrade and retrograde flows of IMA, and clinical applications of the use of proximal and distal IMAs as recipient arteries for breast reconstruction with bipedicled TRAM or DIEP flap from our experimental and clinical studies.

2. Anatomic study

Materials and Methods: The cadavers (3 males and 7 females) fixed with formalin were used in the study. Sixteen sides of abdomino-thoracic wall were dissected and four sides were made into morphological transparent specimen [8]. How the vessels were running, the relationship of vessels and the vessels' diameter were recorded by photo and measured by vernier caliper.

Results: 1) The IMA was found originating from the subclavian artery, then running along the sternum, and segmentally connecting to the intercostal arteries from the aorta. It was divided into two ends at the sixth intercostal space as the deep superior epigastric and musculophrenic arteries. The musculophrenic artery was found linked to the abdominal aorta by anastomosed with superior and inferior phrenic arteries. This is the anatomic basis of distal end of IMA as one recipient supply artery, which means that, if the IMA was cut off near the third intercostal space during the clinical procedure, the retrograde IMA flowed distally from the extensive anastomoses among the intercostal, musculophrenic and deep superior epigastric arteries.[Fig.1].

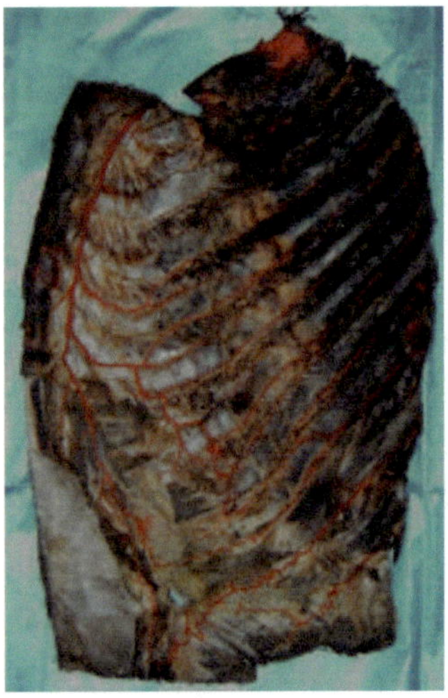

Figure 1. The anastomoses among DSEA,m.p.a. and i.c.a;

http://dx.doi.org/10.5772/56612

2) There were two accompanying veins found with communicating branches. No valve had been found inside the internal mammary vein, intercostal vein and communicating branches. The IMV retrogradely drained distally from two direct ways, via the communicating branches to the other IMV and then to the subclavian vein and via the intercostal vein to the posterior intercostal vein and then to the vena azygos [Fig.2].

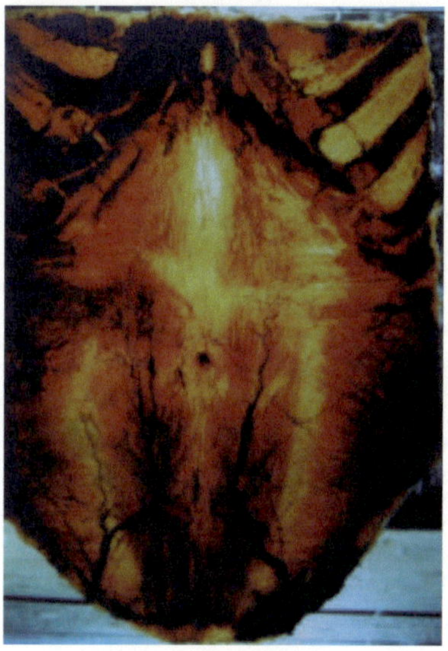

Figure 2. Transparent Morphology specimen of the Thoracoabdominal Wall

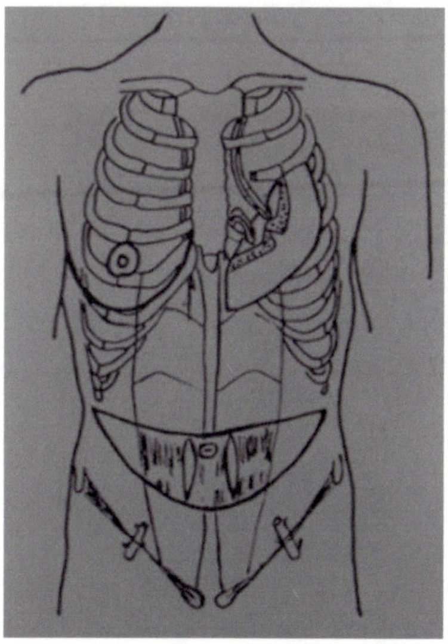

Figure 3. Operative Technique Demonstration

3) The mean diameter and standard deviation of the IMA at the third intercostal space was 2.79 ± 0.15 mm. The diameter of the IMV ranges from 1.50 to 3.94 mm.

4) The Deep Inferior Epigastric Artery (DIEA) was found originating from the external iliac artery under the middle of the inguinal ligment, and then running up medially between peritoneal and transverse abdominal fascia. Under the posterior sheath of rectus abdominal muscle above the semicimular line, it ran up inside the muscle, and connected with the deep superior epigastric artery (DSEA) with "spirial chock anastomosis" at the nearest tendinous intersection above the umbilicus.

5) There were two accompanying veins to the DIEA. The mean diameter of the larger vein was 2.14 ± 0.05mm, while the DIEA was 2.42 ± 0.06mm at their original points of inguen [9].

3. Pressures in a canine model

Materials and Methods: Ten dogs (weight 6-8kg) were given general anesthesia and monitored. After the anterior thoracic wall was opened along the middle line, in the third intercostal space, the pressures at the two ends (proximal and distal) of IMA were measured in twenty sides (both right and left sides using Eight Channel Physiologic Instrument 6400 Japan).

Results: The mean pressure at distal end was 86/77 ± 0.02 mmHg (left sides) and 87/78mmHg ± 0.03(right sides). It was 63-71% of the proximal end ($p<0.05$). There is no statistical significance ($p>0.05$) between the pressure of left side and that of right side [10].

4. Arterial pressures measurement in patients

Patients and Methods: Between 1988 and 2010, 50 cases of unilateral breast reconstructions were performed using the free TRAM, muscle sparing TRAM or DIEP flaps including bilateral deep inferior epigastric vessels as the pedicles. Both pedicles were anastomosed to the two ends of internal mammary vessels (proximal and distal) all by end-end. Here, the procedures of the arterial pressures from both proximal and distal and skin Perfusion Units on different points of flap were measured in two cases. Case 1: A thirty-six-year-old woman was hospitalized for right breast reconstruction, five years after radical mastectomy. Case 2: A fifty-year-old woman wanted her left breast reconstructed, eleven years after radical mastectomy.

4.1. Surgical technique

Pre-operative planning: The diameter and flowmeter of IMA, IMV, DIEA, DIEV were checked by colour Duplex scanning (Acuson 128*P). The flaps were measured 13 cm in height and 42 cm in width. From the middle line, four points were marked cranially and laterally from each side for the measurement of the Perfusion Units. The pressures of both sides DIEA were measured with the same method described above before they were transected.

Preparing of IMA, IMV and the measurement of pressures: 2 cm length of 3rd or 4th rib cartilage was removed. About 4 cm of IMA, IMV was exposed well. Before transection, a needle that had been connected with Multifunction Monitor (HP 6112 U.S.A.) was punched inside the middle point of IMA. The IMA was clamped at the proximal end for pressure measurement of the distal end and vice versa.

Skin Perfusion Units with bilateral DIEA, DIEV pedicles: The Perfusion Units on different points of TRAM flap were measured with Laser Doppler Flowmeter (PEREFLUX PF3 Sweden) with different conditions: before flap incision; on both pedicles and with right or left pedicle only.

Preoperative MDCT: Since 2006, *MDCT* has been used to help pre-operation planning, harvesting the perforaters. Both donor site (deep inferior epigastric artery and vein) and recipient site (internal mammary atery and vein) can be evaluated. [12]

Vascular Anastomosis: After transection of the pedicle, the flap was weighed, photographed and transferred to the chest wall. The flap was bent 90° so that the donor vessels close to the recipient vessels are without tension. The flap was then fixed to the chest wall skin. Next, four conventional end-to-end anastomoses were performed among the arteries and vein. The immediate rate of blood flow of the arteries anastomosis site was measured with Electromagnetic Flowmeter (3200 Japan). Then, the PU was monitored under different conditions.

Shaping of the breast: With bilateral pedicles (two arteries and two veins) the whole flap could be used safely. The flap was positioned in a U-shape, lateral part of the flap ending up laterally de-epithelialised and placed under the local flap to recreate a natural looking anterior axillary fold.

Post-operation monitoring and follow-up: The Perfusion Units on different points of TRAM flap were measured from the first to seventh day, and on the fourteenth day after the operation.

4.2. Results

The flap survived 100% with satisfied contour. The two anastomosis sites were followed up by colour Doplex scanning (Acuson 128*P) five years after the operation on one patient. Both, the flowmeter of the proximal and distal anastomosis stomas were similar. One flap failed due to the artery thrombosis during and after operation, despite several re-anastomosis. 48 hours after the operation, the flap was removed and skin graft was performed. Every part of remaining 49 flaps survived completely with satisfied breast contour.

4.3. Typical cases

Case 3: A fifty-six-year-old female, 12 years after the radical mastectomy and radiation therapy. Verticle and long incision scar was noticed. Not only that the left breast was lost, but serious deformity of chest wall including an unstable scar in part below clavian, axillary fold and axillary area was noticed. Her right breast was big and a matched felt reconstructive breast was desired. Middle vertical infraumbilical caesarean scar was noticed on her abdominal wall. Free bilateral deep inferior epigastric vessels TRAM flaps (12*42cm*), anastomosed to the two ends of internal mammary vessels (proximal and distal) all by end-end was performed for left breast reconstruction. Upper and lateral part of the flap were de-epithelialised and placed under the local flap to recreate a natural looking chest wall and anterior axillary fold. Six months after the operation, nipple reconstruction with modified "arrow" flap was made. [Fig 4,5]

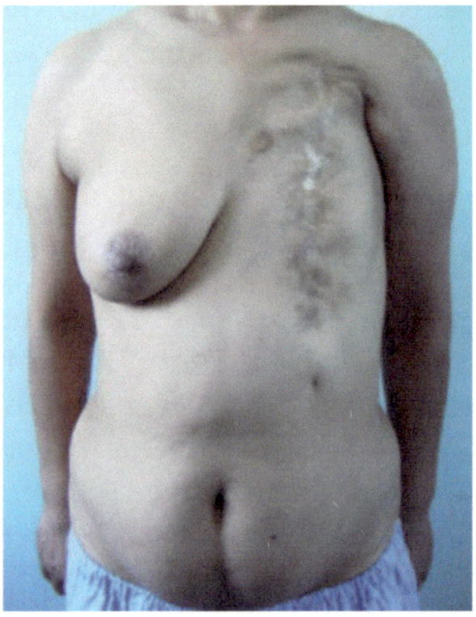

Figure 4. Pre-operation

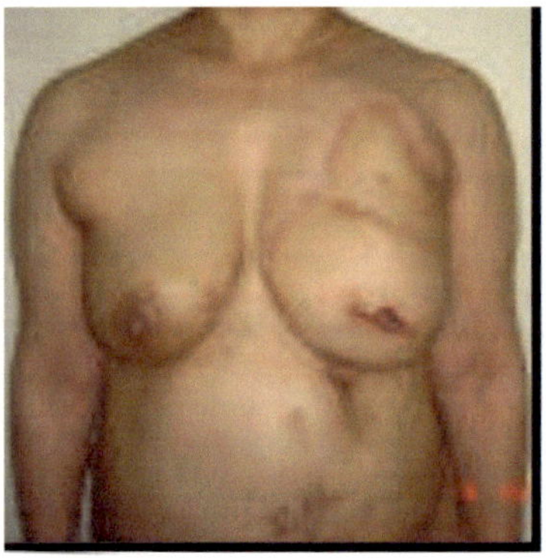

Figure 5. Post-operation

Typical case 4: A fourty-two-year-old female, five years after the left modified radical mastectomy and radiation therapy. Her right breast was big, with abdominal wall not thick enough having a transverse Caesarean scar.

Free bilateral deep inferior epigastric vessels DIEP flaps (10*30cm*), anastomosed to the two ends of internal mammary vessels (proximal and distal), all by end-end were performed.

Upper and lateral part of the flap were de-epithelialised and placed under the local flap to recreate a natural looking chest wall and anterior axillary fold. New nipple was reconstructed with modified "arrow" flap, and the areolar was made by a tattoo. [Fig 6,7]

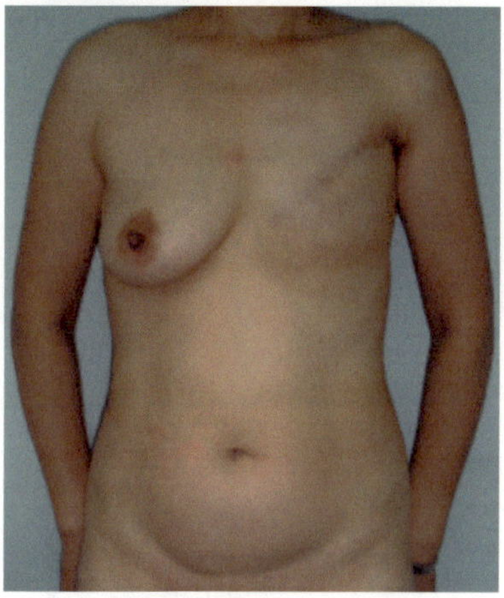

Figure 6. Pre-operation

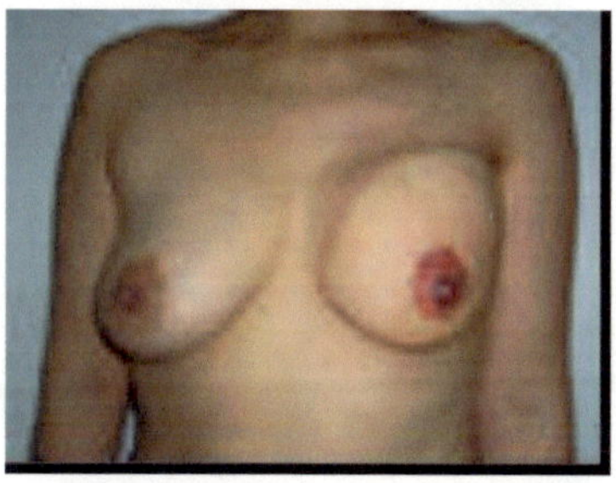

Figure 7. Post-operation

Typical case 5: A fifty-one-year-old old female, ten years after a radical mastectomy and radiation therapy with verticle scar. Even though her right breast was big, her abdominal wall was thin. Free bilateral deep inferior epigastric vessels DIEP flaps (9*28cm*), anastomosed to the two ends of internal mammary vessels (proximal and distal),all by end-end were performed. Upper and lateral part of the flap were de-epithelialised and placed under the local flap to recreate a natural looking chest wall and anterior axillary fold. New nipple was reconstructed with modified "arrow" flap, the areolar was made by tattoo, bilateral for symmetry [Fig 8,9,10]

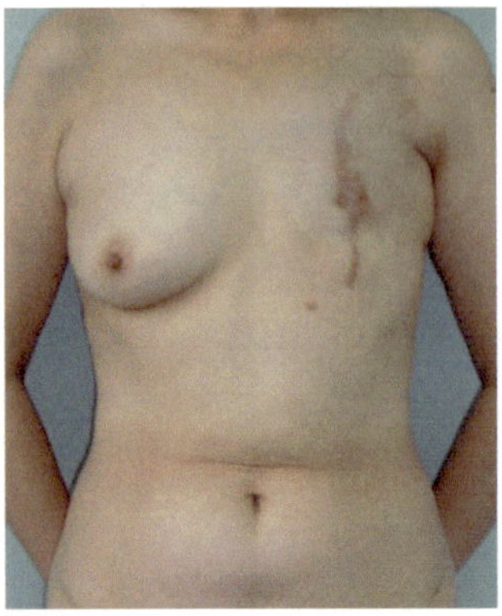

Figure 8. Pre-operation

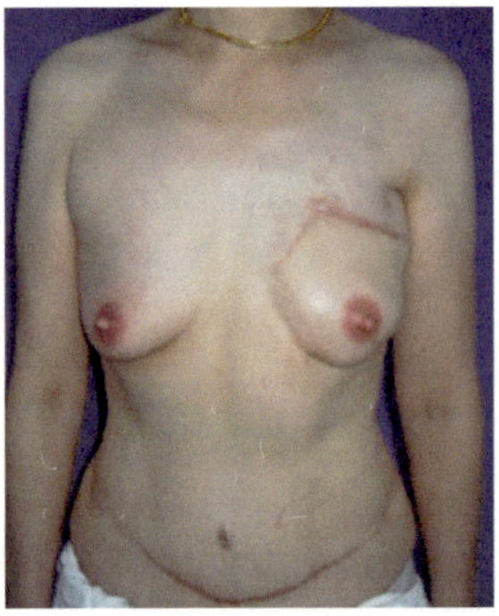

Figure 9. Post-operation

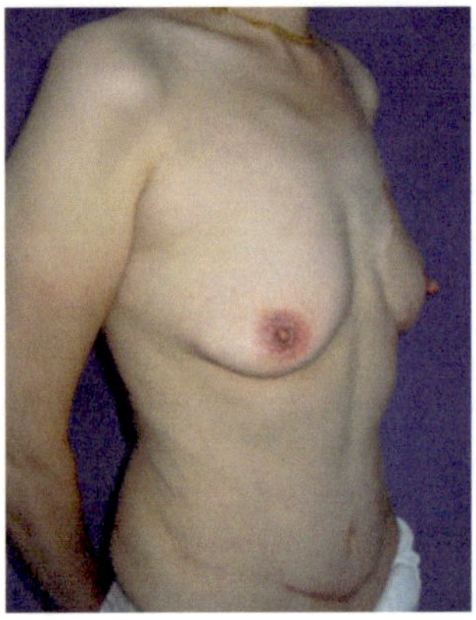

Figure 10. Post-operation

5. Discussion

Owing to its anatomic position, the internal mammary artery (IMA) has been popular in coronary artery myocardial revascularization since 1968 [13]. Studies on its histology, histochemistry, immunohistochemistry, morphology and hemodynamics have shown that the IMA has many advantages such as: thin intima with endothelium-derived relaxing factor (EDRF), fine compliance, relative freedom from arteriosclerosis, and decreased thrombosis or arteriostenosis after coronary bypass operation. Both, the early and late patency in patients are higher than that with vein bypass. In order to reduce the anastomotic tension, some authors proposed that the coronary artery myocardial revascularization could be made by means of retrograde IMA flow. So far, this theory has been only proved to be feasible in animal experiments by Folts (1981) [14] and Wang Zheng(1987) [15]. Paletta (1994) [16] described the extensive anastomoses among the IMA, DSEA, intercostal arteries, musculophrenic arteries in dogs. It is similar to that of human being.

This chapter confirmed the feasibility of using the distal ends of the IMA as recipient vessels for free flaps simultaneous by using the proximal ends. In patients, the pressure at distal end was 66 and 58 mmHg. It was 75-77% of the pressure of the proximal ends. When the flap was supplied only by distal ends of IMA, IMV, the Perfusion Unit of ipsilateral flap was 4.0-6.0, and the Perfusion Unit of contralateral side of flap was 1.4-1.8. When the flap was supplied only by proximal ends of IMA, IMV, the perfusion unit of ipsilateral flap was 3.0-15.0, and the perfusion unit of contralateral side of flap was 1.8-2.1. When the flap was supplied by distal and proximal ends of IMA, IMV simultaneously, the Perfusion Unit of flap with distal side was 4.0-6.5, and the perfusion unit of flap with proximal side was 4.0-16.0. The blood flow at the two anastomoses sites were similar to each other in a later stage (measured five years after the operation). This indicated that, at the beginning, the pressure of the distal end of IMA are lower than the pressure of the proximal end. However, over the time, they have reached a balance. The vascularity in all territories of revascularized bipedicled (proximal and distal) TRAM flap is very good. 49 cases survived completely with satisfied breast contour.

This technique has been popularized in China [17,18],Canada [19],U.S.A. [20],UK and Italy [21].

6. Conclusion

Free bipedicled deep inferior epigastric TRAM /DIEP flap is needed for radical mastectomy deformity or big breasts and can be performed on thin patients or patients with vertical midline scar.

Internal mammary vessels can provid double recipient vessels (proximal and distal ends) for anastomosis to both DIEA, DIEV anastomosis.

Our clinical and experimental studies showed that the distal IMA has reduced perfusion pressure but it provides excellent flow and flap perfusion. This allows reliable use of two pedicles for the survival of the entire flap.

Acknowledgements

We wish to thank Dr. William W Shaw, Dr. Robert J Allen and Dr. Feng Zhang for their refinements in this chapter and their kind suggestions.

Author details

Lan Mu* and Senkai Li

*Address all correspondence to: Lanhu_mu@yahoo.com

Aesthetic and Reconstructive Surgery Center of Breast,Plastic Surgery Hospital, Peking Union Medical College, Chinese Academy of Medical Sciences, China

References

[1] Fujino T,Harashina T,Aoyagi F.Reconstruction for aplasia of the breast and pectoral region by microvascular transfer of a free flap from the buttock.Plast reconstr Surg 1975;56:178-81.

[2] Fujino T, Harashina T, Enomoto K. Primary breast reconstruction after a standard radical mastectomy by a free flap transfer. Plast Reconstr Surg.1976; 58: 371-5.

[3] Shaw W W. Breast reconstruction by superior gluteal microvascular free flaps without silicon implants. Plast Reconstr Surg.1983; 72: 490-501.

[4] Senkai, Li, Yangqun Li, Jun Xu, et al: Breast reconstruction with free superior gluteal microvascular flap (one case report.) Chin J Plast Surg Burns.1990;6(3):228- 229.

[5] Blondeel PN, Boeckx WD. Refinements in free flap breast reconatruction:the free bilateral deep inferior epigastric perforator flap anastomosed to the internal mammary artery. Br J Plast Surg.1994 Oct.47(7):495-501.

[6] Lanhua Mu, Jun Xu,Yuanbo Liu, et al.Breast Reconstrction with the Free Bipedicled Inferior TRAM or DIEP Flaps by Anastomosis to the Proximal and Distal Ends of the Internal Mammmary Vessels. Seminars in Plastic Surgery.2002,16(1):61-67.

[7] Senkai Li, Lanhua Mu, Yangqun Li, et al.Breast Reconstrction with the Free Bipedicled Inferior TRAM Flap by Anastomosis to the Proximal and Distal Ends of the Internal Mammmary Vessels. J Reconstru Microsurg 2002,18(3):161-167.

[8] Lanhua Mu, Yiping Yan, Senkai Li et al.Transparent Morphology of the Thoracoabdominal Wall.J Reconstru Microsurg 2001, 17(8):611-614.

[9] Lanhua Mu,Yan Yiping,Li Senkai,et al. The anatomy study of superior and inferior TRAM. Chinese Journal of Plastic Surgery and Burns.1998;14(2):122-123.

[10] Lanhua Mu, Li Senkai, Li Yangqun, et al. Pressure measurement of the Two Ends (proximal and distal) of Internal Mammary Artery. Chinese Journal of Plastic Surgery and Burns.1999;15(6):427.

[11] Lanhua Mu,Li Senkai,Li Yangqun, et al. Breast reconstruction with TRAM by anastomasesed to the internal mammary artery.Chinese Journal of Plastic Surgery and Burns.1997;(13)2:100-101.

[12] Minqiang Xin,Lanhua Mu,Jie Luan et al. The Value of Mutidector Row CT Angiography for Pre-operative Planning of Breast Reconstruction with Deep Inferior Epigastric Arterial Perforator Flaps. The British Journal of Radiology, 2010 ,83:40-43.

[13] Green GE, Sterzer SH, Reppert EH. Coronary artery bypass grafts. Ann Thorac Surg 1968;5:443-46. Cardioangiol.1995 Jan-Feb;43(1-2):21-7.

[14] Folts JD, Gallagher KO, Kroncke GM, et al. Myocardial revascularization of the canine circumflex coronary artery using retrograde internal mammary artery flow without cardiopulmonary bypass. Ann Thorac Surg.1981:31:21-7.

[15] Zhen Wang, Yuanzhong Shen, LiangHua Zhang,.et al. Experimental study of bypass surgery with retrograte flow of internal mammary artery anastomosed to right coronary artery .1987;4(2):75-7.

[16] Paletta CE, Vogler G, Freeman B. Viability of the trctus abdominis muscule following internal mammary artery ligation. Plast Reconatr Surg 1993;92:234.

[17] Dong Jiasheng, Wang Tao, FENG Reizheng, et al, Breast Reconstrction by Using Transverse Rectus Abdominals Flap with with Deep Inferior Epigastric Perforator (DIEP) .Chinese Journal of Tissue Engineering and Reconstructive Surgery.2005,1(3): 154-156.

[18] Lanhua Mu. Needing a large DIEAP flap for unilateral breast reconstruction: Double-pedicle flap and Unipedicle flap with additional venous discharge. Chinese Microsurgery 2010, 30 (2): 111-117.

[19] Zenn MR, Heitmann C. Extended TRAM flap: feasibility study on fresh human cadavers. Ann Plast Surg. 2003 Mar;50(3):256-62.

[20] Bergeron L, Tang M, Morris SF.A review of vascular injection techniques for the study of perforator flaps. Plast Reconstr Surg. 2006 May;117(6):2050-7.

[21] Marzia Salgarello,Liliana Barone-Adesi,Marcella Sturla, et al, Corespondence to Lanhua Mu. Needing a large DIEAP flap for unilateral breast reconstruction: Double-pedicle flap and Unipedicle flap with additional venous discharge. Microsurgery 2010, 30 (2): 111-117.

Chapter 12

Getting Out of a Tight Spot in Breast Reconstruction — Salvage and Saving Techniques for DIEP, SIEA, and Lymphatic Flaps

Rebecca Studinger

Additional information is available at the end of the chapter

http://dx.doi.org/10.5772/56642

1. Introduction

In performing perforator flaps, there are several obstacles that can arise that can limit your success. In this chapter, I will discuss some of the common problems that can occur with flaps. These can be difficult to navigate and are not always clearly illustrated in books or journal articles. However, some of the ways to successfully address these issues have been through experience and through advice from other experts.

1.1. Patient selection

When evaluating patients for perforator flap reconstruction, there are certain things to keep in mind. In the forefront is the assumption that most patients are candidates, but their overall health must evaluated. A large population of patients with breast cancer are medically stable and the ones that are seeking tissue reconstruction usually fall into this category. Multiple factors should be explored to aid in the selection of a microsurgical flap patient. (Table 1)

The patient's overall health should be taken into evaluation. A younger population of breast cancer patients is often seeking reconstruction with perforator flaps. Usually, there are no other medical problems present. If this is the case, then nutritional, exercise level, and lifestyle habits can help optimize outcomes. Those that maintain healthy eating with a balanced diet often heal more quickly with fewer wound complications. Exercise can help prepare a patient for the rigors of a surgical recovery. It is helpful to determine if the patient's lifestyle habits or work/home situation can accommodate the time and postoperative restrictions that may apply. A patient who is thriving is more likely to do well postoperatively.

Patient Selection	
• Overall health	• Psychology
• Age	• Grieving process/increased susceptibility to illness
• Conditions for anesthesia	• Ability to follow direction
• Cardiac	• Home situation
• Cardiac function permits surgery (i.e. ejection fraction)	• Resilience vs. overwhelmed or overanxious
• Able to tolerate high fluid volumes	• Patience/Understands may be a multistep process
• Able to maintain blood pressure without the use of intraoperative pressors	• Other relative risk factors
• Lung	• Diabetes
• Able to ventilate/intubate easily	• Hypertension
• No presence of pulmonary process that would inhibit large fluid volumes	• Obesity
• Conditions for flap	• Radiation
• Absence of clotting disorders	• Chemotherapy timing
• Atherosclerotic disease	• History of multiple infections
• IV access issues	
• Smoking	
• Absence of tobacco use for 3 months prior	
• Absence of nicotine use for 3 months prior	

Table 1. Factors to be addressed in patient selection for breast reconstruction with free flaps.

The age of a patient may or may not play a large factor into surgical decision making. A person of advanced age may not be able to tolerate a flap reconstruction due to other medical issues. Some surgeons will have a mandatory cutoff of age, for example 65 years, in order to streamline the screening process. There are always exceptions to this rule, and plenty examples can be made of patients who are older than 65, being in better health than some 35 year olds. Age is a relative factor in patient selection.

There are anesthetic conditions that should be evaluated prior to surgery. These mainly include cardiac and lung functions. Patients should have preoperative cardiac clearance prior to surgery. Occasionally young patients with breast cancer have had cardiotoxic chemotherapy, and will not tolerate microsurgery. In having clearance assessed, a patient who may be a candidate for other procedures may not necessarily be one for a flap, knowing that fluid loading is the mainstay of cardiac output in microsurgery and not vasoconstricting inotropes. This is not always clear to physicians who are providing cardiac clearance, so a discussion with them or their primary care physician can be vital in understanding this situation. [1, 2]

Pulmonary screening questions can be useful to determine if a patient is able to oxygenate well, has a good intubation history, and is able to handle fluid volumes. Maintaining oxygen

http://dx.doi.org/10.5772/56642

saturation post procedure increases the viability of the flap. Adequate pulmonary excursion is helpful for relief of postoperative atelectasis and prevention of pneumonia. It is helpful to have a smooth extubation after a case finishes to decrease pressure spikes and possible bleeding. Patients with a history of a difficult airway can alert you to possible complications in wake up. Patients who have a diminished pulmonary function may run into difficulties with large fluid volumes leading to postoperative flap or patient compromise.

Bleeding and clotting disorders are helpful to know in patient selection. Both abnormalities can affect the success of the flap. Based on the degree of severity, both can be accommodated for with the aid of a hematologist. If there is a family or personal history of either of these conditions, then a preoperative consultation should be obtained. Laboratory tests such as CBC, PTT, INR, fibrinogen levels for bleeding and protein S and protein C, antithrombin III, Factor V leidin, prothrombin 20210A, antiphospholipid Ab, and homocysteine levels can be checked to diagnose a hypercoaguable state. (Table 2) [3]

Coagulation Disorders
• Coagulation-promoting conditions
– Procoagulantafibrinogenemia/dysfibrinogenemia
– Protein C deficiency
– Protein S deficiency
– Antithrombin III deficiency
– Factor V Leiden deficiency
– Activated protein C resistance (aPCR)
– DIC
• Coagulation-impeding conditions
– Anticoagulant afibrinogenemia/dysfibrinogenemia
– Factor V deficiency
– Factor VII deficiency
– Factor X deficiency
– Factor XI deficiency
– Factor XII deficiency
– Factor XIII deficiency
– Hemophilia A
– Hemophilia B

Table 2. Coagulation disorders to keep in mind prior to flap performance. (3)

Diseased blood vessels with atherosclerosis and calcifications can make anastomoses of the vessels difficult. It can also be a cause for a later failure with occlusion of the anastomosis. A strong history of vascular disease may be an indication to not perform the surgery. A personal or strong family history of coronary arterial disease may be a reason to select axillary vessels rather than the internal mammary arteries.

A poor peripheral vascular supply does not immediately indicate poor internal vessels. The presence of poor peripheral vessels in the breast cancer population can sometimes be explained by exposure to chemotherapy or multiple venipunctures. If the patient still has a chemotherapy port in place, this can be useful for emergency access throughout the patient's hospital stay. Other central vascular access routes can be predetermined if peripheral access is a known problem.

Tobacco use has been shown to increase complications in microsurgical flap procedures. For breast reconstruction, smoking has been shown to increase donor site complications as well as increased complications in mastectomy skin flaps during immediate reconstruction. Cessation of smoking with a delayed reconstruction has been shown to help decrease these complications. Differences in anastomotic failure have not been shown to be significant. Tobacco cessation at least 4 weeks prior to surgery has been shown to help decrease the risk. Those with an extensive history of smoking are more likely to have complications (10 pack year or greater). Nicotine tests (urine cotinen tests) can be performed to assess if the patient has stopped smoking. These are easy to perform in the office. If the patient is taking nicotine supplements, it can create a positive result. [4, 5, 6, 7]

The psychological/emotional state of the patient should also be assessed. This can be done rather informally in the office by observing the patient's affect, interactions and response to questions. If there is strong concern that the patient is in a state of severe depression or other illness, a psychiatric evaluation should be performed.

The diagnosis of breast cancer comes with a grieving period for patients. This may happen immediately or delayed. When people are in a state of bereavement, their immune system can be compromised, lending them to a poor healing condition. [8, 9, 10] The patient's ability to understand and cope with a possible surgical complication can be crucial to the success of the flap. Their ability to follow direction, anxiety level, and possible resilience needs to be gauged. Breast reconstruction is a multistep process which some patients can find overwhelming.

Oftentimes patients are in a state of emotional flux, grieving about a recent cancer diagnosis or the loss of a breast. This is sometimes seen as a good opportunity to do reconstruction with a tissue transfer to decrease psychological stress. I have found, however, that patients who have gone through the entire cancer process tend to do remarkably well, if not better overall, than their immediate reconstruction cohorts. This is not always the case of course and there are many different views on immediate reconstruction versus delayed, but I have moved from a position of immediate is always less traumatic to now screening my patients when they come in initially to see how emotionally fit they seem to be.

A lot of times delayed reconstruction patients are more compliant and will already have a good support system in place partly due to having the experience from prior mastectomy surgery and treatment for cancer. When doing immediate reconstruction, it can sometimes be difficult to find out about home life and the patient's current psychological state. Some studies show that patients in a state of grieving have a vulnerability to physical illness and this can sometimes predict poor adjustment post surgically. If the patient is incredibly overwhelmed already and appears to be unable to handle any more stress than they are already in, I would recommend starting with a tissue expander reconstruction. The potential for a loss of a flap or post op complications with a tissue reconstruction might be too much for them to bear. A study by Metcalfe et al. looked at the psychosocial functioning of women up to one year later with no significant difference between those with immediate, delayed or no reconstruction. [11]

For other health complications such as diabetes, as long as the condition is under control there should be minimal complications. Complications associated with diabetes can be related to wound healing. It can also be associated with poor vascularity. Hypertension can also be an indication of damaged vessels, depending on the length and severity of the hypertension. Postoperative pressure management and prevention of bleeding can be challenging in this situation.

Patients who are overweight can be candidates for flap reconstruction. In fact, Garvey et al. found that obese patients do better with tissue reconstruction than they do with implant reconstruction. [12] That being said, obese patients are prone to more complications and failure with flap reconstructions than an ideal weight population. [13] Sometimes patients who are larger have larger vessels to work with as well which can help with anastomoses.

Prior radiation is usually a reason to perform a free flap reconstruction. For breast cancer patients, this may be more of an issue with skin availability rather than the availability of recipient vessels, especially if they are internal mammary arteries. Patients that need postoperative radiation and desire immediate reconstruction may benefit more from tissue expander reconstruction until the radiation is finished, and then they can bridge to tissue reconstruction. This preserves the reconstructed tissue from radiation damage, and allows for reconstruction throughout the process. Implants do not necessarily work well with radiation, and so fully expanded breast skin prior to radiation may increase complications as the skin changes.

Patients with a history of tissue expander and implant reconstruction with multiple infections may have difficult recipient vessels dissections as well. This can be an important part of preoperative planning, in order to come up with a backup plan for recipient vessels.

2. Preoperative imaging

Currently, the trend has moved to preoperative imaging to aid in the planning of perforator flap reconstruction. MRI, CTA, Lymphoscintigraphy study, ultrasound, doppler and nuclear medicine are all very useful in helping to determine if a patient will be a good candidate. MRI can image on several planes with no radiation. CTA's have clear images which are excellent for evaluating the body in vessel reconstruction. Nuclear medicine helps with functional tracing of lymphatics. MRI can give functional with additional structural and physical characteristics of lymphatics. [14-19]

The use of preoperative imaging has become a mainstay for many practitioners of perforator flaps. Initially, a handheld Doppler to mark out the perforator signals was a useful way to help assess the presence of a perforator. However, the location of a perforator signal and the location of the actual perforator could vary immensely, and therefore, the limitation to finding the perforator of choice. The trend toward preoperative imaging has helped in intraoperative planning, patient selection and execution of the flap.

2.1. MRI

MRI studies have been very useful as an adjunct in perforator flap imaging. The main advantage is to provide imaging of the vessels and muscular course while limiting the patient's exposure to radiation. In comparison to CT scans, the images are not always as clear. Also, some patients have a harder time with the test itself than a CT scan test for them. Motion artifact can be a factor in the final views. I have had a few cases where the vessels were not present in the DIEP system but were read as and reviewed by myself and the radiologist as being present with motion artifact crossing the view. In actuality, the vessels really were transected from a previous surgery at the point that looked like artifact only to be weakly reconstituted at a later point. This caused a change in operative plan on the table that in retrospect was easily seen. I have had other examples of times when a dominant vessel was damaged or did not show well in this type of study either due to the motion artifact or the slight lack of clarity of the images. (Figure 1.)

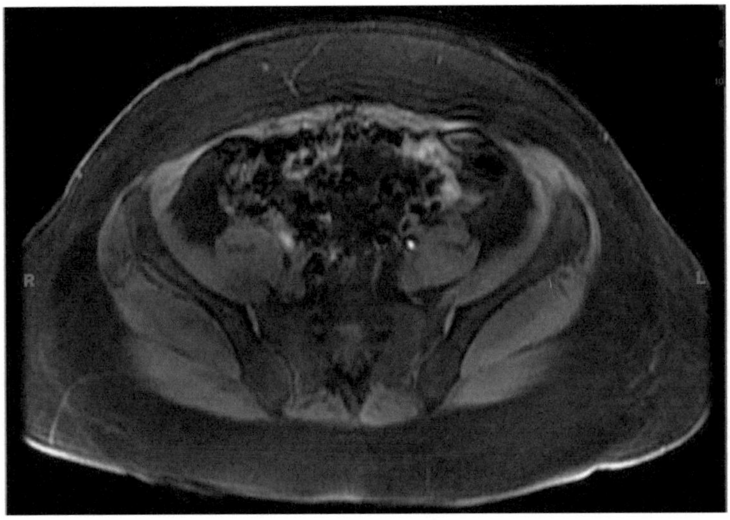

Figure 1. MRI axial view illustrating a perforator vessel of the right abdominal wall.

2.2. CT scan

A CT angiogram of the vessels can be very helpful as well. It has the imaging capabilities to have clear imaging of the position and course of the vessels. It does expose the patient to radiation. IV contrast dye allergy is more likely than gadolinium sensitivity. This can be premedicated for, if the patient's reaction is not too severe. This scan I have found easy to read. The vessels show up clearly. The angiogram part which is usually a reconstruction image at our institution can sometimes make the vessels look a little more im-

http://dx.doi.org/10.5772/56642

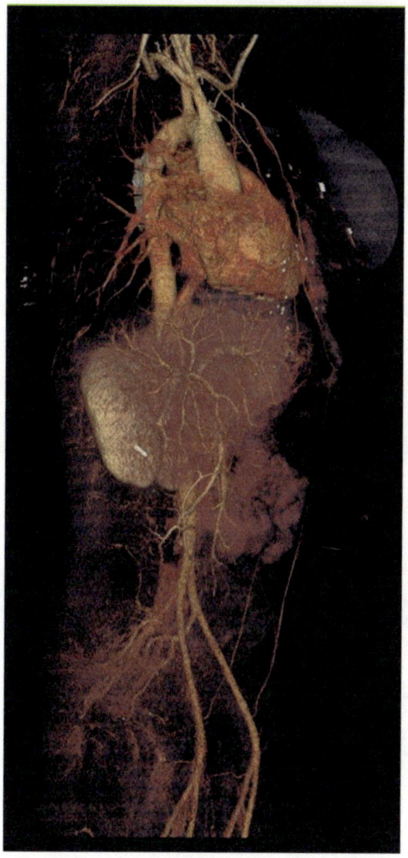

Figure 2. A 3D reconstruction from a CT angiogram illustrates the location of the DIEP vessels as well as the IMA vessels.

pressive than they are, especially if they are quite small. This is apparently due to the layering technique that is present in the reconstruction process of the images. So in order to get an immediate overview of the vessels of the chest and the abdomen, a quick swing through a regular axial series is helpful to get an idea of the strength of the vessels. Then, once viewed, the angiogram reconstruction is invaluable for the muscle path or other anatomical travel that it does. As far as imaging the vessels in the chest, I prefer the coronal view to help with vessel placement near the sternum. Again, I will assess the vessels at the axial view first without the reconstruction images and then go to the coronal view. I have found that the axial reconstructions of the chest vessels are somewhat difficult to get a good read, due to the almost 3d view of the curved ribcage. (Figure 2.)

2.3. Lymphoscintigraphy

A nuclear medicine lymphoscintigraphy study is very helpful to determine the function of the lymphatics in all the extremities. Performed by injecting a tracer isotope in the web spaces of the hands and feet, the uptake of the isotope into the lymph nodes is tracked and followed. This provides a map of which areas are functioning well. This is useful to see if there is another injury to a set of lymph nodes elsewhere which would restrict the harvesting of the nodes in that area. It is to be expected that the area in question would not function well. This test can be a confirmation of that, although it does not always correlate with the physical severity that is noticed clinically, and the images can over and underrepresent the clinical picture. (Figure 3.)

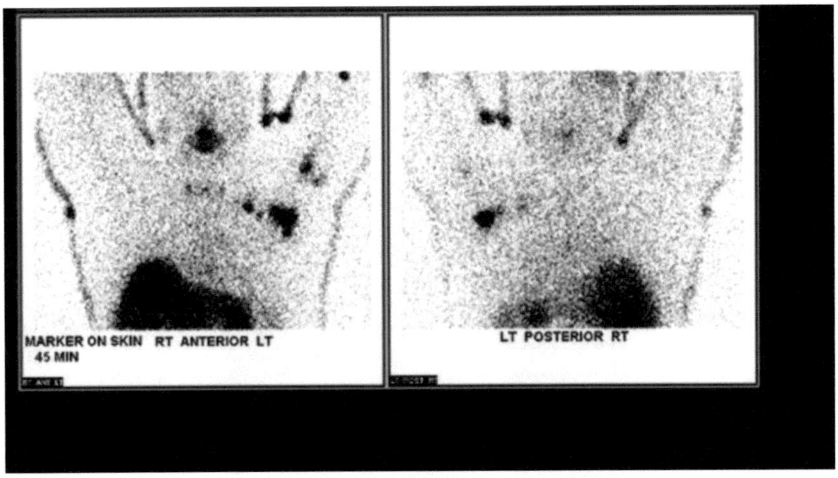

Figure 3. A lymphoscintigraphy study illustrates the absence of lymphatic activity in the right axilla due to prior lymph node dissection and scarring. The left shows evidence of lymphatic activity.

A CT scan and MRI can both be useful for lymph node imaging. They can each show the path and anatomical locations of the lymphatics. With certain software technology, MRI can give a good functional lymphatic result without the use of injections which is very helpful. (Figure 4.)

2.4. Evaluating the Imaging

Preoperative imaging of the chest, abdomen and pelvis gives the most information for operative planning. Whether it is done by MRI or CT, the ability to see the vessel placement in relation to physical structures and landmarks can increase the efficiency of intraoperative vessels selection and completion of the procedure. A systematic review of the study is helpful.

Initially, looking at the recipient vessels in the chest is a good place to start. A coronal view shows the internal mammary arteries in relation to the sternal edge and rib spaces. Thoracodorsal vessels, branches and their relationship to the dissection area are seen in this view. Axial views help to show perforator vessels in the breast tissue that can be preserved during an immediate reconstruction. The internal mammary veins are also easier to see in this view. Frequently on the left side of the chest the veins are smaller than may be helpful. This can also

http://dx.doi.org/10.5772/56642

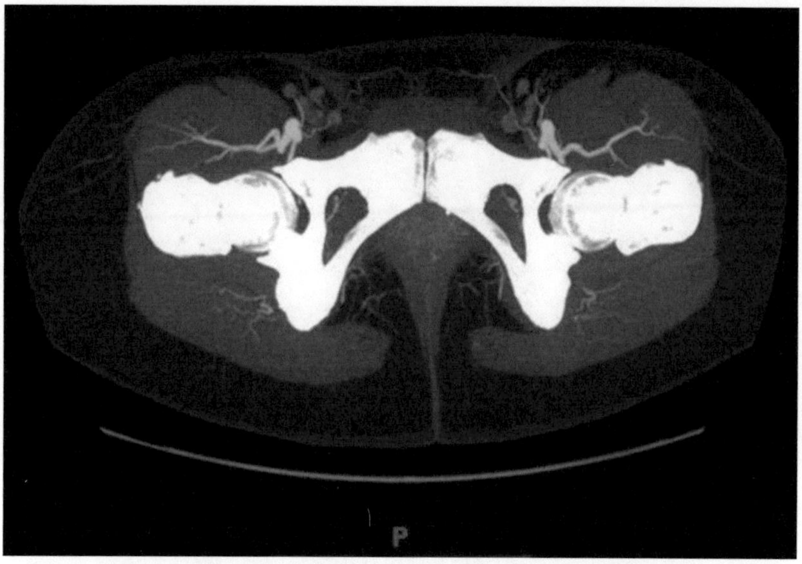

Figure 4. CT scan showing the lymph nodes and vessels present in the groin area.

help to show continuity of the vessels in the axilla, and the amount of axillary compression due to scarring in a delayed case. (Figure 5.)

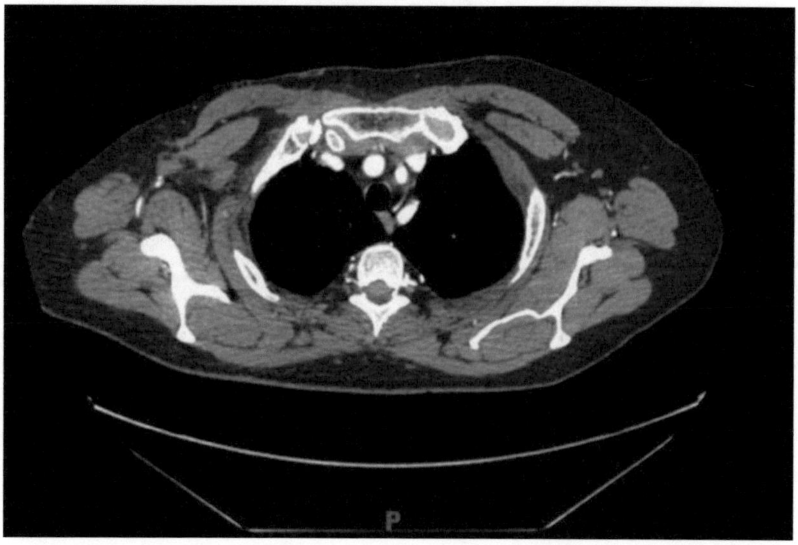

Figure 5. The axillary vessels are seen clearly on the left side of the patient. On the patient's right (left side of image), the CT shows the compression of the axilla due to scarring from prior lymph node removal and scarring.

After evaluating the chest vessels, the abdominal vessels are visualized in a similar fashion. Coronal views can show branching of the deep inferior epigastric vessels. This is helpful in planning for double pedicled or stacked flaps. Also the perforators and superficial vessels can be viewed in relationship to each other to help select DIEP or SIEA flaps. (Figure 6.)

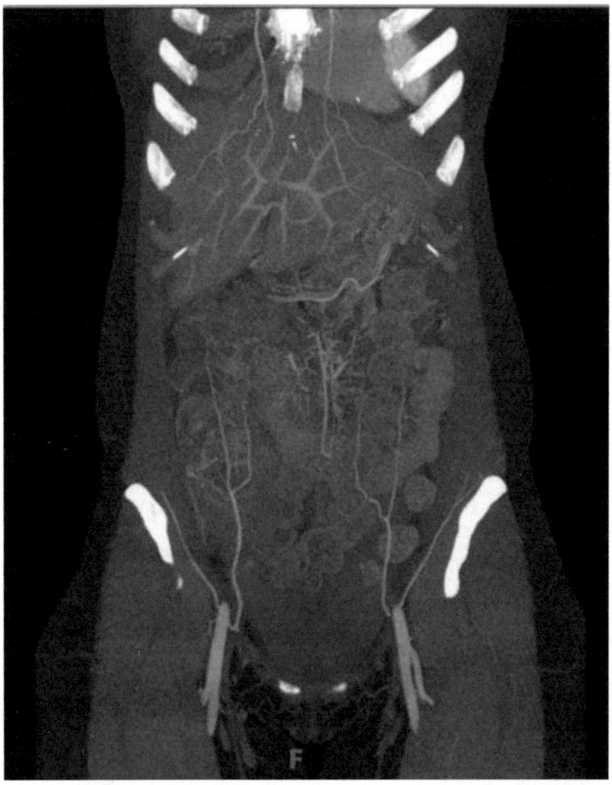

Figure 6. In this view, the deep inferior epigastric and superficial inferior epigastrics are visualized. The internal mammary vessels are also seen. The superficial and deep vessels can be compared to evaluate which are more appropriate in size to use.

Axial views of the abdomen are viewed approximately 4 cm above the abdomen, all the way down to the bottom of the pelvis. Looking for the perforators along the way, the vascular branching is traced superiorly and inferiorly to see which direction the branches are going. Once the vessels are identified, then the pathways are traced through or around the muscles, and a comparison is made to the superficial system to see what appears to be dominant. At this time, the caliber of the vessel is compared to the recipient vessels seen in the chest. (Figure 7.)

If a lymphatic flap is going to be included, then the functionality of the lymph nodes are visualized. The donor sites must be functioning without any evidence of delay or diminished signal. This is seen with the lymphoscintigraphy study. Anatomically, a CT or MRI study can show the location of the lymphatics. This can help plan the flap in relation to final placement. (Figure 8.)

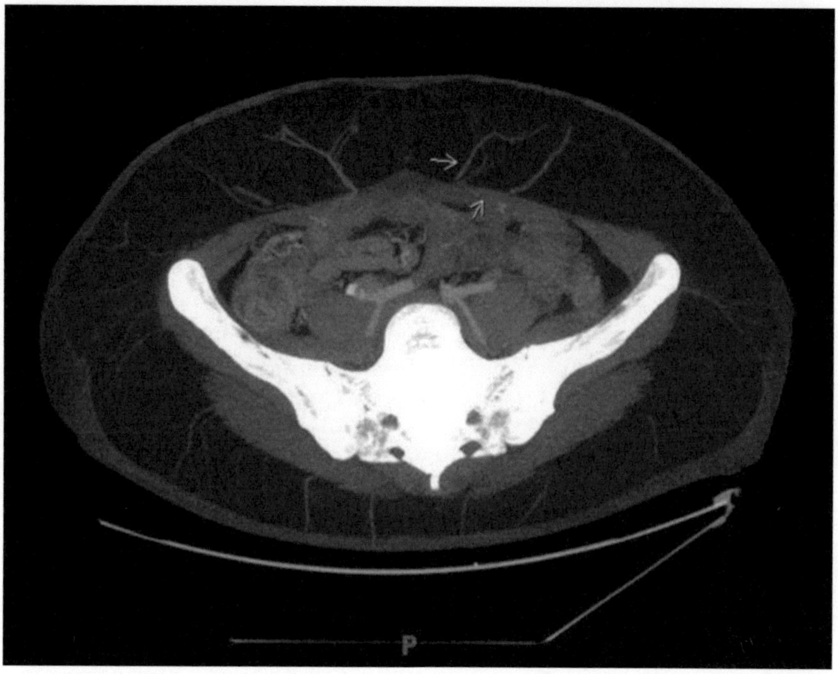

Figure 7. The perforator vessels are marked with arrows. These are located near the umbilicus. Using this view, and scrolling up and down, the vessels can be traced throughout their course to the pedicles. This can help in planning to select the lateral or medial vessels based on the size of the perforators, presence of a vein as well as minimal disruption to the muscle.

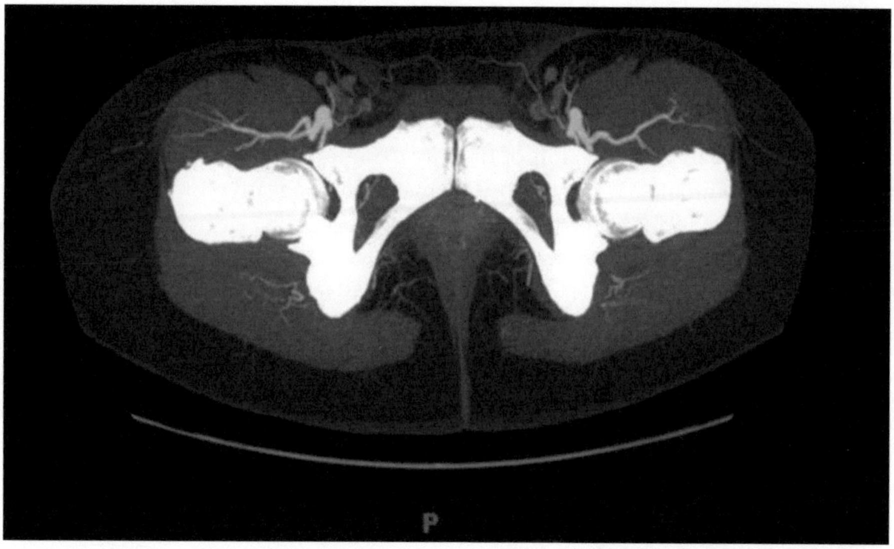

Figure 8. This CT angiogram illustrates both the lymph nodes located at the groin area as well as the vascularity that is associated with the nodes. This can be used in flap planning for the area and proposed vascular planning.

3. Approaching the DIEP flap

The design of this flap is going to be based on two factors: where the blood supply is located, and the amount of tissue needed to recreate the defect. Using preoperative imaging, the vessel location of the flap is easier to determine. Adjustments to the positioning of the flap will be made accordingly. In general, a design not unlike an abdominoplasty procedure is selected for the superior, lateral and inferior incisions. Check with the patient in an upright position if it seems as if the tissue can be closed by pinching the skin together. If you need more tissue, then have the patient bend forward slightly and then mark the area where the skin edges can be closed from this point on. Remember, if this is the case, you will need to have an OR table that will flex the patient into this position, and to check the functionality of the table prior to the start of the case if this is the design that you are committed to.

One way to calculate the amount of tissue to remove is to measure the contralateral breast if present, or the current breast if going to be removed, and determine how much skin is needed and how much of the fat is needed to balance the two breasts. If doing bilateral reconstructions, and there is no premeasured size, then an approximation can be made with a measuring tape, but curving it in the air to assess the size. The skin quality of the chest tissue can be checked as well. If doing an immediate reconstruction, it can be difficult to predict how much of the skin tissue will be left or how strong it will be depending on the breast tissue itself and general surgeon's mastectomy technique. Once the skin flexibility is determined, an approximate second measurement can be made of possible additional fat that can be harvested beyond the skin envelope. This may result in a contour deficit of the abdomen but may allow the skin to be initially closed with a revision to help the scar later. (Figure 9.)

Once the approximate size of the area is determined, then the radiographic study of choice can illustrate where the vessels are positioned relative to the umbilicus. Usually they are at the level of the umbilicus or slightly below. In this instance, the flap design can be made superiorly to just above the umbilicus, allowing for a moderate inferior scar. If the vessels are located further below the umbilicus, or if they appear to be a superficially dominant system, a change to an SIEA plan can be made, or a shift of the flap design lower in the abdomen can be made to yet lower the abdominal scar, for a more cosmetic postoperative look. If the vessels are at the superior edge of the umbilicus or higher, then the flap can be shifted cephalad, depending on how much further up the vessels are. In this instance, the inferior flap will also be shifted closer to the umbilicus, making it more difficult to disguise postoperatively in abdomen revealing clothing. (Figure 10.)

Laterally, the flap design can be made with the patient's habitus in mind, allowing the natural folds of the skin to help design the lateral edges. A point to remember, oftentimes a distant lateral edge will not be adequately supplied by the DIEP vessels, and so will be removed to prevent necrosis at inset. Because of this, I do not plan for long lateral extensions, unless doing so is purposeful for the flap, is based on the vascular supply placement, or is a way to prevent lateral scar deformities or "dog ears."

There are several ways to approach elevating the flap. One such way is to start at the umbilicus and separate it from the surrounding tissues using a 15 blade scalpel (or surgeon's choice).

http://dx.doi.org/10.5772/56642

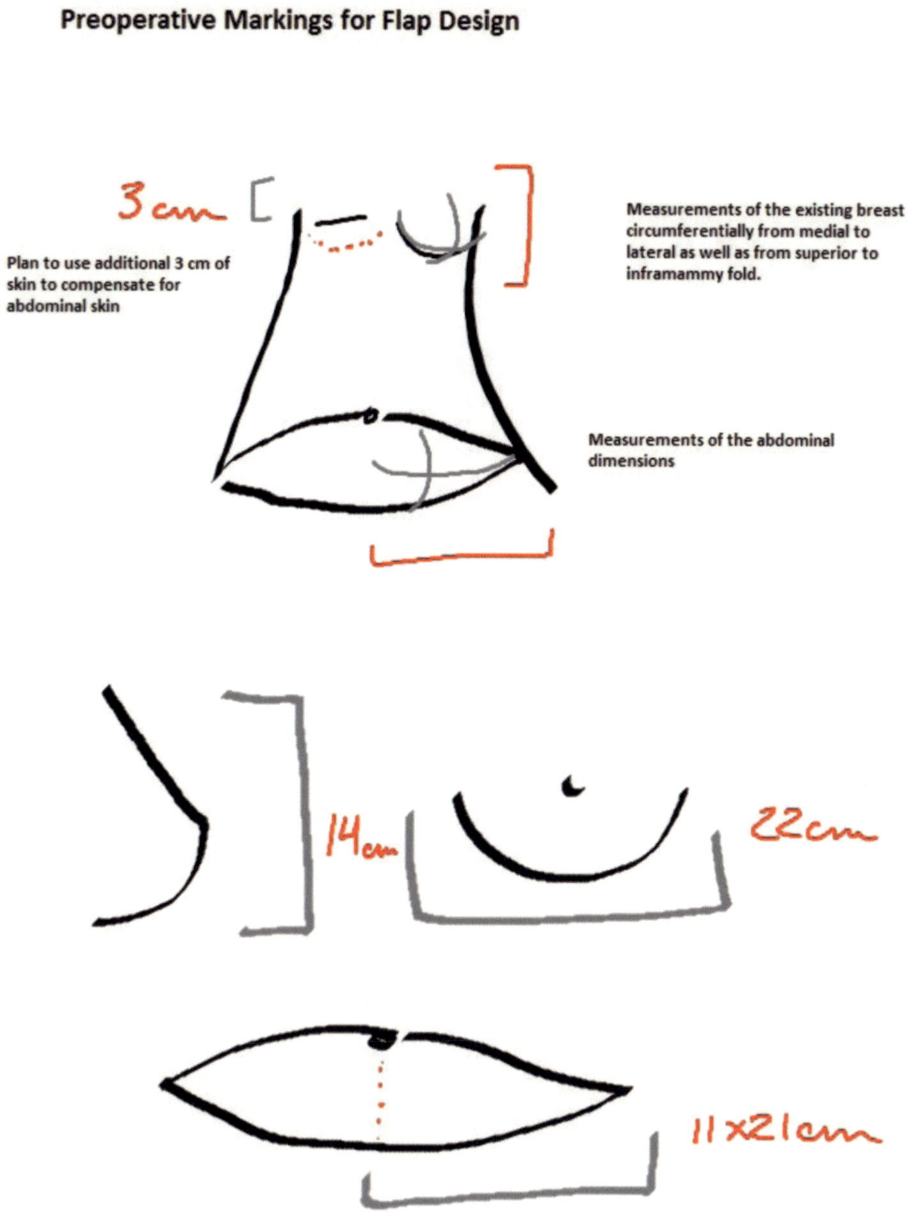

Figure 9. Planning of the flap measurements can be made by measuring the width and height of the existing breast tissue if it is present. This can help to determine if more or less skin needs to be taken. This is particularly useful if the patient has an incredible excess of tissue, and the flap is designed to be smaller, or can help to illustrate sizing to a patient if there may not be enough tissue to match the opposite side.

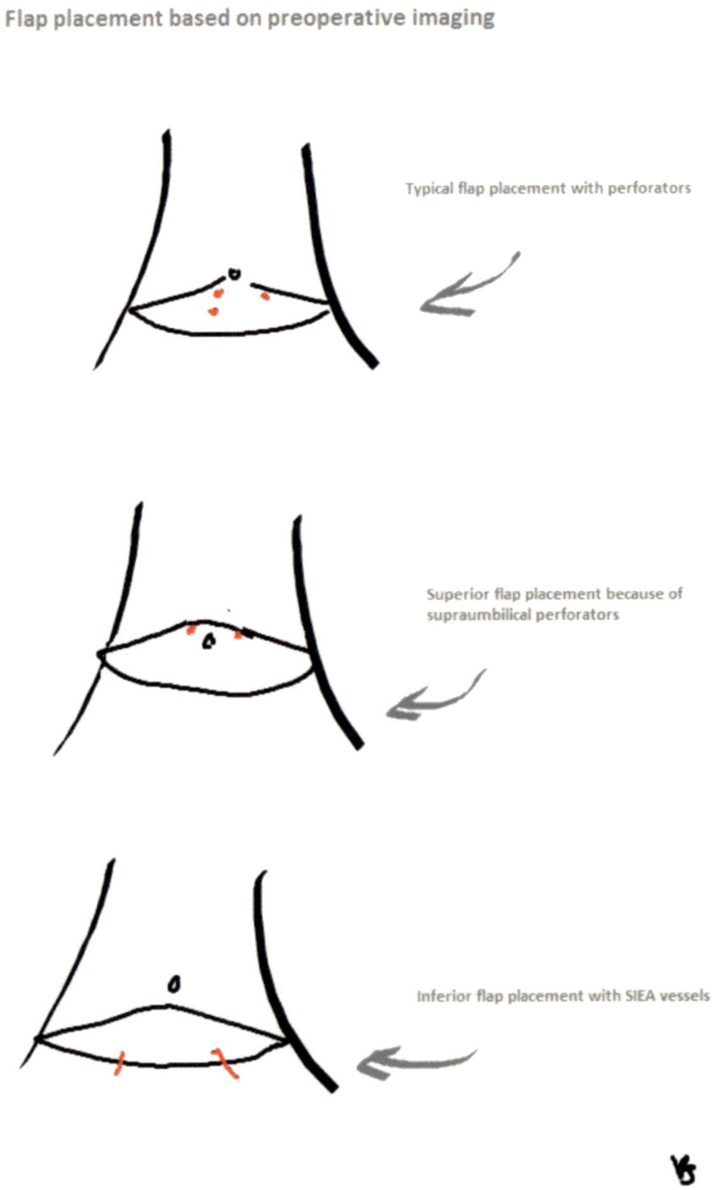

Figure 10. Placement of the flap design can be tailored to the presumed location of the perforator vessels. This can be determined by preoperative imaging. This can be especially useful if the vessels are located at the edges of the initial flap design. Changing the location of the flap to center it more around the vessels can improve the survival of the flap

Once the umbilicus has been freed, then the markings are incised with a scalpel blade. Prior to incision, another helpful technique is to draw marks perpendicular to the incisions, and then

http://dx.doi.org/10.5772/56642

put tacking staples at these areas both superiorly and inferiorly to help match the abdominal skin edges together, and prevent dog ear deformities.

Once these are incised, then electrocautery dissection is used to dissect the subcutaneous tissues down to the fascia superiorly and inferiorly. If the plan is to include more subcutaneous tissue than skin, dissect down to the scarpas layer in a perpendicular fashion from the skin. Once below the fascial layer, then the dissection can bevel out to include more tissue. It can be done directly under the skin as well, but it makes for a more difficult final closure of the abdomen with a greater risk of contour deformity and widened scar. The additional fat harvest is usually performed in a superior fashion. Laterally, the initial dissection is not always done to the depth of the fascia often because the fascia is not located as far laterally as your incision may start. In this instance, a dissection of a presumed equal depth to that of the main abdomen is performed, leaving subcutaneous tissue underneath the dissection until the actual fascial location is reached.

Inferiorly, the dissection can be done a little differently to maximize success. The superficial inferior epigastric arterial and venous systems are located in this area. Initial dissection with a scalpel can be performed in this area to get through the dermal layers. Once this is finished, then bipolar cautery with microhemostat dissection can be performed to locate the superficial vein(s), and the artery with venous commitantes. There are several ways to do this. One method of locating these vessels is to use the electrocautery on cut mode, and gently push the tissue over to see if there is something located near it, and then cauterize those areas which have nothing, or use it with microsurgical or fine tipped hemostats to lift the tissue and then cauterize. Usually there will be a vein located towards midline which is fairly sizeable. This is usually visualized on the preoperative scans, and so the location and depth can be approximated by these. Usually more laterally, the arterial system can be located. Even further laterally a second venous system is often noted and travels towards the midline. In order of depth, most commonly I have found that the more medial the vessel is located, the less deeply it lies. (Figure 11.)

These vessels are important in this dissection because they can: help you in times of venous congestion to provide a second or third draining vein; can convert your flap from a DIEP to a SIEA if the artery appears to be suitable; and give you some information about the perforator occasionally by the size of the vessels (veins especially) versus the size of the perforators. (Figure 12.)

The vessels in this area have a tendency to spasm often and early. It is very helpful to use a vessel loop around the vessels as soon as they are found in order to keep them safe during dissection. Usually the best view that you will have of them is the first view. If you think you saw a large shadow for a vein or a system and then it disappears, leave that particular area and come back to it. Even veins that are 3 mm in diameter I have seen collapse to look like a fibrous attachment. They can often stay in this state, and until you follow them down a little to areas undissected, can look inconsequential. Papaverine can be useful to help them relax, but time is usually best.

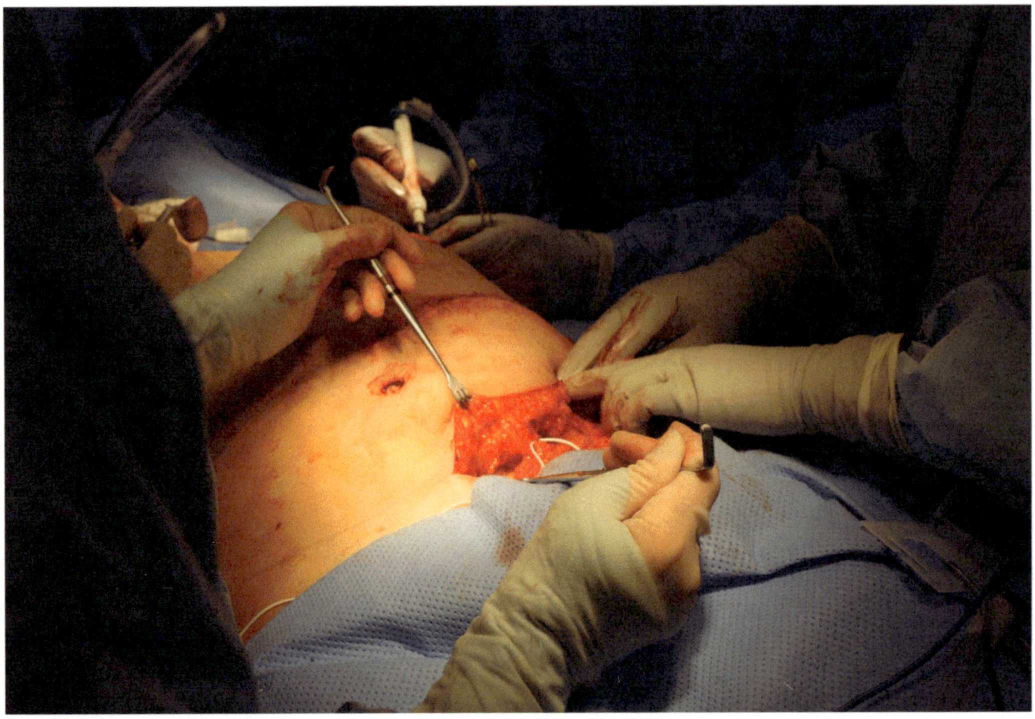

Figure 11. Initial dissection of the superficial vessels. Inferior dissection is done on the flap to find the more medial superficial vein, as well as a possibly useful superficial artery. It is helpful to use a vessel loop under the vessel when it is first found, as these vessels have a tendency to go into a hard spasm, making it very difficult to see and very easy to injure.

Once the vessels have been found and isolated, then the rest of the inferior area of subcutaneous tissues can be further dissected using electrocautery or bipolar cautery, ensuring that the vessels that are isolated are not damaged. At this point, if the arterial system does not seem adequate for an SIEA flap, then dissection of the veins, usually the more medial one can be performed. This is done by gently dissecting around the vessel, using small clips (i.e. gem clips) to clip the branches. Branches can also be tied. Bipolar cautery can also be used with caution to perform this portion of the dissection. The risks with that are getting too close to the main vessel and having thermal injury to the portion of the vessel that you would use, having the bipolar "meld" to a small branch and in removing it, avulsing the branch off the main portion of the vessel damaging it and shortening the usable length or creating more work for you to repair it and possibly creating a stricture by doing so. Once a sufficient length has been obtained, and this varies too as far as how much of a sense that you have that you would need to use it in the future, then it is clipped or tied and divided and reflected back towards the flap. Another way to dissect is to go until the vein starts to dive down, and then transect it after it has curved. Usually at this point you will need a little retraction of the subcutaneous tissue that you did not dissect with a small retractor such as an army navy or Richardson retractor, senn retractor a lone star (a silastic tube with a curved hook, sharp or dull).

http://dx.doi.org/10.5772/56642

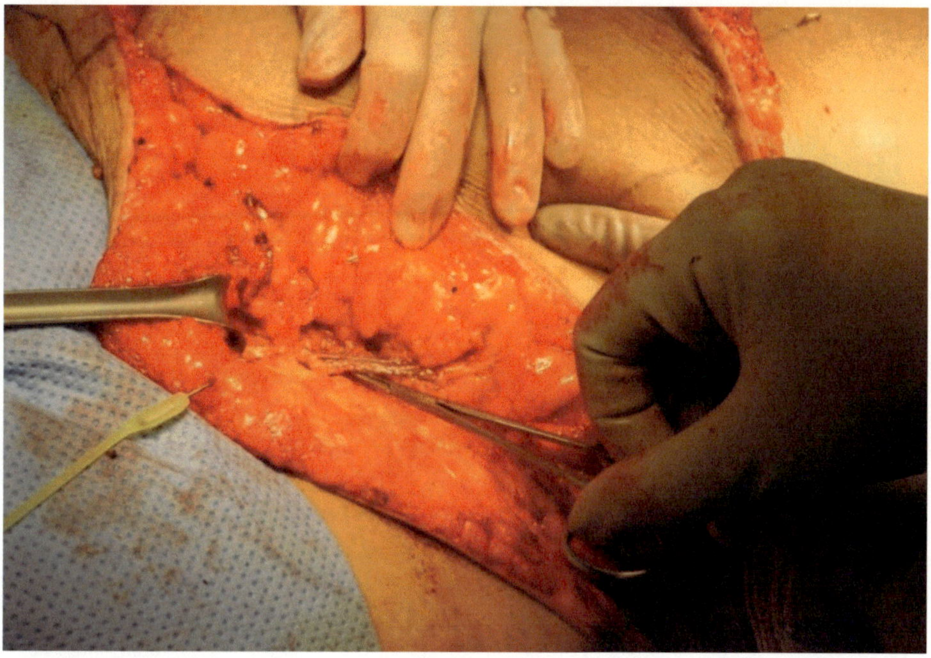

Figure 12. Dissecting the superficial vessels. Using fine blunt dissection, and bipolar cautery to help, the superficial inferior epigastric vessels are evaluated for a SIEA flap potential, or use of an accessory vein if necessary for additional drainage.

Once the subcutaneous tissues have been dissected to the fascia on all edges of the flap, then the flap can be raised to locate the perforators. One of the ways to do this is to go from lateral to medial. This can be done while sitting down, having an assistant on the opposite side of the table. The assistant will support the flap up and away from you as you start to raise it. This can be done with electrocautery. I will usually use the cut mode for this with a setting of 30/30. The cut mode of cautery tends to give a cleaner separation from the fascia making it easier to see. Most dissections have a "clean" suprafascial layer to it. This makes the visualization of the perforators easier. Others have fatty tissue or scar tissue that makes an adherent or "sticky" plane to dissect. In these instances, then the dissection is done much more slowly in order not to damage anything. You may run into perforating vessels long before you reach the rectus muscle. Unless there is a clear indication from preoperative imaging that these travel superficially under the fascia and then join the DIEP system, they will not usually be adequate for use. These can be cauterized or clipped on the way to the perforators. (Figure 13.)

If it is unclear as to where the rectus muscles are located, electrocautery stimulation of the muscles can be performed to see where they are. This is done by gently and quickly stimulating the fascia with the cautery. The fascia can remain intact during this test if it is done quickly. If the direction of contraction is vertical, then the rectus muscle is below, if diagonal, then you are in the territory of the obliques. Once in the rectus muscle territory, a safe dissection mode is to switch to bipolar cautery and hemostat dissection to find the perforators.

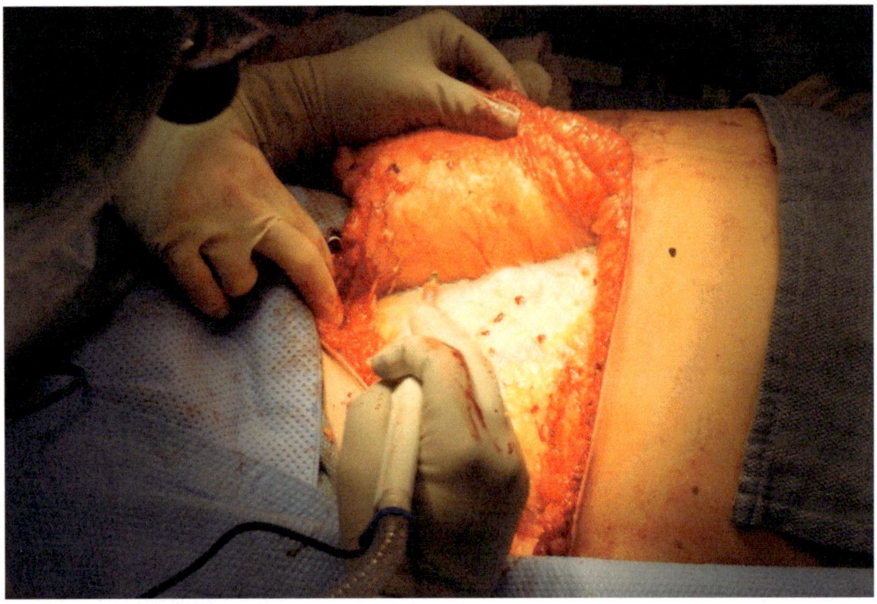

Figure 13. Dissecting the abdominal flap from laterally to medially using cautery. The perforator branches initially can look like branches of a tree. Once this is seen, then careful dissection can lead to the "trunk" of the perforator branches.

As you are lifting the flap away from yourself, small vessels will usually start to appear, as if the tops of a tree. As you continue medially, these start to condense into thicker branches or a single trunk. At this point a perforator is usually underneath. Another way to see one is by looking for "shadowing" underneath the tissues, it will usually be the vein. A third way is to notice a small opening in the fascia. Usually the perforators are located in small oval gaps in the fascia and sometimes the edges of these gaps will be visible before the vessels are.

There are lateral and medial row perforators, meaning that some will be closer to the umbilicus and some will be closer to the obliques. Once you locate the lateral perforators, you can use a vessel loop to go around them, and then start the dissection from medial to lateral, or superiorly to inferiorly or inferiorly to superiorly. This is to locate the medial perforators. Once these are located, then the planned vessels based on studies are confirmed or an alternative is chosen. If there is a question about the actual flow provided by these vessels, Doppler skin signals can be used to assess which is supplying the overlying skin. Vessel clamps can also be used to determine if one has better flow or venous return than another. Another technique is to use a fluorescein injection and monitor the flow to determine the dominant perforator. Oftentimes, the grouping that has a larger vein and a similar artery size is the one to choose. Radiographic studies can also determine the selection by viewing the pattern of distribution into the subcutaneous tissues that each has, as well as its subfascial course.

The majority of the main selected perforators are around the level of the umbilicus. These can be medial or lateral. There are also areas where a grouping of vessels with a larger nerve are located. These can initially look to be ideal, but on further inspection will be fairly useless for a vascular supply. Two locations where these are commonly found are just on the superior medial aspect of the umbilicus and midway through the flap between the umbilicus and pubis, often located between the medial and lateral row. Another temptation can be to select multiple medial perforators in a row to use. The lateral row often can be coordinated with more than one perforator as the branches follow a linear path through the rectus muscle. Medially, the perforators can cross through the muscle at several points resulting in transection of the muscle transversely in order to connect the systems.

Once selected, then the dissection to release the perforator is performed. If you have an assistant who is holding the flap for you, they must be extremely careful to make sure that they are not pulling the flap in such a way to avulse or create a stretch injury to the perforator vessels at this time. Separation of the vessels from the fascia can be done by directly going to the fascia that is surrounding the pedicle and using blunt/fine tipped scissors (i.e. Wescott) splitting the fascia further cephalad and caudad to follow the path of the perforators. Another way to do this is to start indirectly by scoring the fascia with a scalpel superiorly and inferiorly to the pedicle, catching the edge of the fascial opening or going slightly lateral or medial to it. Once this is incised or scored, then scissor dissection can open the fascia up at a little distance inferiorly to the perforator. At this point, usually the vessels are not directly underneath the fascia (although radiographs do help to see this), and the fascia can be gently split and retracted until the perforators are visualized. This can be a helpful way to avoid cutting into a branch or the actual vessel at your initial dissection. (Figure 14.)

Once the perforator has been visualized under the fascia, then it is dissected down to the deep inferior epigastric artery and veins. This is done with microhemostat dissection and bipolar cautery to dissect the tissue freely from the vessels. Branches can be tied or clipped and divided. Careful attention is paid to crossing nerve branches in order to spare them during the dissection. During the dissection of the branches through the muscle, it is important to keep the bipolar tips clean, otherwise they can stick to the cauterized tissue, and especially if it is a small branch of the vessels, can cause tearing and damage to them. We use lubricant on the bipolar tips to keep them from sticking.

Occasionally it is not clear what branch of the perforator vessel is going to the deep vessels. If this is the case, then dissection through the muscle to find the pedicle can be performed and then the dissection work its way cephalad towards the perforator. Once this has been done, then the branches can sometimes be easier to separate from the main branch point. Do not assume that if a perforator branch initially goes medially or laterally that it is not going in the right direction. It can often travel from side to side and then dive down. It is possible to transect what looks like a branch, only to have nothing left underneath at all. Superior to the perforator, there is often a continuation of the vessel. Occasionally the deep vessels will terminate at the perforator but this is less often the case. Finding the vessels that are travelling superiorly and are not curving back to join the pedicle, these can then be clipped or tied and then divided. Harmonic scalpel is also useful for this purpose. Once these are divided, then it can free the perforator to see branch points as well. This can be a useful maneuver to aid in dissection, as well as one of safety to prevent the perforator from getting tethered and injured by stretch during dissection.

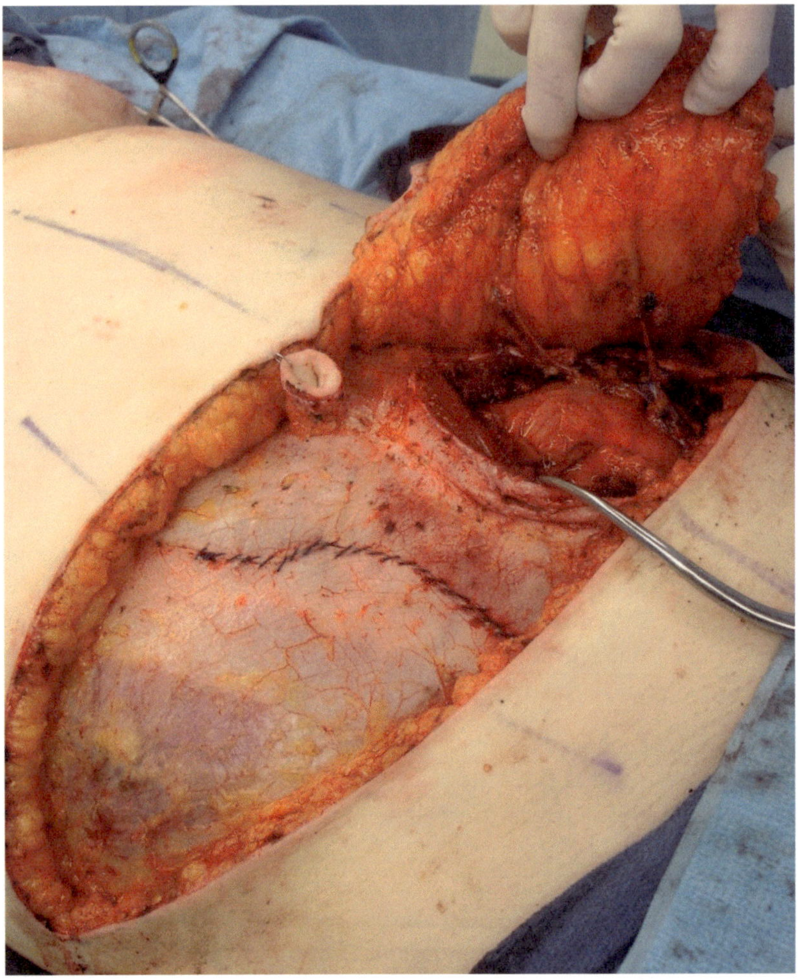

Figure 14. Two perforator branch points can be helpful for flow if they are in the same dissection plane. Retraction in the plane can help to visualize the pedicles.

A place where the radiological studies can come in helpful is in viewing the course of the vessels. This is viewed by scrolling through the cuts of the vessel in question. This has helped on more than one occasion where a vessel appears to be a main branch off the pedicle, but is actually travelling through the muscle and is hidden. If a muscle sparing TRAM technique was to be employed in this situation, then the vessels would be transected and the flap would not be viable. (Figure 15)

If the perforator is traveling through an inscription point, it can be a short course to the pedicle, but it is often difficult to dissect because of the fibrous nature of the structural attachments in the area. It is best to go slowly in this dissection, being aware that the tethering effect seen at this area can cause the vessels to appear smaller than they are, making it less clear as to where they are travelling. Sometimes it is only after they are released that their full size is appreciated.

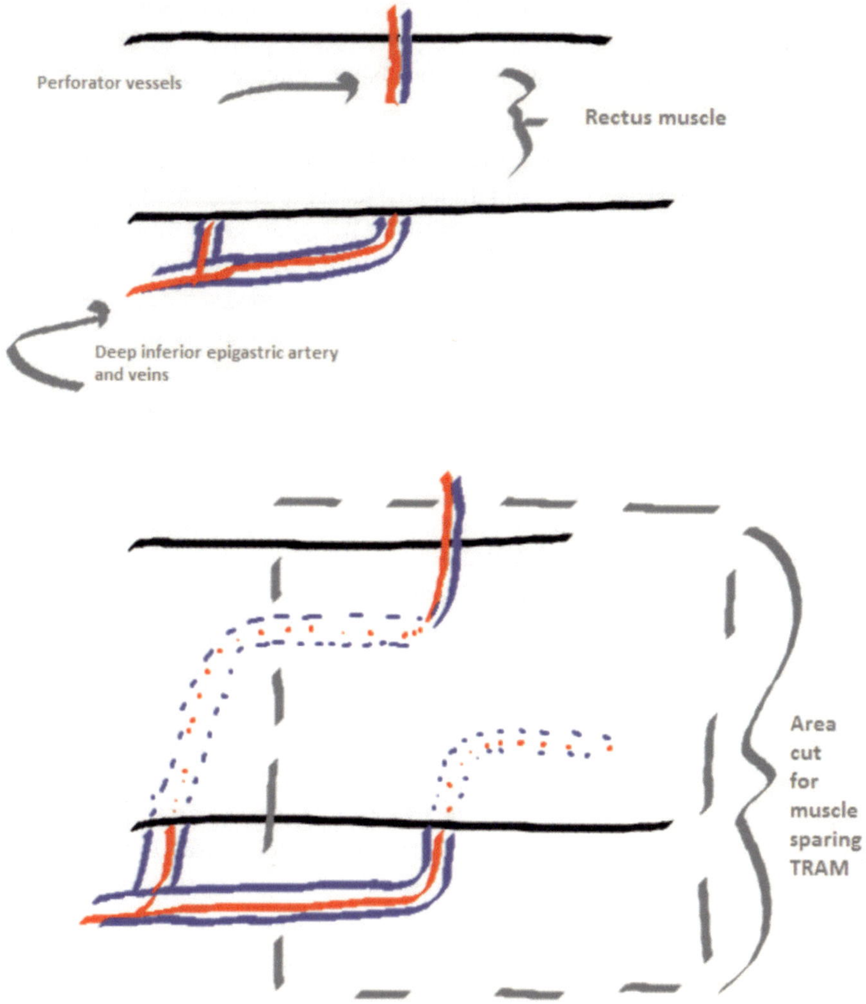

Figure 15. Diagram image of external physical perforator and pedicle branch image which can be misleading. Treating this as a muscle sparing opportunity can lead to a total transection of the actual communication between the perforator and pedicle. Prior imaging can be useful if it shows the intramuscular course clearly, as well as fully dissecting the vessels out as the ultimate test.

Loupes are often used in the dissection of the vessels. The most common I have seen is 2.5x for the dissection of the abdominal vessels, and 6x for the IMA dissections. Other surgeons do not use loupes at all. The benefit to using loupe magnification is in seeing small branches or tethering material that can rip or damage the vessel inadvertently during the dissection or can help to show a path that the vessel is taking. A different source of damage can occur, though, in the inadvertent neglect of other factors in dissection by the inability to see them through the loupes. An example of this would be tethering or pulling and damaging the perforator because that portion of it is not in the loupe dissection window. This is when not using the loupes or looking around them is better. If this is difficult to do, then a good assistant who can watch the dissection plane can alert you to impending mistakes or injury. Another way to proceed is to routinely check over the edge of the loupes before making another adjustment in the placement of the vessel.

Once the initial dissection of the perforator is done, then dissection of the pedicle is done in a similar fashion. Branches are secured and divided. Nerves are dissected free from the pedicle in order to preserve them. One of the ways to do this is to gently dissect these off with hemostats, clipping small branching vessels. If they are tightly associated, gently hydrodissect them off the vessels using heparinized lactated Ringers solution on a 22 gauge angiocatheter with a 10 cc syringe. This can show you the actual branches if there are any, versus fibrous attachments which can be transected with scissors.

After the attachments have been released, then an inspection of the vessels to assess the caliber and length of the pedicle is made. If they seem to match the recipient vessels and it seems like there is enough room to maneuver then your dissection is done. Separating the vessels from each other at the area that will be divided can be useful at this point to save time when at the recipient site, create more length If you are at a main branching point for the pedicle, and allow you to see branch points that are evident when the vessels are inflated, but may not be obvious when empty. You can decide to procure extra length by dividing the branches and dissect further down the pedicle, or you can preserve the remaining vessels' direct blood supply route to the muscle.

Branch points can be useful if you preserve them sufficiently. There is no need to randomly take long branches of vessels to incorporate with the pedicle. A risk of doing so is to have a large blind end of the vessel which can clot and then propagate that clot towards the main flow area, and then occlude it. However, if you are planning on doing a large flap, a branch point, particularly the dividing branch of the main pedicle trunks can be an anastomotic recipient for the pedicle vessels of the other half of the abdomen.

Once the vessels have been fully freed from the surrounding tissues, then the Doppler signals on the skin can be confirmed and marked with marking pen (which can often fade or smear away) or a marking suture such as a 5-0 prolene. This will help to find the vessels signals once the flap is inset. If the flap appears to be perfused well (i.e. good skin tone, no sign of congestion, positive capillary refill, and bleeding around the edges), but there is no skin Doppler signal, then an implantable Doppler may be useful post anastomosis to help monitor the flap.

The pedicle can be marked with methylene blue or a marking pen for aid in orientation. One side is marked while the other is left plain. This can help to keep the vessel from being twisted while it is deflated and harder to see. Another way to do this is to clip the branches on one side of the pedicle and tie the branches on the other, leaving a physical reminder of the sides. Usually a marker dipped in methylene blue is sufficient, quick to apply and long lasting.

There are different ways to approach dividing the vessels. One way is to clip and divide the artery first, allowing the veins to drain and then clip and divide them. Another is to terminally clip the smaller of the two veins, and then clip the artery and main vein, leaving those two vessel ends open. A third is to clip across all three at once with a large vascular clip and divide

http://dx.doi.org/10.5772/56642

them, leaving all edges free to drain. At this time, it is helpful to keep track of the ischemic time by having the time recorded when the vessel flow was stopped.

At this point, the flap can be gently removed, watching that the pedicle and perforators are not caught on a nerve or any unnoticed attachment. The flap can be weighed and then placed onto the recipient site. The weight can be useful, especially in cases of bilateral reconstructions, or immediate reconstructions when a size match is anticipated. Once at the recipient site the flap is secured with sutures, or staples or a combination of the like to allow full attention to be paid to the anastomosis and prevent avulsion of the vessels with a shift in the flap placement.

4. SIEA

There are similar dissection points for the SIEA with a couple of differences. The dissection of the flap can be shifted inferiorly a couple of centimeters if this makes a difference in final closure. Shifting the flap too inferiorly can result in a shorter pedicle length. The initial dissection can be done similarly to that of a DIEP flap. Once the inferior portion of the dissection is performed, then the vessels are carefully dissected to find the arterial and venous systems.

The venous systems are located medially and laterally usually. The medial vein can be fairly close to the midline or up to a third of the length of the flap away. The arterial system can be located close to the medial vein or much further laterally. Once the vessels are located, a similar method of isolating the vessels with vessel loops can be performed. The main goal in the assessment of the vessels at this point is the arterial flow. A couple of points can be made here. The artery should be clearly visible at this point. This can be deceiving because it will usually be surrounded by two veins. The veins can vary from being small and unusable on either side of the artery, to being large and mimicking the artery itself with a small hair of an artery causing a signal and maybe a small pulsation in one of them. A nice rule of thumb is to have the artery be at least 1 mm in diameter at the initial dissection point, visibly pulsatile and/or palpably pulsatile. If the artery is tethered by tissue or branch attachments it may not initially pulsate visibly until these are removed. Also, it may be difficult to distinguish the surgeon's own digital pulse from the pulsations of the patient's vessel.

As dissection proceeds further, the artery should increase in apparent size and strength. The veins are often quite large and sometimes will join with each other if you have the patience to continue to dissect toward each other. This can be useful for drainage purposes especially if a lateral vein is the dominant drainage vein for half of the flap and the medial for the other half. As the dissection gets closer to the fascia, there is often increased branching of the artery. This can be confusing as the branches can look equally as dominant and the directions can look similarly logical as far as the next dissection area. In this instance proceed with caution and try a different angle to view the posterior side of the dissection. Another trial is to gently clamp the branch that appears to be the main trunk and see if the pulsations decrease markedly and/or the signals change. If not, then this branch can be divided and dissection continues usually with a branch underneath.

Once at the fascial level, the artery and veins may be of sufficient length and size. Dissection to remove the rest of the connecting tissues and branches is performed. Keeping a vessel loop around the lowest portion of the dissected vessels can help keep you out of trouble at this point. If the vessels do not appear to be large enough (and the artery can often be a 1mm or 1.5 mm at the largest), then the fascia can be split (to be repaired after), and the vessels can be carefully followed further down. Usually, there is not a large gain in distance at this point but there may be a small gain in size. Branch points often will abound in this area which may be useful but may also get in the way because of their proximity to the future anastomotic site.

Prior to the final dissection to length of the SIEA vessels, dissection of the flap off of the fascia is performed to free it up and to do a final assessment of the choice of flap. If there is a possible perforator choice that seems better, then gentle clamping of each of the vessel sets with visualizing of the flap and Doppler monitoring can help determine which of the two has an advantage.

The arterial recipient vessel for the SIEA flap may need to be much smaller than a DIEP vessel recipient. These recipient vessels can be selected ahead of time by using perforators, branch points, axillary vessels or the IMA more caudad on the ribcage. This will help with a final size match and flow.

5. Lymphatic flap

If performing a combined flap of lymph nodes and SIEA or DIEP flap breast reconstruction, preoperative planning for which abdominal side to transfer should be made. The lymphatic flap design is created in order to keep the lymphatics harvested above the inguinal ligament. The most medial lymph nodes are left in place to help prevent donor site lymphedema.

The dissection is performed sharply at the inferior edge of the breast reconstruction flap. Vessels are clipped if not being used, or dissected out to length if going to be the main donor vessels. The lymphatics can be located underneath the superficial inferior epigastric vessels. Once the vessels have been found, then dissection for the lymph nodes are performed below the Scarpa's fascial layer and down to the abdominal fascia. Once the dissection has been performed to the inferior aspect of the flap, then the rest of the flap can be raised by dissecting from the lateral portion of the flap to the inferiormedial portion of it until the flap is free.

If the flap will be resting for a while before harvesting, be cautious of stuffing the lymphatics back into the pocket and having the vessels kink as you can get hidden vascular congestion of the flap until you extract it again. Careful handling of the lymph nodes is important to keep them functional. Avoiding electrocautery appears to help the lymphatic channels to reconnect with the recipient lymphatics by preventing the sealing of the edges of them.

5.1. Postoperative plan

The postoperative management of the free flap patient can be as important as the surgery itself in the final success of the flap. There are several acceptable ways to manage the flaps. Deciding

http://dx.doi.org/10.5772/56642

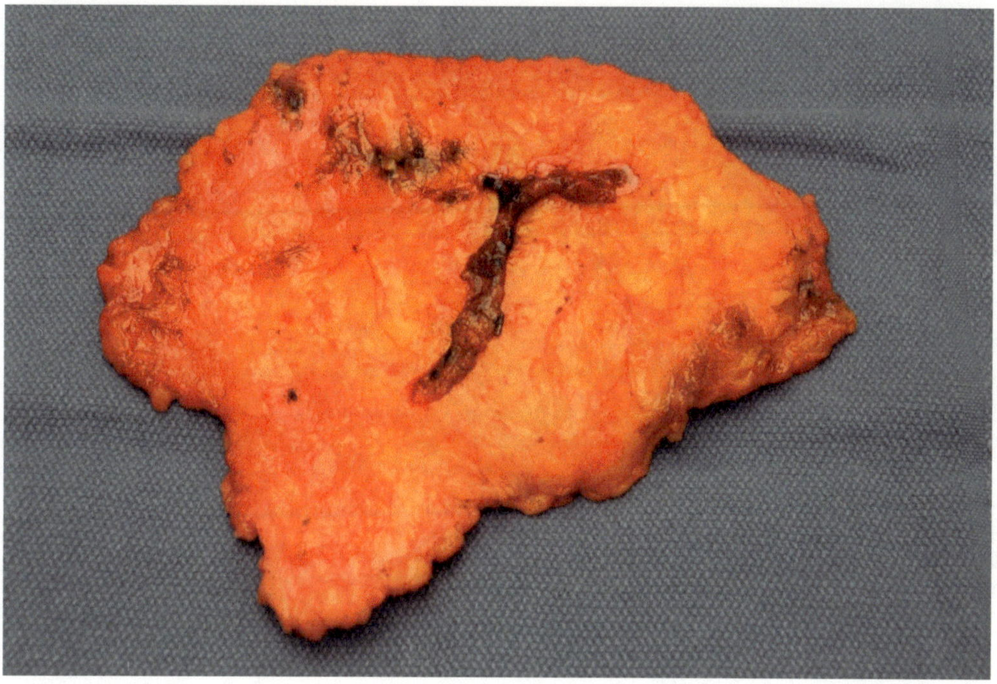

Figure 16. Subcutaneous view of DIEP flap with lymphatic composite flap.

on a plan, and being flexible with it when necessary will lead to better outcomes. As part of the plan, the support staff who help to monitor the flap are just as vital as the protocol, if not more so, as they are who will alert you to the changes that can be fixed by going to the operating room.

Initially the patient will be in the post anesthesia care unit. It is important that the nurses there know what you are looking for in flap evaluation. Clinical evaluation points should be addressed every hour immediately postoperatively. Some evaluation parameters can include the patient's vital signs, the temperature of the flap, Doppler signals on the surface of the flap, internal Doppler signals, firmness of the flap and capillary refill. Once the parameters are established, having a flow sheet for the nurses to record their findings can illustrate trends of the flap. If trends are changing, then the surgeon should be alerted as to the next course of action.

Once the patient has been recovered, the patient is moved to the floor. This can be an ICU setting or a regular floor. If in the intensive care unit, the flaps can be monitored every hour. On the floor, every hour checks may be more difficult to do over a prolonged period of time. In the ICU, the patients are less likely to be able to be ambulatory. If other patients in the unit are unstable, then it is possible that the flap patient will get less monitoring for a period of time. On the floor, the patient is more likely to be able to ambulate more quickly. Also, patients are usually more comfortable in a less intensive setting.

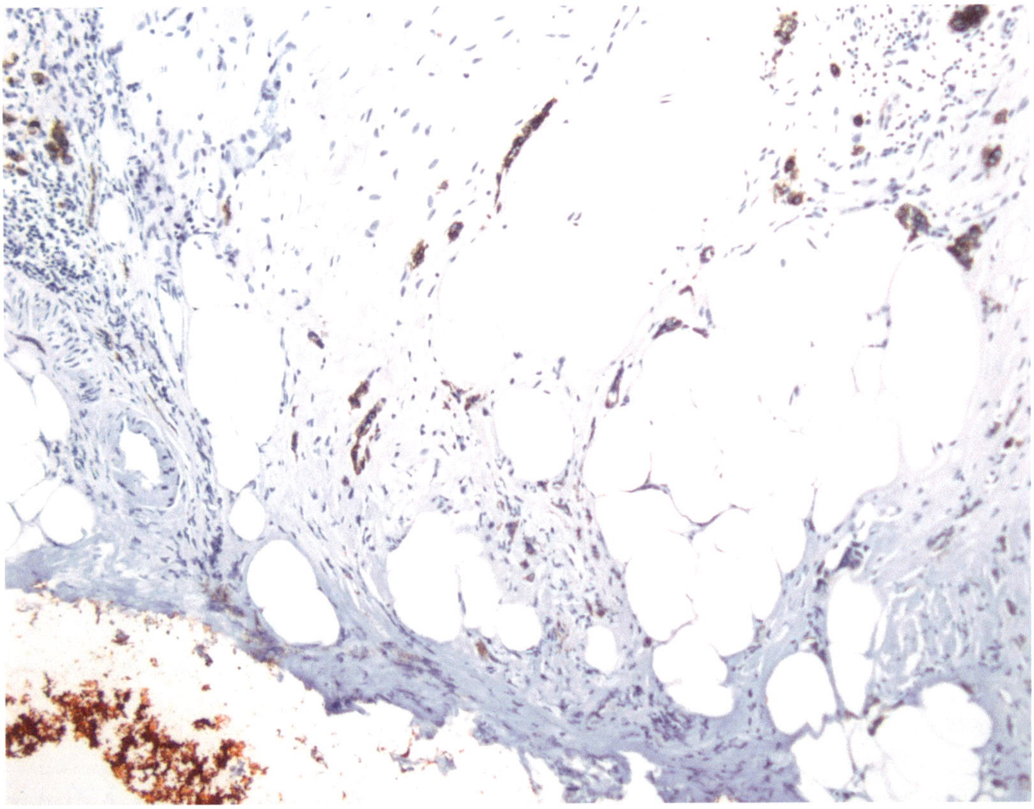

Figure 17. Microscopic image of cauterized tissue at the inferior portion of the slide, as compared to the normal cell structures of the more superiorly based cells. It illustrates how in order to create new connections between cells, keeping cautery damage away from these surfaces can maximize the cells' chances for this.

The simplest postoperative plan that I have seen and which has been just as effective as more elaborate plans is to have the patient evaluated every hour for 4 hours in recovery, and then they go to a regular floor with q 2 hours for the remaining 8 hours of the first 12 hours postoperatively, and then q 4 hours evaluations until the end of their stay. There is no warm room or overheating of the patient. The patient is heplocked on postoperative day 1. They are given a regular diet, with no additional anticoagulants. The labs are not checked, and the patient is expected to ambulate and void on their own. The patient is monitored for two more days and as long as they are doing well, they are discharged home, possibly with or without drains. That being said, it depends on the comfort of the surgeon, and the reliability of the staff that they work with, which may dictate what postoperative protocol they fill comfortable with.

Postoperative monitoring variables which are simple are often the best. Temperature monitoring using temperature strips can indicate changes in flow of the flap. Softness of the flap can indicate changes in congestion, capillary refill indicates congestion vs arterial inflow loss. Skin Doppler signals can help find a diminishing signal. Several methods to evaluate flaps are utilized, some more technologically advanced than others. [21]

Whatever method is chosen, communication with the staff is key. Early detection of problems with early intervention will have better postoperative salvage. Communication with nursing staff has evolved through time, now including phone technologies. [20]

5.2. Troubleshooting the flap

Occasionally, there will be a change in the flap that requires some intervention, operative or nonoperative. This possibility should be discussed with the patient preoperatively in order to give them a sense of what they will be asked to do. If they have an understanding about this, then they are much more likely to stay calm and follow directions.

The monitoring techniques that are employed will give you information on what course of action to follow next. Often, intraoperative and immediate postoperative incidents can help you start your plan. If the patient had a rough wake up in the operating room, is vomiting postoperatively, or has sustained high blood pressure in recovery, then a change in signal may be because a hematoma is accumulating from a disruption of a vessels and the flap will need to be opened to reverse a failure due to the compressive nature of the process. Oftentimes, the signs will be a change in flap temperature (cooler), firmness (firmer), quicker capillary refill (congestion), or change in color (pink to purple indicating congestion). If the arterial signal becomes lessened or is lost, then the anastomosis may be closed by a clot. Initial changes can be addressed by a release of pressure at the bedside, and if they are resolved, a small drain can be placed to help ensure further drainage if necessary and to monitor the flow, or an operative exploration can be performed to stop any further bleeding if it seems to be an active process.

If the patient is wild in recovery, and thrashes quite a bit, or just changes position often, with a pedicle that is either quite long or quite short, then a change in the flap can indicate that the vessels have become kinked or twisted due to movement, or that the flap itself has shifted position, resulting in tension of a vessel which may be resolved with repositioning and support of the flap.

Generally speaking, most issues with the flap will be from venous congestion. This could be because the flap is dependent on a superficial vein for additional drainage, or the vein is easily kinked before it has healed into place. These issues can be treated with direct and indirect interventions such as positioning, temperature therapy, leeches, direct venous drainage, and operative anastomosis. (Figure 18.)

It can sometimes be difficult to know when it is a time to intervene with a flap and when it is time to let the flap continue to adjust.

If in the operating room the flap is normal skin colored/pale, moderate temp, possibly cool, possibly warm, if the capillary refill is absent, or 3 seconds or more, flap is soft, skin tissue may be firm or soft, and Doppler sounds are fine on the flap skin, then everything should be fine. If the Doppler signal is staying strong or stronger, hearing sounds on more areas than just the initial areas, capillary refill is showing up and still 3 seconds or more, the temperature is getting warmer or feels the same as the rest of the skin, then the flap is still doing well

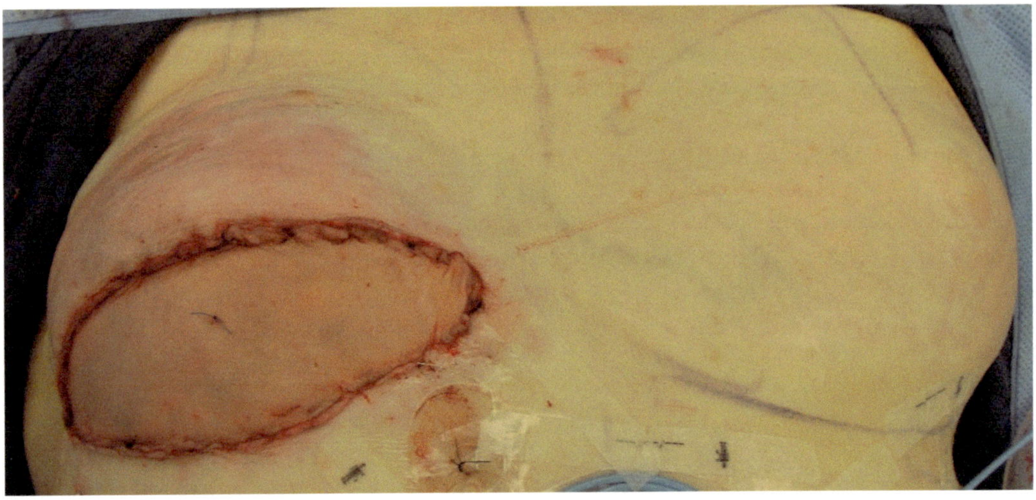

Figure 18. An illustration of venous congestion in a flap, the most common cause of flap failure. Congestion can manifest in varying colors of pink to purple hues. Distinguishing between hyperemia and congestion can be done by the speed of capillary refill. Capillary times of 3 seconds or greater usually indicates adequate drainage even in the presence of hyperemic coloration. Capillary refill that is 2 seconds or less, or is becoming quicker even in the presence of very mild coloration or almost normal skin tone can indicate that a precipitous congestion process will follow.

If the capillary refill was quicker and now getting slower, skin color is pink but capillary refill is slow (just around wake up or initial hook up), observe for a little while, while closing or in the or for 30 minutes or so. If it is not improving but the capillary refill is still slow, then it is generally ok to wake and go to recovery especially if the Doppler sounds are strong or improving, temperature is improving, and capillary refill time is getting longer. Then in recovery, the initial color should start to improve. This color change can happen to a single flap, to both flaps of a bilateral reconstruction, or to just one of the two flaps in a bilateral reconstruction, even if the vessels sizes seem similar. One of the things to check to help determine the patient's skin reactivity is to look at other areas of the body. Check the patient's native skin on the upper chest area, (neckline flushing), and check for refill, oftentimes is quick as well, or look at the incision lines to see if handling the tissues of the abdomen is causing a similar reaction to gauge if this is unique to the flap and requires a re-exploration or if you can wait on it.

If the capillary refill is quick and seems to be getting quicker, (1-2 seconds), open the incisions and observe, if it resolves then too much pressure with closure is possible. Repositioning the flap can be helpful, or reducing the size of the flap, loosely closing the skin for a delayed closure, or doing further dissection of the pocket to allow for more room may be necessary. If after opening the incision there is still a problem, take the flap out of the inset and observe the flow and flap color changes/Doppler signals with the anastomosis intact. If the flow improves then it is a positioning issue.

If the superficial veins are dilated, and the tissue looks congested (purple), then open the superficial vein and let it drain, if the anastomotic vein looks functional. Make sure to check the anastomosis and position of vein to make sure it is flowing and not twisted. Undo the vein if that doesn't work, let the native vein drain a little to return it to its regular positioning if it was twisted. You can open the costal cartilage above the space if the vein path is not easily seen to make sure there is no tethering or hidden twisting. If additional drainage is necessary, you can anastomose the accessory vein of the comitants, if there is a second IMV available or a branch of the first, or anastomose the second vein into a branch of the first.

The superficial venous system can be used to drain into a branch of the main pedicle. You can anastomose it to the IMV, anastomose it to another branch or vein found in the field, or drain it with a catheter. If the superficial vein is long enough to reach the original anastomosis or a branch then it is easy to anastomose to aid in drainage. If it won't reach around the edge of the flap, then you can dissect the vein back into the flap for a distance and then split the flap underneath it, i.e the fat and scarpa's fascia, to allow the vessel to reach the IMV or the original pedicle. Make sure you open scarpa's fascia to keep it from tethering at this point. More easily done with couplers, this can be attached to a branch point along the way in case you need it.

Arterial insufficiency can present as loss of signal, paleness of the flap and loss of tone. The treatment for this is returning to the operating room to inspect and repair the vessel, possibly using thrombolytics as well. If there is a loss of arterial signal, change the Doppler batteries. Make sure the blood pressure is normotensive. Hydrate the patient with an IV bolus if necessary or if blood loss is suspected and/or CBC confirms, a blood transfusion, to return to a normotensive state. Confirm that the patient did not receive vasoconstricting inotropes which may be causing spasm of the vessel. We also restrict the use of certain migraine medications (such as Imitrex) for possible similar effects. If this is not the case, explore quickly. An arterial salvage intervention is usually successful if caught early enough.

If you need to return to the OR to explore the flap, communicate with the team (equipment is readily available) and the anesthesia staff (avoiding pressors on intubation, especially with a bilateral flap in order to avoid damage to the other side). Once prepped and the incisions are opened, then gently secure the flap with either staples or sutures, so that if while exploring the flap there is less help in the OR, or in trying to evaluate the vessels, there is not an inadvertent avulsion injury performed. If it is strictly positional and everything is flowing well but the vein appears to be open but clotted, then TPA can be used. This can be done in several ways, including disconnecting the arterial side of the flap and injecting arterially, injecting the accessory vein, or disconnecting the anastomosed vein and flushing through that. Mainly, it is important that after the TPA is used, that the vessels be flushed with heparinized saline to help move the clotting process out of the main system and hopefully the TPA into the microcirculation where more damage can occur if this is not properly flushed. It is tempting to try to rush through this step, however, if there is an internal vessel blockage that you can release this way, your chances of success postoperatively will be higher.

Troubleshooting the flap is done in a systematic fashion. Determining when to operate and when to treat conservatively can take experience in judgment. If in doubt, an exploration will allow you to visualize the actual flow of the vessels and will allow you to see if there is a physical problem that can be repaired in order to have a successful flap.

Sometimes there is a nonoperative fix for a problem such as congestion, or sensitive positioning. In these cases, prolonged nonoperative interventions may be the only way to fix the issue. Some of these are prolonged bed rest for positional changes, cool or warm therapy for the flap, and/or leech therapy. If all the venous avenues are maximized that are possible, the vein is working and flap is draining but slowly, or unable to provide enough drainage to the whole flap or the area in question, then, ice the flap to slow the arterial flow down, and keep changing it to keep the flap cool. Patient positioning to help with drainage, by keeping the patient flat in bed may be needed. Trendelenberg positioning may be useful but difficult to maintain. Keeping the patient in bed for up to a week is hard to do but can be helpful. If the patient is in bed, make sure that pressure areas are protected to avoid decubitus ulcers, especially the posterior scalp.

Leeches are another way to address venous congestions. Medicinal leeches may be stored in the pharmacy or a unit floor may keep them in a refrigerator. Leeches are usually kept in two containers, the first inside the second and the second or first taped, as they are maneuverable creatures and love to escape. They are not supposed to be reused, but used as a one time application, and may not be released due to the biohazard of blood borne pathogens. They like a warmer environment, so if initially they don't want to feed, warm the flap first with a warm blanket or wash cloth. Then if they still won't, make a small prick in the skin with a needle to get them to attach to that area. Hold them with plastic pincers or plastic covered/rubber shod covered instruments. It is not always easy to tell which side is head first. If it really won't attach, then try another leech. If there is congestion and not enough arterial flow (i.e. congestion has progressed too far and the flap has or is shutting down) the leeches will not attach or will not stay long. Barriers and making sure that the flap is secure is key. Oftentimes, a flap will be opened first to relieve congestion. Make sure that the flap area is reclosed and/or sealed with tissue glue before applying leeches. They will want to crawl into a dark space. Make sure the patient is on antibiotics, and check a CBC. Do a pediatric stick as time goes on and check q6 at first to make sure they don't drop too far. When using leeches, keeping a Hgb of 10 is a good guide because there will be some shifting and this way it won't drop too far. If you let them drop, and they will, the flap will shut off due to low flow.

After leeches are finished, they will often want to "wander." This can be stressful for the patient and the staff. Make sure room cleaning is available often if they travel across the floor. Again, with surgery, and as surgeons, we are used to so many anomalies of the human condition that this can be seen as a minor issue. Sometimes patients and their families handle it extremely well, sometimes not at all. Sedation is helpful for the patient if their blood pressure tolerates it. Keeping the area clean helps the family. Frequent checks, at least q 1hour is helpful to corral rogue leeches. Social work support and counseling for the patient can be helpful. Usually the process is around 3-7 days in all. Other means to help are frequent washes and changing of the sheets, occlusive dressings as a barrier, and reiterating the temporal nature of the intervention as a helpful alternative to keep their flap for the rest of their lives. Scarring can be permanent from where the leeches latched. Smaller skin paddles are harder to get good drainage from.

Leech therapy, Hirudo medicinalis, has a longstanding presence in microsurgery. The gut flora of the leech, Aeromonas hydrophila, can cause infections in 2-20 of patients not treated prophylactically with antibiotics. Ciprofloxacin is the drug of choice for prophylaxis, but there can be resistance to this as well. Monitoring hemoglobin levels closely and replacing with blood products as needed is vital. Giving the patient psychological and social support during this period is sometimes a forgotten but vital part of the treatment. [22-29] (Figure 19.)

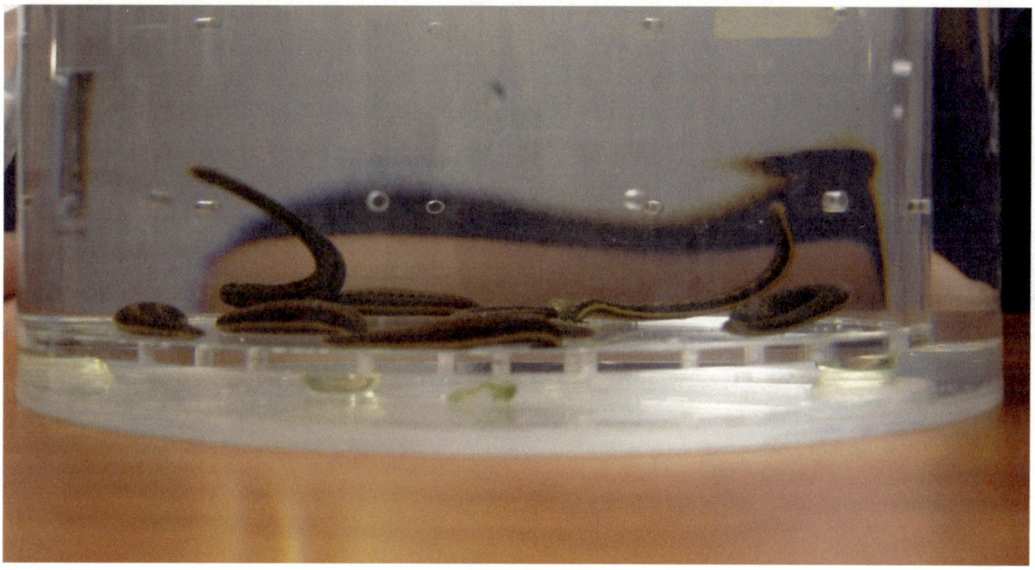

Figure 19. Medicinal leeches in storage ready for application.

Currently, I prefer to catheterize a vein if possible or ice the flap versus using leeches. And of the two, I like icing. It avoids the loss of blood, the patient can easily participate as it is a commonplace remedy, it can be continued at home and it is very effective. Catheterizing the flap can be done by inserting an angiocatheter into a vein that was preserved in the initial dissection (superficial inferior epigastric). The angiocatheter can be secured with a 3-0 silk tie to the vein. This is then connected to arterial line tubing which in turn can be secured to the skin with a suture or occlusive dressing to keep it from avulsing the catheter from the flap. This can then be accessed by gently drawing off blood from the catheter to help prevent congestion. This can be done if there is no other alternative. A difficulty I have found is if the line coagulates. Flushing with heparinized saline post draw is helpful. If it becomes too blocked TPA can be used as well judiciously. Also, connecting the catheter to an external ventricular drain (CSF monitor) to calibrate a constant drip rate can aid in a measured release of pressure as well as prevention of clotting. Hemoglobin levels must be checked and addressed with this intervention. (Figure 21.)

Using ice to cool the flap and treat congestion can be done in the operating room, using sterile ice in sterile bags, or on the floor using ice packs or cold gel packs. Have the nursing staff

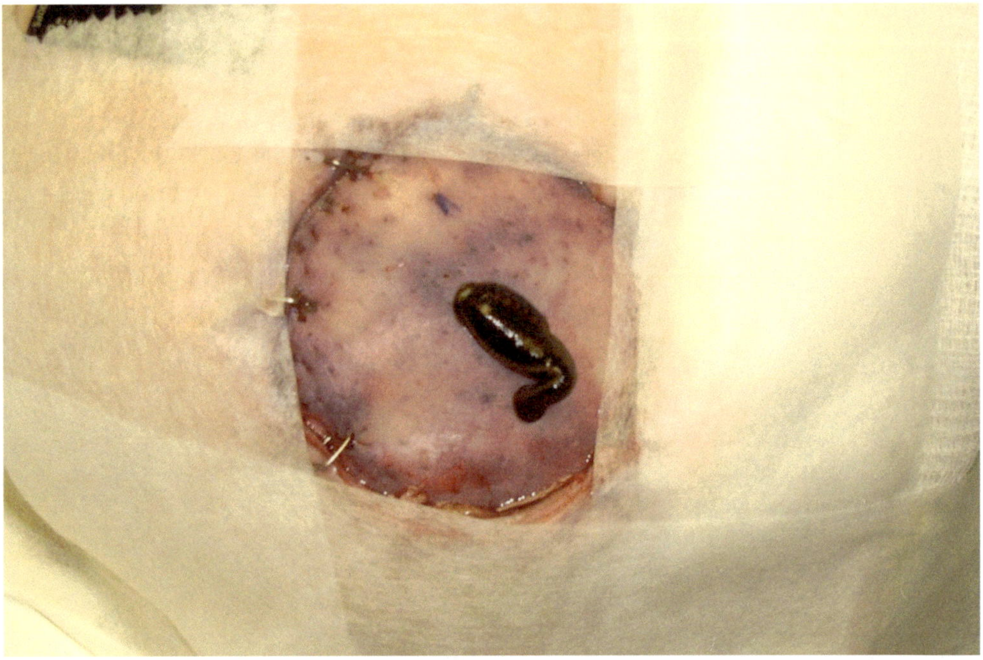

Figure 20. Application of leech for congestion therapy. In this instance, surgical paper tape was applied to help prevent leech attachment to mastectomy flap skin.

continuously change them to keep things cool. Continue to use the ice until the capillary refill time has improved, then you can increase the time interval between the ice applications gradually, using the capillary refill as a gauge. The skin color will usually be hyperemic and so you cannot always rely on a pink color of the flap as being a sign of congestion. Capillary refill is the most accurate measurement of this. If the patient is able to monitor the refill times accurately and is reliable, then you can discharge the patient home using ice packs as well.

If there is firmness with upright positioning, put the patient back down, give it a day or 12 hours and try again slowly. If the flap is cool after the surgery has finished, then warm the flap with a blanket in recovery. If it is functioning, it should be able to maintain the temperature as long as it is covered and not exposed for extended periods of time. I don't like forced air blankets (Bair huggers) as they falsely elevate the temperature but if a warm blanket is placed and then the flap maintains that temperature, then most likely all is well. Sometimes the temperature will drop if the flap is exposed to examine it, if so then continue to keep it covered quickly after examination. If it continues to improve then it is doing well, if it continues to fall, you may have arterial insufficiency or impending congestion.

If one flap is congested slightly and the other is cool with a quieter arterial signal, then warm one and cool the other. Even though it may be a bilateral reconstruction, treat each flap individually. If a flap looks mottled at the edges then it is likely will lose that skin especially if it gets worse. However, you can also cool it down to see if those areas can be preserved and continure to observe. If the flap has a black eschar, go in and debride to healthy tissue, and

http://dx.doi.org/10.5772/56642

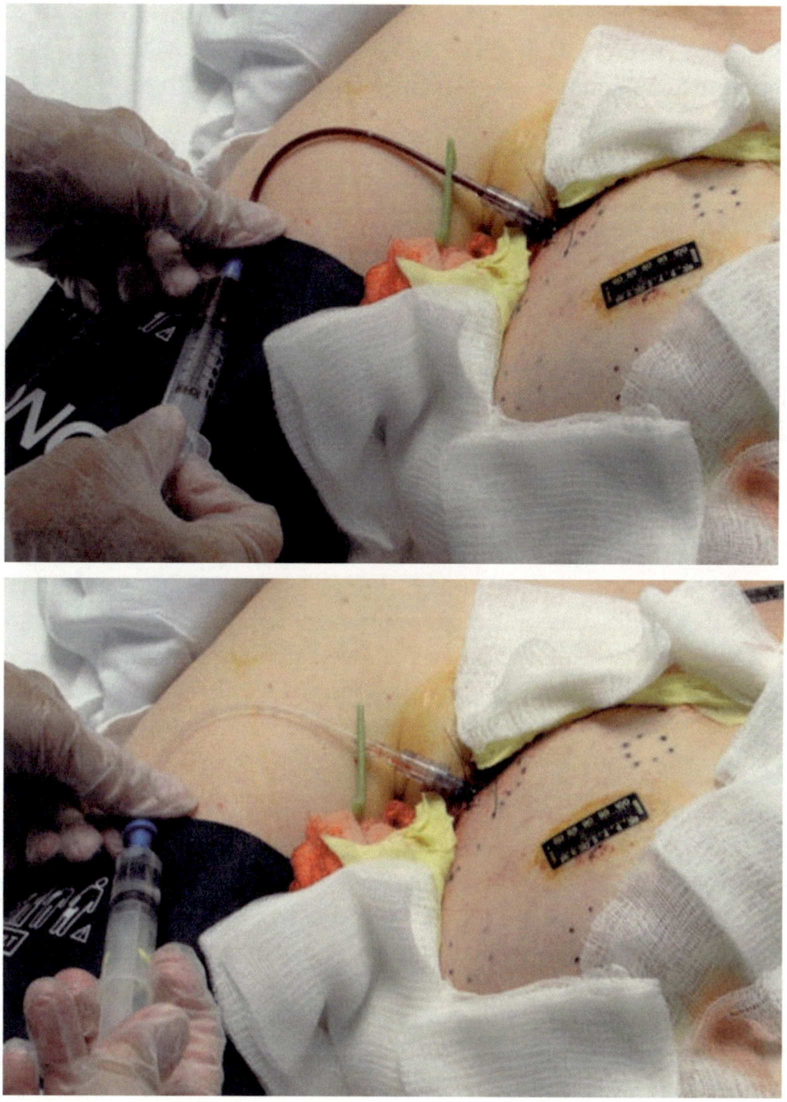

Figure 21. Catheterization of the superficial inferior epigastric vein. In this instance, catheterization of the superficial vein with an 18 gauge angiocatheter had been hooked to sterile arterial line. This was secured with sutures to the skin. A 10 cc syringe was used to gently draw blood back every half an hour until the flap coloration improved, or at longer intervals depending on the signs of congestion. After each draw, heparinized saline was flushed into the tubing to help keep the catheter open. This time interval for the process was extended over each 12 hour period. After 2 days, the drainage was discontinued. CBC's were used to assess the patient's possible need for transfusion.

cover with skin if possible. Integra may or may not be helpful if there is no skin coverage, and no granulation tissue.

Flexibility in times of trouble to shift therapy, or continue to change modalities as the flap progresses is key. Usually a flap will declare itself as salvaged within the first week or two postoperatively. During these times, discussions with the patient can help to keep them positive and willing to participate in an intervention that may only need a couple of extra days to work. Persistence and attentiveness to detail can salvage many flaps.

6. Solo surgeon

Performing flap surgery as a solo practitioner has its own challenges. To do so as part of your career will take dedication and some extra work at first. It can be successfully done and can be a rewarding part of your practice. There are several arrangements that need to be made initially and then during the growth phase of the process to ensure success. This is both on a professional level as a practitioner and with the hospital, including support from administration in time and materials, as well as support staff.

If unfamiliar with perforator flaps, and/or free flaps in general, it is highly recommended that you get some training in these procedures first before branching out. Even if familiar with free TRAMS, there can be a significant amount of difference with a DIEP that can make this less likely to succeed. If at all possible, spend some time with a surgeon who performs these to get a better idea of how they work. If these have not been a part of residency training at all, and you are just starting out, then a fellowship is recommended. Even performing as a resident and making the leap to doing them in practice can have unexpected stressors that may impact the success of the operation.

If working at a community hospital, it is likely that they may not be set up for flap reconstruction surgeries. If this is the case, you will want to discuss the matter with the operating room director and or surgical administrator to ensure their support with this venture. You will want to have at least a couple microsurgery sets of equipment and a team of people who will be initially assigned for training and working with you in the operating room, postoperatively in recovery and on the floor. You may want to discuss billing with the hospital, as these can initially be very costly for the hospital if the times are long, but can work out much better as the operative times are condensed.

6.1. OR setup

I would recommend at least two set of microsurgery instruments and possibly three. One is the backup for the first in case anything is damaged. A note here, sometimes in cleaning, if the sterile processing is unfamiliar with microinstrumentation, the instruments can be ruined by rough or improper handling. Make sure the team is inserviced on the handling of these instruments. Often, the company will send someone to help with this step. I will usually use a partial set for the harvest dissection and a full set for the anastomosis. A second set is there for backup as well as for a bring back cart. The main thing here is to have a set that you are comfortable working with, that will handle the tissues appropriately and that is in enough supply so that if something is damaged, or being processed, there is another set to use in case of emergency, or take back.

6.2. Instrumentation

When ordering instruments there are some practical items to consider. Medium and long length instruments are useful. Sometimes the recipient vessels are located in a deep pocket and you will need the length to get there. If it is not possible to get both sets, I opt for the long one, as I can reduce the length of grip on the long ones if need be, and still have access for the deeper vessels.

It is very useful to have fine tips for small vessels. I consider a dilator to be indispensable for this, as well as for pulling vessels through tight spots (i.e. small couplers). They are not textured that I have found and this is a limitation in the grip. Oftentimes I am able to position something quickly with these, but then immediately move to a textured forceps to actually maneuver the tissue in the place I would like it to be.

Textured instruments are a must, both for needle drivers and for pickups. These help when there is loose tissue nearby that is slipping and you would like to trim, or if the vessel itself is slipping, this is helpful to get a good bite on it. Needle drivers can slip and roll the needle especially if the needle is rounded throughout its construction. Again, anything that can help to keep the position, and allow force to be applied without losing the angle of the needle or positioning will continue to speed the process up.

A fine tipped, blunt-tipped instrument is very helpful in dissection. A scissors that is sharp and one that is blunt tipped is helpful in these maneuvers. The blunt edges allow for dissection through the muscle and loose tissue without inadvertently cutting branches or the vessels of interest. Sharper scissors can be nice for trimming vessel edges prior to anastomosis.

A coupler anastomosis system is helpful while operating as a solo surgeon. Their use is simple enough to have limited to no assistance from another person, the handling can be done one handed while stabilizing the other hand, and the closure helps to prevent leaking of the anastomosis thereby preventing the solo maneuvering of the vessel to get a posterior wall bleed. Also, you can observe the lumen throughout the process so that you know that it is open. The coupler instrumentation is something I recommend having two or three of in case one has failed. Instruments that can be useful with this process are dilator, textured forceps, j-hook and curved forceps. A wide range of couplers is useful, but usually a range from 1.5 mm to 3 mm will get you through most of what you need. With couplers, less assistance is needed for both the artery and vein. Suturing is still useful but placement, tying, and cutting without assistance can result in a lot of steps that add time to the case.

Retractors- Anything that will help minimize variability in positioning, or possibly supporting staff expertise is useful for success. Self-retaining retractors such as gelpies, or wheatlaners (I prefer blunt), are useful in the dissection and positioning of tissues. Staples can help as well, when a flap is swaddled in a lap sponge or on its own. The most useful retractors I have found are a hook with a silastic tubing or silicone tubing attached to the end. They can be sharp or dull tipped. I prefer the dull. They are called several names, including lone stars, fish hooks or urinary retractors. They hook on to the tissue edge, can be pulled back and secured with a hemostat. These can be used during any part of the procedure and are easily repositioned. (Figure 22.)

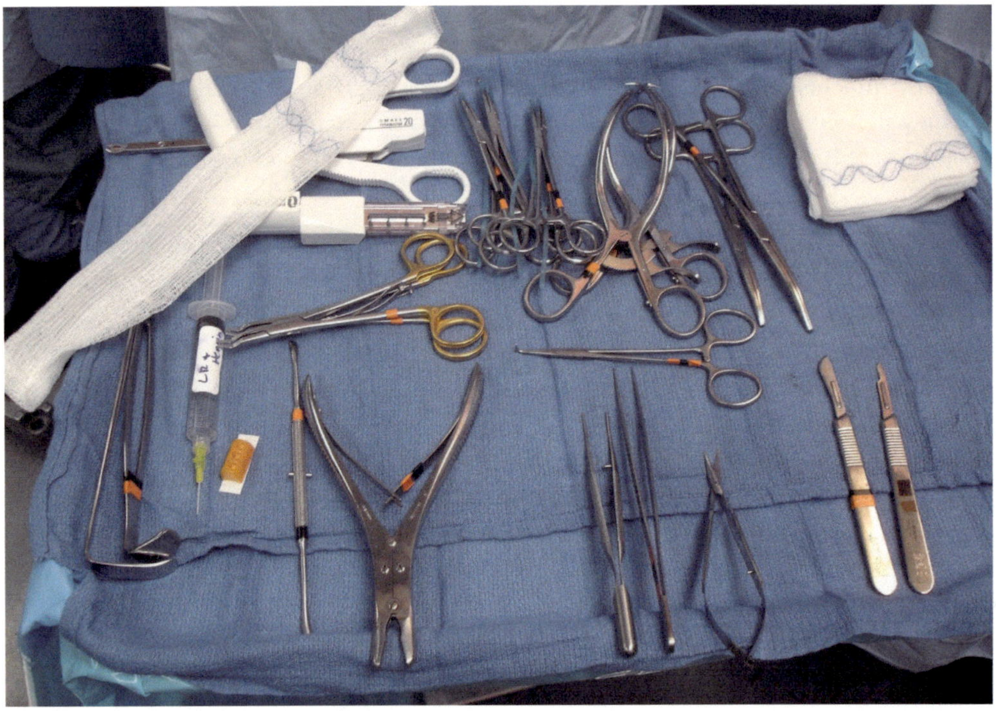

Figure 22. A tray of useful items for retraction for the solo surgeon. These include self-retaining gelpi retractors, lone star elastic retractors, army navy retractor, as well as surgical staplers and clamps.

Knowing the instruments-It is important to have the staff learn which are textured which are not, how to load a coupler, how to handle instruments, whether you want them to load suture or not, etc. how to work the microscope, positioning, prep work, tucking the arms, etc. crucial and noncrucial times of the case. Good communication in these areas is the best way to keep your cases running smoothly and to decrease frustration of the surgeon and of the support staff.

Assistance- if you are able to, utilize a first assistant or an RNFA, PA or resident. This type of help can be useful for items, such as retracting- when is too much, how to keep you out of trouble, how to handle the tension on the perforators, irrigating, getting a global view; closing-closing the abdominal wall, putting in drains, closing the abdomen itself, closing the skin on the flaps, depending on skill level and future training, de-epithelializing the flap, finding the superficial veins, dissecting the initial superior, and lateral borders of the flap, raising the chest skin flaps, (fellows only for me-dissecting out IMA/axillary vessels). If this option is possible, then you may find a reliable assistant to be invaluable in these cases to expedite the process.

6.3. Anesthesia

The importance of working with anesthesia cannot be overstated. A well informed anesthesia team is worth so much in this case. Having anesthesia on board, with the goals clearly stated and the parameters understood is paramount to success. "The intraanesthetic basic goal is to maintain an optimal blood flow for the vascularized free flap by: increasing the circulatory blood flow, maintaining a normal body temperature to avoid peripheral vasoconstriction, reducing vasoconstriction resulted from pain, anxiety, hyperventilation, or some drugs, treating hypotension caused by extensive sympathetic block and low cardiac output." [1] Communication with anesthesia can help in planning for the case at hand and for unexpected issues. [2] A postoperative extubation that is deep, preventing the bucking phenomenon can help maintain appropriate flow patterns for the flap and the new anastomosis. Finishing a case and then having the patient buck and blow a branch, or having pressors given throughout the case, can either ruin the flap or cause you to reexplore. As a solo surgeon, additional time for preventable trouble shooting can be less and less productive as you may become fatigued. Without a partner to help carry the additional burden, it is important to keep all aspects of the case running as smoothly as possible.

7. Floor and postoperative care

Training the nurses to follow up flaps can take a large investment of your time. Presentations are helpful especially when illustrated. Your physical presence during the monitoring of the cases is extremely useful. Initially you may find that staying overnight at the hospital for the first 25 or 50 cases is useful until the teams understand what you are looking for. After a core team is trained, they can help to train others. Making yourself available 24 hours a day for phone calls, or with direct contact is extremely useful, especially in instances where there is a question about the viability of the flap.

8. Personal OR time

In the operating room if you will be practicing by yourself with or without first assistants who are not physicians, you will need a plan to approach the flaps. If there will be an assistant who can help retract, etc, and you are able to know who they are, then go through the procedure with them a few days in advance in order for them to think of questions and rehearse the plan before the actual procedure. If you are by yourself entirely, then it is good to come up with a timing plan. By yourself, plan to take a 10-15 minute break every 2 hours except at the time of the anastomosis. This allows for a small intake of nutrition and a chance to let your mind relax. Microsurgery is a surgery of finesse, and as you get worn out, it can turn a simple dissection into a nightmare by a small judgment error or a rougher handling of the tissue. This in turn can lead to extra hours in the case, to first fix the issue that was made, and then continue with the case. As a resident, I have witnessed a competent surgeon destroy the vessels at the final hour of anastomosis because he was mentally fried, and so the hours of prior dissection and careful handling were lost in a matter of minutes. Again, this can seem like an odd concept, but if you are going to be working alone, you have no one else to help you so you need to make sure that you are as sharp and relaxed as you can be. If you do have help, such as an RNFA or

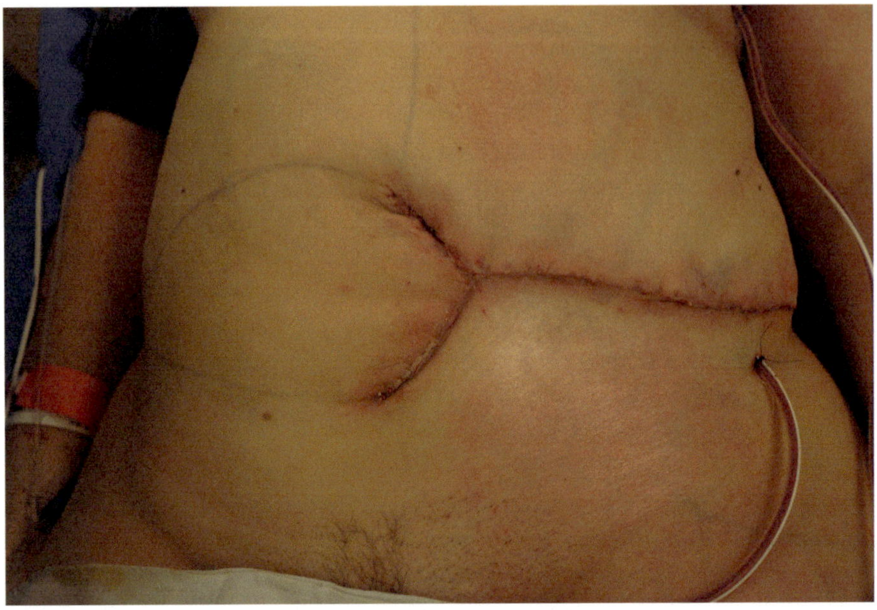

Figure 23. Use of hemiabdominal technique when needing to delay for a double flap reconstruction if operating solo, or for a backup if the vessels fail for a unilateral, or a source of fat for fat grafting in a thinner patient who does not need the full effect of a double pedicled flap.

PA, you might want to take a break every 4 hours, or at least just before the anastomosis in order to perform that portion in a rested fashion. Nothing is more frustrating than trying to save time by plunging ahead for the anastomosis and keep the ischemic time as limited as possible and then find that you are inadvertently taking twice or three times as long as you usually do because you are slightly fatigued and you hadn't realized it. Once the vessels are transected and the flap is ready to be anastomosed, then I consider it not a time to break at all until it is flowing, unless there seems to be a chain of events that is making the condition worse every time you try to repair it. In that instance, make sure that the bleeding is controlled, clamped or whatever, that the patient is stable, that you step out for a second to get a different perspective and again, something to eat or drink, and/or a chance to telephone another expert to ask for advice.

When it comes to reconstruction with the patient's tissue, a factor to keep in mind is that there is a limit to how many opportunities a person has to use their body as a source for reconstruction. Once it is successful, it lasts for a lifetime. A delay, a prolonged recovery, a second surgery, while not easy for the patient or the surgeon, is relatively miniscule in comparison to the rest of the lifetime, versus rushing a procedure for convenience or determination, and then losing that opportunity for the patient and having to come up with a second option which is likely not as optimal as the one you had selected. (Figure 23.)

When working alone, you want to modify the variables during the operation and postoperatively that may impede the success of your efforts. The procedure will be challenging enough

http://dx.doi.org/10.5772/56642

on its own. These techniques can be useful to help create a rhythm for you regardless of who you have to help. Once you find your own level of comfort, then you can plan accordingly and with success. If the case is really bad, stop, close and cover, talk to the family, and come back the next day. A lot of these things may seem to be a waste a time, but in the scheme of things, 12 hours or 24 hours later can make a difference between salvage and failure and the design of something completely different.

Although working alone, if it is possible, have a group of colleagues, or meet other physicians who perform these surgeries regularly and who may be available to you by telephone or other immediate communication. When you are in the middle of surgery and you are not sure why something is not working, it is useful to have the opinion of someone who has experience and who is not fatigued or emotionally involved in the case to help you come up with a different solution or to confirm your own judgment.

In conclusion, performing perforator flap reconstructions is a challenging and rewarding way to help those have had breast cancer. It can be done as a group or in a solo practice. There are many techniques to make the initial dissection successful, and then if running into difficulty, tricks to salvage the flap to result in a successful perforator flap reconstruction.

Author details

Rebecca Studinger MD, MS*

St. John-Providence Hospital, Ascension Health, Novi, MI, USA

References

[1] Hagau N, Longrois D. Anesthesia for free vascularized tissue transfer. Microsurgery. 2009;29(2):161-7.

[2] Scholz A, Pugh S, Fardy M, Shafik M, Hall JE. The effect of dobutamine on blood flow of free tissue transfer flaps during head and neck reconstructive surgery*.Anaesthesia. 2009 Oct;64(10):1089-93.

[3] Richard K Spence, MD; Hemostatic Disorders, Nonplatelet. Medscape reference Updated: Jan 12, 2010

[4] Chang LD, Buncke G, Slezak S, Buncke HJ. Cigarette smoking, plastic surgery, and microsurgery. J Reconstr Microsurg. 1996 Oct;12(7):467-74.

[5] Reus WF 3rd, Colen LB, Straker DJ. Tobacco smoking and complications in elective microsurgery. Plast Reconstr Surg. 1992 Mar;89(3):490-4.

[6] Chang DW, Reece GP, Wang B, Robb GL, Miller MJ, Evans GR, Langstein HN, Kroll SS. Effect of smoking on complications in patients undergoing free TRAM flap breast reconstruction. Plast Reconstr Surg. 2000 Jun;105(7):2374-80.

[7] Vandersteen C, Dassonville O, Chamorey E, Poissonnet G, Nao EE, Pierre CS, Leyssale A, Peyrade F, Falewee MN, Sudaka A, Haudebourg J, Demard F, Santini J, Bozec A. Impact of patient comorbidities on head and neck microvascular reconstruction. A report on 423 cases. Eur Arch Otorhinolaryngol. 2012 Oct 19. [Epub ahead of print]

[8] Schleifer SJ, Keller SE, Camerino M, Thornton JC, Stein M. Suppression of lymphocyte stimulation following bereavement. JAMA. 1983 Jul 15;250(3):374-7.

[9] Zisook S, Shuchter SR, Irwin M, Darko DF, Sledge P, Resovsky K. Bereavement, depression, and immune function. Psychiatry Res. 1994 Apr;52(1):1-10.

[10] Biondi M, Picardi A. Clinical and biological aspects of bereavement and loss-induced depression: a reappraisal. Psychother Psychosom. 1996;65(5):229-45.

[11] Metcalfe KA, Semple J, Quan ML, Vadaparampil ST, Holloway C, Brown M, Bower B, Sun P, Narod SA. Changes in psychosocial functioning 1 year after mastectomy alone, delayed breast reconstruction, or immediate breast reconstruction. Ann Surg Oncol. 2012 Jan;19(1):233-41. Epub 2011 Jun 15.

[12] Garvey PB, Villa MT, Rozanski AT, Liu J, Robb GL, Beahm EK. The Advantages of Free Abdominal-Based Flaps over Implants for Breast Reconstruction in Obese Patients. Plast Reconstr Surg. 2012 Nov;130(5):991-1000.

[13] Chang DW, Wang B, Robb GL, Reece GP, Miller MJ, Evans GR, Langstein HN, Kroll SS. Effect of obesity on flap and donor-site complications in free transverse rectus abdominis myocutaneous flap breast reconstruction.Plast Reconstr Surg. 2000 Apr; 105(5):1640-8.

[14] Greenspun D, Vasile J, Levine JL, Erhard H, Studinger R, Chernyak V, Newman T, Prince M, Allen RJ. Anatomic imaging of abdominal perforator flaps without ionizing radiation: seeing is believing with magnetic resonance imaging angiography. J Reconstr Microsurg. 2010 Jan;26(1):37-44. Epub 2009 May 18.

[15] Pennington DG, Rome P, Kitchener P. Predicting results of DIEP flap reconstruction: The flap viability index. J Plast Reconstr Aesthet Surg. 2012 Nov;65(11):1490-5. doi: 10.1016/j.bjps.2012.05.015. Epub 2012 Jun 14.

[16] Keys KA, Louie O, Said HK, Neligan PC, Mathes DW. Clinical utility of CT angiography in DIEP breast reconstruction. J Plast Reconstr Aesthet Surg. 2012 Oct 18. pii: S1748-6815(12)00564-5. doi: 10.1016/j.bjps.2012.09.025. [Epub ahead of print]

[17] Smit JM, Klein S, Werker PM. An overview of methods for vascular mapping in the planning of free flaps. J Plast Reconstr Aesthet Surg. 2010 Sep;63(9):e674-82. Epub 2010 Jul 31.

[18] Greenspun D, Vasile J, Levine JL, Erhard H, Studinger R, Chernyak V, Newman T, Prince M, Allen RJ. Anatomic imaging of abdominal perforator flaps without ionizing radiation: seeing is believing with magnetic resonance imaging angiography. J Reconstr Microsurg. 2010 Jan;26(1):37-44. Epub 2009 May 18.

[19] Vasile JV, Newman TM, Prince MR, Rusch DG, Greenspun DT, Allen RJ, Levine JL. Contrast-enhanced magnetic resonance angiography. Clin Plast Surg. 2011 Apr;38(2): 263-75.

[20] Hee Hwang J, Mun GH. An evolution of communication in postoperative free flap monitoring: using a smartphone and mobile messenger application. Plast Reconstr Surg. 2012 Jul;130(1):125-9.

[21] Luu Q, Farwell DG. Advances in free flap monitoring: have we gone too far? Curr Opin Otolaryngol Head Neck Surg. 2009 Aug;17(4):267-9.

[22] Patel KM, Svestka M, Sinkin J, Ruff P 4th. Ciprofloxacin-resistant Aeromonas hydrophila infection following leech therapy: A case report and review of the literature. J Plast Reconstr Aesthet Surg. 2012 Oct 18. pii: S1748-6815(12)00578-5. [Epub ahead of print]

[23] Hermansdorfer J, Lineaweaver W, Follansbee S, Valauri FA, Buncke HJ. Antibiotic sensitivities of Aeromonas hydrophila cultured from medicinal leeches. Br J Plast Surg. 1988 Nov;41(6):649-51.

[24] Lineaweaver WC, Hill MK, Buncke GM, Follansbee S, Buncke HJ, Wong RK, Manders EK, Grotting JC, Anthony J, Mathes SJ. Aeromonas hydrophila infections following use of medicinal leeches in replantation and flap surgery. Ann Plast Surg. 1992 Sep;29(3):238-44.

[25] Elyassi AR, Terres J, Rowshan HH. Medicinal leech therapy on head and neck patients: a review of literature and proposed protocol. Oral Surg Oral Med Oral Pathol Oral Radiol. 2012 Jul 20. [Epub ahead of print]

[26] Whitaker IS. Josty IC. Hawkins S. Azzopardi E. Naderi N. Graf J. Damaris L. Lineaweaver WC. Kon M. Medicinal leeches and the microsurgeon: a four-year study, clinical series and risk benefit review. Microsurgery. 31(4):281-7, 2011 May.

[27] Elyassi AR, Terres J, Rowshan HH. Medicinal leech therapy on head and neck patients: a review of literature and proposed protocol. Oral Surg Oral Med Oral Pathol Oral Radiol. 2012 Jul 20. [Epub ahead of print]

[28] Porshinsky BS, Saha S, Grossman MD, Beery II P, Stawicki S. Clinical uses of the medicinal leech: A practical review. J Postgrad Med 2011;57:65-71.

[29] Nguyen MQ, Crosby MA, Skoracki RJ, Hanasono MM. Outcomes of flap salvage with medicinal leech therapy. Microsurgery. 2012 Jul;32(5):351-7.

Section 4

Lymphedema

Chapter 13

Treatment of Breast Cancer-Related Lymphedema Using Combined Autologous Breast Reconstruction and Autologous Lymph Node Transplantation

Corinne Becker

Additional information is available at the end of the chapter

http://dx.doi.org/10.5772/56465

1. Introduction

Lymphedema can appear after lymphadenectomy and radiotherapy for cancer treatment of the breast. The reported incidence of lymphedema, which can occur many years after the initial treatment, varies due to different methods of long follow-up. Patients requiring more extensive breast cancer treatment with axillary lymph node dissection and radiation have the greatest risk for development of lymphedema.[3,4]

In a study of 20 years follow-up of breast cancer patients [3], 49% of patients reported having lymphedema and 13% (33 of 263 women) had augmented measurements of the affected arm. The incidence of lymphedema following breast cancer treatment ranges from 24% to 49% after mastectomy, and 4% to 28% after lumpectomy. [1]. It appears that removing lymph nodes around the axillary vein is responsible for the development of lymphedema. Lymphangitis is an inflammation of the lymphatic channels that occurs in response to a distal infection such as paronychia, an insect bite, or secondary infections in the inter-digital spaces. Erysipelas may require hospitalization in acute cases. Then, the skin becomes progressively more fibrotic and thick, and transformation in elephantiasis may be observed. Lymphangiosarcoma is a rare malignant tumor that occurs in long-standing cases of lymphedema. The sarcoma first appears as an ecchymotic mark, or a tender skin nodule in the extremity. Stewart-Treves syndrome (STS), defined as lymphangiosarcoma arising from post-mastectomy lymphedema, has an extremely poor prognosis, with an overall mortality rate of 70-90% even following limb amputation. this is why it is particularly important to treat the lymphedema. Physiotherapy is essential in managing the edema, but it will not be effective if there are no remaining lymphatic channels. The most effective form of physiotherapy appears to be manual lymphatic drainage and multilayer bandages. Physiotherapy must be combined with the other techniques. The major drawbacks of conservative treatment are: significant time commitment, labor intensive, requirement for specialized therapists, and lifelong commitment by the patient.

This pathology destroys the quality of life of the patients both functionally (lost of work in 70% definitively) and psychologically and the cost to insurance companies are increasing (infections, physiotherapy for life, etc.)[2]

2. Surgical treatment in iatrogenic upper extremity lymphedema

The surgery is divided in 2 groups: debulking techniques and the reconstructive techniques.

1. Debulking techniques include lipoaspiration and excisions:

   - excisions of fat and soft tissue were used in cases of severe elephantiasis, but rarely:

   - lipoaspiration performed for fatty lymphedema often required continuous compression garments for life. This technique is used for fatty and soft tissue lymphedema and is mostly used in Sweden (cold climate).(Brorson)

2. reconstructive techniques are more sophisticated and attempt to reestablish the anatomy:

   - The autologous lymph node transplantation (ALNT) may provide an effective solution by replacing the scarred tissue with new lymphatic pathways because the transplanted nodes contain lymphatic growth hormone.[7] The incidence of infections decreases because the nodes contain immune cells.

   - The combination of this lymph node flap with the DIEP or SIEA (and even TRAM) provides simultaneous treatment for lymphedema and breast reconstruction. The lymph node flap can also be added as a second free flap with the other flaps for breast reconstruction such as the TDAP, SGAP, TUG, PAP and even with more traditional techniques such as the latissimus dorsi flap.

   - The quality of lymphovenous anastomosis (supermicrosurgery) is improved thanks to the improved quality of microsurgical materials. However, the pressure within the lymphatic system must be maintained above the venous pressure (normally, the venous pressure is higher than lymphatic pressure) to avoid collapse of the tiny anastomosis. This is achieved by permanent external compression. This may explain the poor long-term results of this surgery, but this technique can be used as an adjunct to ALNT.

   - lympho-lymphatic grafts are technically extremely difficult. This procedure results in large donor site scars in the lower extremities with inconsistent results. [8]

For each individual patient, combinations of these procedures may be indicated to achieve improved results.

http://dx.doi.org/10.5772/56465

3. Clinical evaluation and indications of surgery

Patients are evaluated by a multidisciplinary team (oncologist, physiotherapist, surgeon, pain management specialist, neurologist, radiologist) to understand the etiology of the lymphedema, and/or pain and paresthesias.

The patient must be oncologically cleared and free of cancer recurrence. Appropriate physiotherapy must by applied preoperatively. The clinical exam is essential: fibrotic areas, folds, compression, sequelae of radiotherapy, type of pain, evaluation for the neuroma, palsy or paresthesia, quality of the skin, and skin lesions are all components of the pathology that must be evaluated.

Radiologists are now performing lymphatic MRI which allows us to visualize a map of the lymphatic system of the arm and thorax. Specific pathology can be identified such as hypoplasia of the vessels due to chronic infection, lack of lymph nodes and/or vessels in the axilla following lymphadenectomy, radiotherapy and chronic infections, and collateralization of lymphatic vessels. If these pathways do exist [6], surgery should be delayed following satisfactory physiotherapy. In some cases, lymphangioisotopy combined with the scan, provides more dynamic information, but is less useful.

EMG can be used to identify the site of nerve compression or degeneration along with the affected muscle (useful for tendon transfers in plexitis). The pain specialist can help diagnose the cause of pain, provide appropriate medical treatment if necessary and help determine if there is an indication for surgery.

In subclinical cases, if the patient desires breast reconstruction, the indication for an adjunct autologous lymph node flap will depend on establishing the presence of lymphatic pathology by using preoperative mri (or isotopic lymphoscintigraphy). If the lymphedema is present, the DIEP or SIEA will include the lymph node transplant.

4. Operative technique

4.1. Autologous lymph node transplantation for upper limb lymphedema

The dissection begins at the axillary region. The fibrosis is dissected and the thoracodorsal vessels are identified. This part of the operation can be extremely difficult, because normal anatomy may be severely distorted due to scar contracture from surgery and radiation. The location of the axillary artery, vein, and brachial plexus are often changed because of radiotherapy-related contracture. The plexus and axillary vein can be compressed by large fibrotic bands and the surgeon must be particularly cautious during dissection in these areas. Vascular branches with suitable sizes for microanastomosis are prepared. Neuromas may be encountered around these vessels which are treated when present. If paresthesia or palsy is present, external neurolysis is performed and the thoracobrachial space must be decompressed. The dimensions of the flap requirements will then be estimated as well as the need for fat and skin.

The superficial inguinal lymph node flap starts with an incision performed over a line located between the iliac crest and the pubis. The length of the incision depends on the flap size needed to fill the defect. The subcutaneous tissue is incised to the depth of the fascia cribiformis, where a superficial diagonal vein can be found. The fatty tissue located deeper to this superficial fascia and superficially to the muscular aponeurosis contains 4-5 lymph nodes that can be transferred based on the superficial circumflex iliac vessels. This pedicle is dissected and the flap is elevated around these isolated vessels. Inferiorly, the inguinal crest is a very important limit of the dissection, and preserving the deep lymph nodes is critical in preventing secondary lymphedema at the donor site.

The flap is then transferred to the axillary recipient site with microsurgical technique.

4.2. Extended abdominal flaps

The inguinal lymph nodes flap can be incorporated into the flap of the adjacent skin and fat in the lower abdomen, based on the superficial inferior epigastric vessels (SIEA) or the deep inferior epigastric vessels (free TRAM or DIEP). To harvest the nodes, the incisions of the abdominal flap must be lowered to the level of the iliac crest, including the inguinal lymph node flap previously described (subcutaneous tissue containing the nodes, vascularized by the circumflex iliac vessels). If the microsurgical anastomosis of the flap are made to the internal mammary vessels, the lymph node extension should be harvested at the opposite side of the pedicle. If the flap is reattached at the thoracodorsal system, the nodes can be harvested at the same side. The lymph node flap should be placed in the axillar region. It has to be inserted around the axillary vein, where the lymphatic tissue was first resected.

The need for a second set of anastomosis will be assessed during surgery. SPY imaging can be used intra-operatively to evaluate the perfusion of the transferred nodes and the flap

4.3. Lymphovenous anastomosis

LVA can be performed in the proximal and/or distal regions of the limb, depending on indication (elevated pressure in the lymphatic system). PDE is a mapping device of the superficial lymphatic pathways, useful to determine the locations of the LVAs. These are performed under big magnification, with 11-0 or 12-0 (where available) nylon sutures.

4.4. Selective external liposculpture

After 6 month min, the water disappears but the fat remains sometimes because the lipocytes were not circulated for many years. A special Mercedes canula is more convenient, the fibrosis can still be important. The liposuction is only performed on the external part of the arm and very softly on the forearm (post part also).

http://dx.doi.org/10.5772/56465

5. Complications and concerns

Lymphocele at the donor site can be avoided with the use of a drain on the initial post-operative period (48h) and local compression. If the deep lymph nodes beyond the inguinal ligament or in the axilla are not disturbed, no iatrogenic lymphedema of the donor limb should be noted. Local infections and delayed wound healing are rare, even in irradiated tissues. The autologous lymph node flap is a buried flap. Flap monitoring is difficult. Vascular thrombosis is believed to occur in 2% of the cases, in which no improvement is perceived. For enlarged flaps, thrombosis will lead to exploration of anastomoses, and eventually flap loss. When 2 sets of anastomoses are performed, the ALNT part of the flap can remain viable. Infection risks are present in chronic infected patients, but prophylactic antibiotic therapy limits their occurrence (no exceed 2%).

Scars can become enlarged, and even hypertrophic, but they are concealed under a the slip or bra.

6. Clinical outcomes

On a series of more than 2.500 patients operated in 20 years, with stage 1,2 and 3 lymphedemas (International Society of Lymphology), 98% of patients present some degree of improvement, and 40% of the stages 1 or 2 lymphedemas have complete remission and do not need additional physiotherapy treatment. Follow-up of at least 3 years are included. Elephantiasis is never completely healed and patients will still need physiotherapy. 95% state some kind of amelioration. Only 2% of patients keep having infection episodes. Results will depend on the longevity of the lymphedema and the presence of fibrotic tissue. Bilateral lymphedemas will have worse outcomes. Generally, the patients do loose 2 cm /months, and this during 2 years, progressively.[9-10]

The results are better for short duration and less severe lymphedemas. In moderate cases, MRL shows new lymphatic pathways, with effective lymph drainage. Even the long-standing lymphedema (over 15y) can show some improvement.

When neuromas of the intercostal nerves are encountered, neurolysis and removal of surgical clips is effective, achieving pain-relief in 98% of patients. For brachial plexus neuropathies, neurolysis of the nerves and coverage with a non-irradiated, well-vascularized tissue (ALNT or enlarged abdominal flap) will be effective. These patients experience less pain and palsy stabilization. Although sensation can be slightly recovered the 2 following years, motor recovery is rare, and can only be expected in young patients. Tendon transfers can be beneficial for some patients with partial palsies, once the lymphedema disappears. We do not advise the use of a tourniquet.

The lymphovenous anastomosis can destroy the remaining lymphatic channels if they became trhombosed. The addition seems not very helpful except in particular cases where the lymphatic vessels are well seen with the fluorescein.

The combination of the autologous lymphnodes transfer with addition of 1 lympholymphatic anastomosis is not necessary because the VGEFc are creating new pathways.

In conclusion, patients resistant to any kind of physiotherapy, showing no drainage of the upper limb, can benefit from the autologous lymph node transfer to restore the anatomy. The nodes containing VGEF3 induce new lymphatic vessels growth. After chronic infctions, it is well known that the vessels becomes obstructed. The patients can expect good results in 98% and normalization in 40% after 2 years. The post operative lymphatic MRI does explain the indications of the surgery, and the results (new ways, transplanted nodes visible....). No morbidity of the donor site is observed if the dissection doesn't pass under the inguinal ligament.

The combination with different free flaps to restore the breast at the same time is ideal.

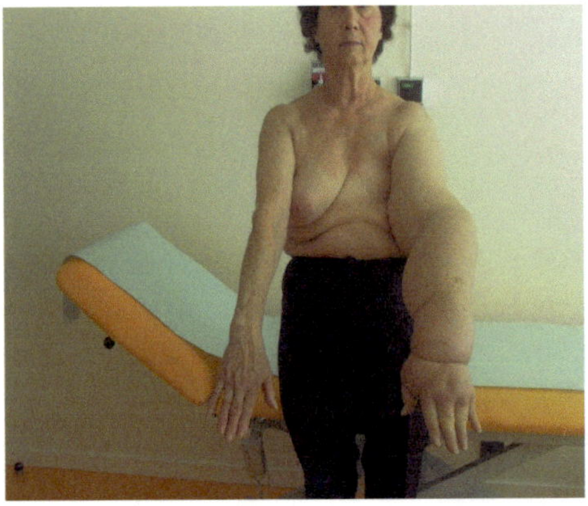

Figure 1. Typical case of lymphoedema

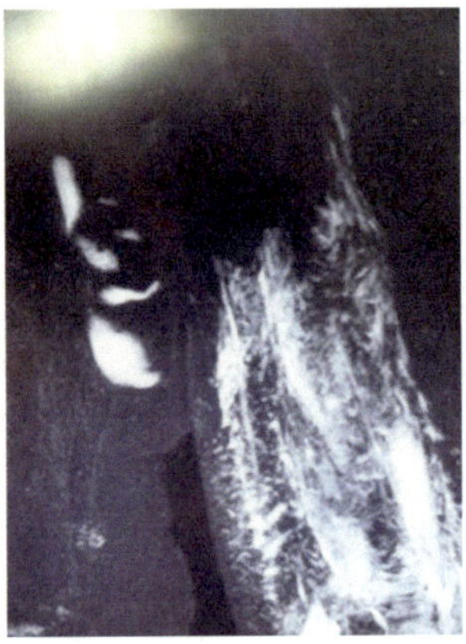

Figure 2. Lymphatic MRI showing lack of lymphnodes ans lymphatic vessels after adenectomy and radiotherapy for-breast tumor. Evidence of complete absence of drainage. Physiotherapy cannot treat such cases.

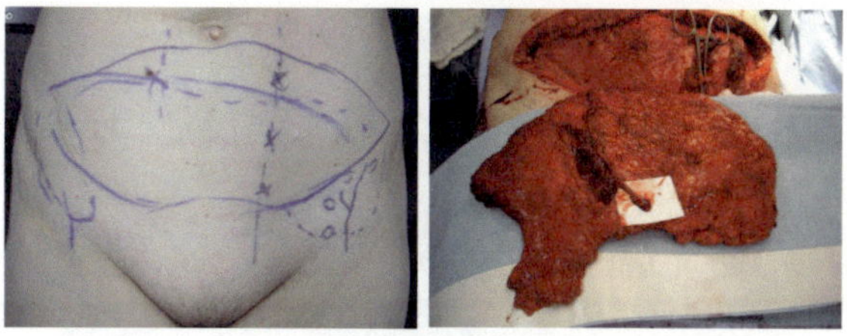

Figure 3. Design of the enlarged DIEP based on the deep epigastric vessels connected with the superficial circonflex iliac art.

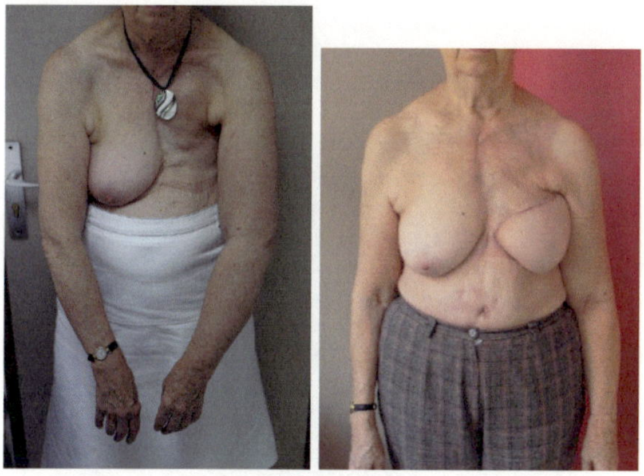

Figure 4. 76-year-old woman operated 25 years ago who underwent mastectomy, adenectomy and radiotherapy. Suffering from lymphoedema for the last 20 years. She was operated post radiotherapy from bypass for cardiac ischemia. Results 6 months later after breast reconstruction by DIEP combined with ALNT.

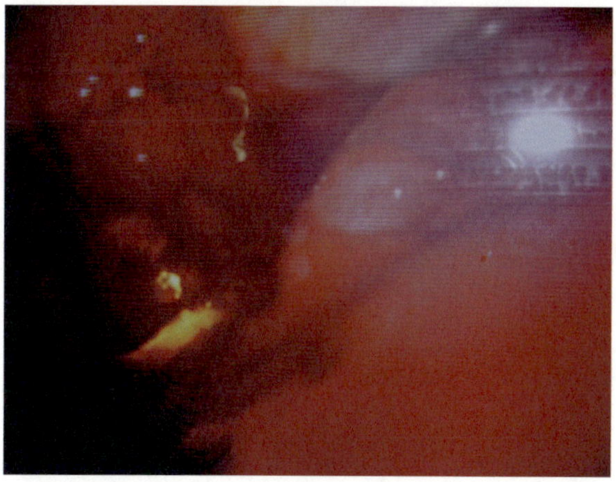

Figure 5. Living transplanted nodes observed by endoscopy

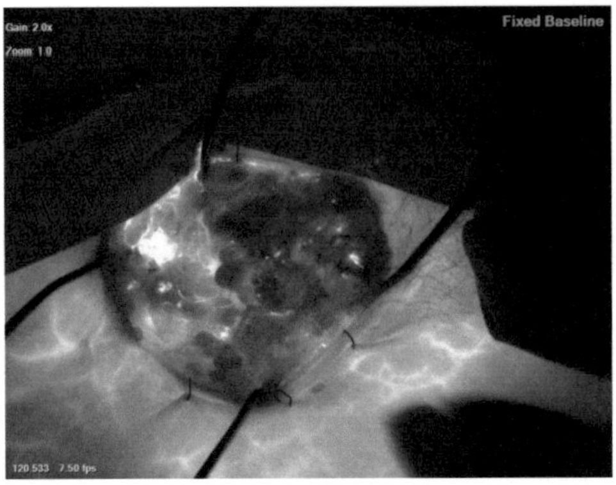

Figure 6. Spy of the flap

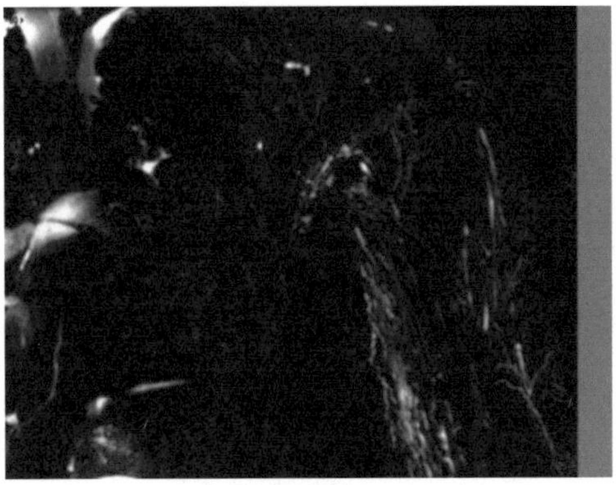

Figure 7. Post operative lymphatic MRI

Author details

Corinne Becker

Lymphedema Center, Paris, France

References

[1] Cormier JN, Askew RL, Mungovan KS, et al. Lymphedema beyond breast cancer: a systemic review and meta-analysis of cancer-related secondary lymphedema. Cancer 2010;116(22):5138-49.

[2] Ahmed RL, Prizment A, Lazovich D, et al. Lymphedema and quality of life in breast cancer survivors: the Iowa women's health study. J Clin Oncol 2008;26(35):5689-96.

[3] Petrek JA, Senie RT, Peters M, et al. Lymphedema in a cohort of breast carcinoma survivors 20 years after diagnosis. Cancer 2001;92(6):1368-77.

[4] McLaughlin SA, Wright MJ, Morris KT, et al. Prevalence of lymphedema in women with breast cancer 5 years after sentinel lymph node biopsy or axillary dissection: objective measurements. J Clin Oncol 2008;26(32);5213-9

[5] Arrivé L, Azizi L, Lewin M, Hoeffel C, Monnier-Cholley L, Lacombe C, Tubiana JM. MR lymphography of abdominal and retroperitoneal lymphatic vessels. AJR. 2007; 189(5): 1051-8.

[6] Saaristo AM, Niemi TS, Viitanen TP, Tervala TV, Hartiala P, Suominen EA. Microvascular breast reconstruction and lymph node transfer for post mastectomy lymphedema patients. Ann Surg. 2012; 255(3): 468-73.

[7] Springer S, Koller M, Baumeister RG, Frick A. Changes in quality of life of patients with lymphedema after lymphatic vessel transplantation. Lymphology. 2011; 44(2): 65-71.

[8] C. Becker ; Linfologia, p.54, August 1996.– Transplantation of lymphnodes ; an alternative method for treatment of lymphedema.

[9] C. Becker, M. Riquet Annals of surgery243 3 and 313-315. March. 2006.- Post mastectomy lymphedemas..

[10] C. Becker E-mémoires de l'Académie nationale de chirurgie, vol. 7, n°1, p 55-64, 2008– La chirurgie du lymphoedème, effet des greffes ganglionnaires..

[11] C. Becker, Ph. Duc Nhat Minh, J. Assouad, A. Badia, Chr. Foucault, M. Riquet - The Breast, vol. 17, issue 5, p 472-476, October 2008. Postmastectomy neuropathic pain: results of microsurgical lymph nodes transplantation.

[12] C. Becker - Perspectives. E-memoires de l'académie nationale de chirurgie. 7 (1) : 55-64, 2008. Traitements actuels des lymphœdèmes.